Textbook of
PSORIAIS

Textbook of
PSORIASIS

Editor-in-Chief

Jayakar Thomas MD DD MNAMS PhD FRCP (Edin, Glasg, Lond, Irel)
FRCPCH FAAD FIAD FIAP
Professor and Head
Department of Dermatology
Sree Balaji Medical College and Hospital, Bharath University
Chennai, Tamil Nadu, India

Editors

Parimalam Kumar MD DD DNB FRCP FIAD
Professor and Head
Department of Dermatology
Government Villupuram Medical College
Villupuram, Tamil Nadu, India

Sindhu Ragavi Balaji MBBS MD
Consultant Dermatologist
Carves Skin Clinic
Chennai, Tamil Nadu, India

Dinesh Kumar Devaraj MBBS MD
Medical Director and Consultant Dermatologist
Vee Care DermatoPlastic
Chennai, Tamil Nadu, India

Foreword

D Prabhavathy

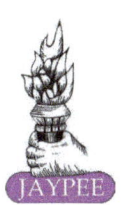

JAYPEE The Health Sciences Publisher

New Delhi | London | Philadelphia | Panama

Jaypee Brothers Medical Publishers (P) Ltd

Headquarters
Jaypee Brothers Medical Publishers (P) Ltd
4838/24, Ansari Road, Daryaganj
New Delhi 110 002, India
Phone: +91-11-43574357
Fax: +91-11-43574314
Email: jaypee@jaypeebrothers.com

Overseas Offices

J.P. Medical Ltd
83 Victoria Street, London
SW1H 0HW (UK)
Phone: +44 20 3170 8910
Fax: +44 (0)20 3008 6180
Email: info@jpmedpub.com

Jaypee Medical Inc
325 Chestnul Street
Suite 412, Philadelphia, PA 19106, USA
Phone: +1 267-519-9789
Email: support@jpmedus.com

Jaypee Brothers Medical Publishers (P) Ltd
Bhotahity, Kathmandu, Nepal
Phone: +977-9741283608
Email: kathmandu@jaypeebrothers.com

Jaypee-Highlights Medical Publishers Inc
City of Knowledge, Bld. 237, Clayton
Panama City, Panama
Phone: +1 507-301-0496
Fax: +1 507-301-0499
Email: cservice@jphmedical.com

Jaypee Brothers Medical Publishers (P) Ltd
17/1-B Babar Road, Block-B, Shaymali
Mohammadpur, Dhaka-1207
Bangladesh
Mobile: +08801912003485
Email: jaypeedhaka@gmail.com

Website: www.jaypeebrothers.com
Website: www.jaypeedigital.com

© 2016, Jaypee Brothers Medical Publishers

The views and opinions expressed in this book are solely those of the original contributor(s)/author(s) and do not necessarily represent those of editor(s) of the book.

All rights reserved. No part of this publication may be reproduced, stored or transmitted in any form or by any means, electronic, mechanical, photocopying, recording or otherwise, without the prior permission in writing of the publishers.

All brand names and product names used in this book are trade names, service marks, trademarks or registered trademarks of their respective owners. The publisher is not associated with any product or vendor mentioned in this book.

Medical knowledge and practice change constantly. This book is designed to provide accurate, authoritative information about the subject matter in question. However, readers are advised to check the most current information available on procedures included and check information from the manufacturer of each product to be administered, to verify the recommended dose, formula, method and duration of administration, adverse effects and contraindications. It is the responsibility of the practitioner to take all appropriate safety precautions. Neither the publisher nor the author(s)/editor(s) assume any liability for any injury and/or damage to persons or property arising from or related to use of material in this book.

This book is sold on the understanding that the publisher is not engaged in providing professional medical services. If such advice or services are required, the services of a competent medical professional should be sought.

Every effort has been made where necessary to contact holders of copyright to obtain permission to reproduce copyright material. If any have been inadvertently overlooked, the publisher will be pleased to make the necessary arrangements at the first opportunity.

Inquiries for bulk sales may be solicited at: jaypee@jaypeebrothers.com

Textbook of Psoriasis

First Edition: **2016**
ISBN: 978-93-5250-165-6
Printed at

Dedicated to

Many devoted practitioners who provide skin health to psoriatics, our committed teachers of dermatology, the millions who suffer from psoriasis, and most of all to our spouses for their care, love, and affection without which this humble piece of work would not have been a reality.

Foreword

The practice of medicine requires the acquisition of knowledge and skills, and the learning of attitudes and behaviors, apart from the manner in which it is disseminated. Professor Jayakar Thomas has exemplified this in his book on psoriasis.

I have many reasons for my pleasure in writing the foreword for this title *Textbook of Psoriasis*. Having known Professor Jayakar Thomas for over three decades stands foremost of all. He is an enthusiastic celebrity in dermatology. I have been reading his several works—original articles, chapters in books, and also his other books.

In this book, he has interweaved clinical, pathological, and therapeutic details of psoriasis in such a reader-friendly manner that represents any international publications. The clinical images are a feast to the eyes and well illustrated.

All the other contributors deserve to share this honor of preparing and putting in volume of effort to publish this book.

It is my opinion that this book can ill afford to be missed out a place in any medical library and the hands of any physician.

I wish Professor Jayakar Thomas and all the contributors to continue their work on similar great titles.

D Prabhavathy MB DD MD
Former Professor and Head
Department of Dermatology
Madras Medical College
Chennai, Tamil Nadu, India

Preface

"Knowledge, if not shared is of no use at all."

Over the years, advances in dermatologic science have been spectacular. We are pleased to present this *Textbook of Psoriasis* as a follow-up to our earlier title *Psoriasis—a closer look*. Bearing in mind that virtually every area of dermatology and dermatology education has evolved remarkably, and that many new concepts have emerged, this book has been written extensively in the light of the varied needs of the book's readers.

This title offers a thoroughly updated presentation of the classic pathophysiology, basics of clinical presentation, and the details of the cutting-edge methods and tools that are now available for the assessment of symptoms and the effective management of psoriasis. The text is supplemented by to-the-point photographs, radiographs, illustrations, and patient-care algorithms and tables.

We wish all readers a happy and fruitful reading.

Jayakar Thomas
Parimalam Kumar
Sindhu Ragavi Balaji
Dinesh Kumar Devaraj

Contents

CHAPTER 1:	Introduction	1
CHAPTER 2:	Epidemiology	4
CHAPTER 3:	Etiopathogenesis	9
CHAPTER 4:	Clinical Aspects	36
CHAPTER 5:	Pediatric Psoriasis	94
CHAPTER 6:	Psoriasis and Pregnancy	132
CHAPTER 7:	Psoriasis and Human Immunodeficiency Virus	145
CHAPTER 8:	Psoriasis as a Systemic Disease	151
CHAPTER 9:	Investigations	174
CHAPTER 10:	Treatment	187
CHAPTER 11:	Complications and "The Psoriatic March"	231
CHAPTER 12:	Psychological Aspects, Course and Prognosis, Follow-up and Rehabilitation	237
	Index	247

CHAPTER 1

Introduction

Psoriasis, a common skin disease which is probably as old as mankind is seen in any age group from the newborn. Psoriatic skin changes have been described since biblical times. The first documented description is found in the Old Testament in the third book of Moses. It was confused with leprosy for hundreds of years, and, therefore, many people with psoriasis were ostracized in the middle age (Fig. 1.1). At the beginning of the 19th century, Robert Willan, an English physician, was the first to clinically describe psoriasis (Crissey and Parish 1998). Humankind suffered and studied this disease for at least 3,000 years, and, naturally, several possible causes for the disease have been hypothesized.[1]

Psoriasis is now classified as an immune-mediated inflammatory disease of the skin. Psoriasis, a T-cell mediated chronic inflammatory disorder of the skin is seen in about 3.5% of the population.[2] One-third of psoriasis cases in a dermatology center are seen in pediatric age group.[3] It is recognized as the most prevalent autoimmune disease caused by inappropriate activation of the cellular immune system and affects people of all age including the newborn. Psoriasis is a lifelong inflammatory disorder of the skin that can vary widely in its presentation, but is characterized by the common features of erythema, thickening, and scaling of the skin. The diagnosis is usually made on clinical grounds by any well trained clinician.

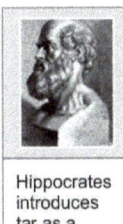
Hippocrates introduces tar as a treatment for skin ailments.
400 B.C.

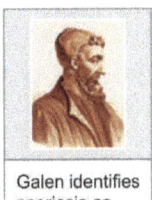
Galen identifies psoriasis as a skin disease; he names it "psoriasis."
150 A.D.

People with psoriasis (and leprosy) warned others of their arrival by ringing a clapper.
1300

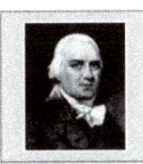
Dr. Robert willan, around 1809, first recognized psoriasis as a specific clinical entity.
1809

Fig. 1.1: History of psoriasis since 400 BC

Despite considerable research into its etiology, there are still no definitive genetic or biochemical markers for psoriasis, and it continues to be diagnosed primarily based on skin manifestations. Its impact on a patient depends not only on the percentage of body surface area of the lesions but also on their location. Involvement of the hands, feet, scalp, and genital areas can have a disproportionate effect on quality of life and disability. Additionally, in a significant subset of psoriasis patients, the disease process involves progressive damage to the articular joints. Up to 30% of people with psoriasis also develop psoriatic arthritis (PsA) which may be over diagnosed or under diagnosed due to the heterogeneity of its expression.

Patients with arthropathy or enthesopathy of various types may be over diagnosed as PsA in the presence of cutaneous psoriasis and the diagnosis PsA may be missed, in the absence of cutaneous psoriasis. Patients with PsA are at increased risk for developing other comorbidities. Moreover, clinical studies have increasingly revealed associations of psoriasis and its treatments with many systemic diseases. Although establishing causality in these associations remains problematic, these associations have immediate diagnostic and therapeutic implications.

The trend of increasing incidence of childhood psoriasis, observed in recent times is alarming. The chance of translating this into an increase in morbidity due to psoriasis during adulthood cannot be ruled out.

Psoriasis not only affects physical well-being but has emotional and relational consequences that go far beyond the skin. Timely diagnosis and appropriate management can not only arrest progression but also minimize the psychosocial burden imposed by this illness. Thereby disfiguring states and its evolution into a metabolic syndrome requiring extensive treatment can well be averted.

Every physician treating a psoriatic patient, must look past the skin and see the patient as a whole, with particular attention to address the associated comorbid conditions. Although there is no consensus regarding screening for metabolic conditions in psoriatic patients, it is strongly recommended that all adult patients above the age of 40 are screened for metabolic comorbidities more so with reference to female patients and those with positive family history of psoriasis or comorbidity.

The role of biomarkers for assessment of disease severity, for prediction of the outcome of therapeutic interventions, and for distinction between the different clinical variants of the disease has been emphasized.[4] Therapeutic options are approached from different angles and an attempt has been made to cover as much recent drugs as possible including the role of monoclonal antibodies targeting interleukin-17 receptor A (IL-17RA) and IL-17A in the treatment of plaque psoriasis.[5] A fair understanding of the disease's underlying inflammatory processes may well improve the management of patients with psoriasis. It is suggested that a holistic approach, including education, counseling and psychological support, regular follow-up is needed for optimal care of psoriatic patients.

This book will cover almost all aspects of psoriasis with particular attention to pediatric psoriasis, including the rare clinical form like congenital erythrodermic psoriasis and present the latest update especially on the etiopathogenesis and treatment options. An evidence based approach has been given while discussing these issues. There is increasing awareness the world over that psoriasis is more than "skin deep" and is now emerging as a systemic disease.

It is attempted to emphasize the role of inflammation as a major factor, leading to multiple organ dysfunction. Similarly, the concept, "psoriatic march" is also thrashed out though it is not yet formally proven. Finally, the reader will accept that a holistic approach, including education, aggressive treatment wherever necessary along with psychological support in the form of empathy rather than sympathy, is all that is needed for care of psoriatic patients. The main aim of the treatment should be to reduce the burden of the disease over time by controlling symptoms, helping the patient to cope with the chronic nature of the disease, limiting psychological and relational consequences, and preventing systemic complications and comorbidity by choosing the right drug at the right moment and keeping a strict vigil on the side effects.

REFERENCES

1. Coimbra S, Oliveira H, Figueiredo A, Rocha-Pereira P, Santos-Silva A. Psoriasis: epidemiology, clinical and histological features, triggering factors, assessment of severity and psychosocial aspects. Psoriasis-A Systemic Disease. Editor: Jose O'Daly; INTECH, Open Access Publisher, 2012. Available at (http://www.intechopen.com/books/psoriasis-a-asytemic-disease).
2. Kurd SK, Gelfand JM. The prevalence of previously diagnosed and undiagnosed psoriasis in US adults: results from NHANES 2003-2004. J Am Acad Dermatol. 2009;60:218-24.
3. Raychaudhuri SP, Gross J. A comparative study of pediatric onset psoriasis with adult onset psoriasis. Pediatr Dermatol. 2000;17:174-8.
4. Molteni S, Reali E. Biomarkers in the pathogenesis, diagnosis, and treatment of psoriasis. Psoriasis: Targets and Therapy. 2012;2:55-66.
5. Gooderham M, Posso-De Los Rios CJ, Rubio-Gomez GA, Papp K. Interleukin-17 (IL-17) inhibitors in the treatment of plaque psoriasis: a review. Skin Therapy Lett. 2015;20(1):1-5.

CHAPTER 2

Epidemiology

INTRODUCTION

True prevalence of psoriasis over the world is difficult to arrive at. There is considerable racial variation in the prevalence of psoriasis from country to country which may be attributable to many factors like climate, genetic susceptibility, and lifestyle. Psoriasis affects 1%–8% of the world population, depending on the country.[1] The prevalence of psoriasis and the comorbidities associated with psoriasis is on the rise. However, according to Basko-Plluska and Petronic-Rosic, the prevalence of psoriasis has not changed with time according to epidemiological studies, in contrast to other autoimmune diseases whose prevalence rates have increased.[2] In the US, psoriasis affects approximately 2% of the population, although rates as high as 4.6% have been reported.[3,4] Bell et al. showed an age-adjusted and sex-adjusted annual incidence of 60.4 in 1,00,000 between the period of 1980 and 1983.[5] More recently, Huerta et al. reported an incidence rate of 14 per 10,000 people.[6] The difference in reported incidence rate can be attributed to the different case definitions used in these studies. Psoriasis is extremely rare to absent in certain ethnic groups, such as Africans, African-Americans, Japanese, Alaskans, Australians, and Norwegian Lapps.[4,7,8]

According to Kurd and Golf, psoriasis is seen in about 3.5% of the population.[9] One-third of psoriasis cases in a dermatology center are seen in pediatric age group.[10] In India, the prevalence of psoriasis varies from 0.44% to 2.8%, it is twice more common in males compared to females, and most of the patients are in their third or fourth decade at the time of presentation.[11]

Psoriasis has a bimodal distribution of age of onset. Those individuals with early onset appear, in general, to have more severe disease and are much more likely to have an affected first-degree relative with psoriasis. One-third of adults with psoriasis, report the onset during childhood. Ethnic variation is not clear, with some studies quoting incidence highest in Caucasians.[12] The prevalence of psoriasis seems to be affected by latitude. It is alarming to note that 40,000 children under 10 years were afflicted by psoriasis.[13] The distribution of psoriasis in children is almost equal in boys and girls. However, female preponderance has been observed by some authors. The occurrence of psoriatic diaper rash in younger children and its inclusion increases incidence of psoriasis in children under two.[12] The exact age distribution is not clear though literature states that nearly 30% of patients with psoriasis develop the disease before the age of 18 years.[14] It is of interest to note that in the age group less than 20 years, the frequency of psoriasis was 20% higher in girls than in boys, in contrast to adults.[15] Compared with 37% in adult-onset patients, 49% of pediatric-onset patients had first-degree family members affected with psoriasis. Some studies have reported familial incidence in childhood cases of psoriasis as high as 89%.[16]

The prevalence of the disease in childhood and adolescence ranges between 0.5% and 2%, while its estimated incidence was reported to be 40.8 pediatric cases/100,000 person-years. Moreover, it has been shown that the prevalence of the disease exhibits a linear increase from the age of 1 year (0.12%) to the age of 18 years (1.2%). Most studies agree that the mean patient age at disease onset for juvenile psoriasis is 7–11 years. There seems to be no male or female predominance among children and adolescents suffering from psoriasis.[17]

Psoriasis can first appear at any age; however, a bimodal distribution of the age of onset is characteristic. The majority of cases, approximately 75%, present before the age of 40 years, with a peak at 20–30 years old. The remaining cases present after the age of 40 years. Patients with early disease onset tend to have a positive family history of psoriasis, frequent association with histocompatibility antigen, [human leukocyte antigen (HLA)]-Cw6, and more severe disease. Those with onset after the age of 40 years usually have a negative family history and a normal frequency of the Cw6 allele.[2]

Involvement of joints with psoriatic arthritis is less prevalent in younger patients; however, it does occur in childhood disease and should be considered in the differential of pediatric arthritis.[18] The heritability of psoriasis is as high as 91% which is supported by many studies, documenting a concordance in incidence of as high as 73% and 20% in monozygotic and dizygotic twins, respectively.[19]

Involvement of multiple genes makes the genetic basis of psoriasis complex and hence, it is difficult to draw a conclusion about the correct heritability of the disease. The heritability of psoriasis has been estimated to be 60%–90%, based on twin studies. Thus, making psoriasis a highly heritable disease, the heritability seems to be highest of all multifactorial genetic diseases.[20,21] Concordance rates as high as 70% have been reported among monozygotic twins, versus 12%–30% among dizygotic twins.[22] According to family studies, it was shown that if both parents have psoriasis, the offspring has a 50% chance of developing the disease. The risk decreases to 16%, if only one parent has psoriasis. The siblings of a psoriatic child with unaffected parents have an 8% risk of developing the disease. Males have a higher risk of transmitting psoriasis to offspring than females, which is likely due to genomic imprinting.[23] HLA studies have shown that psoriasis is associated with several HLA antigens, most frequently HLA-Cw6, which confers a relative risk of 10 for developing the disease in the Caucasian population. However, only approximately 10% of individuals who express the HLA-Cw6 allele go on to develop psoriasis.[24] In addition, HLA-Cw6 influences the age of onset of the disease. HLA-Cw6 is expressed in about 85%–

90% of patients with early-onset psoriasis, but in only 15% of patients with late-onset disease.[25]

Human leukocyte antigens—B13, HLA-B17, HLA-B37 and HLA-Bw16 have also been associated with plaque psoriasis. HLA-B27 is expressed with an increased frequency in pustular psoriasis and acrodermatitis continua of Hallopeau. A significant association between guttate psoriasis and erythrodermic psoriasis with HLA-B13 and HLA-B17 expression has been reported.

Protein tyrosine phosphatase N22 (PTPN22) and its association to psoriasis have been extensively analyzed. There seems to be a positive association between psoriasis and the PTPN22, the significance of which is yet to be proved beyond doubt.[26] Many analytic epidemiologic studies have identified multiple risk factors like smoking, obesity, alcohol consumption, diet, infections, medications, and stressful life events to play an important role in the disease manifestation.

European studies have also confirmed that current smoking and obesity are independent risk factors for developing psoriasis.[27] One of the largest studies estimated that 30% of new psoriasis cases were due to being overweight (body mass index >25).[28] A higher prevalence of psoriasis has been demonstrated in current smokers than never-smokers or ex-smokers.[27] Many studies suggest that alcohol plays an important role in the exacerbation of psoriasis.[29] It was noted that heavy drinkers have a tendency to develop more extensive and inflamed skin lesions.[30-32]

Infections are known factors to be associated with psoriasis. Acute bacterial and viral infections have been associated with the onset or exacerbation of psoriasis.[33] Streptococcal infections are often triggers of guttate psoriasis, especially in children and young adults.[34] There are reports to show the association of HIV infection and psoriasis. Medications, including β-blockers, lithium, antimalarials, tetracycline antibiotics, non-steroidal anti-inflammatory drugs, and steroid withdrawal have been associated with the onset or exacerbation of psoriasis, mostly based on case reports.[35] Antimalarial drugs may exacerbate pre-existing psoriasis in up to 40% of patients by inhibiting the enzyme transglutaminase and causing epidermal proliferation.[36] The role of psychological stress has long been attributed in the exacerbation of psoriasis. Acute psychosocial stress was shown to induce altered hypothalamic-pituitary-adrenal responses in patients with psoriasis, particularly in those who experienced a flare of disease with stress.[37]

CONCLUSION

Psoriasis, an age old disease, occurs worldwide. It is indeed difficult to document the prevalence of the disease due to various factors. Complex genetic and molecular basis make it impossible to study the epidemiology of prevalence and pattern of disease. However, it is clear from the literature that the prevalence of psoriasis is on the rise and in future, children affected by psoriasis and psoriatic arthritis will increase. Variations in climate, genetic susceptibility, and lifestyle will play a major role in determining the epidemiological profile. The prevalence seems to be 1–8% of the world population which will vary from country to country and from place to place even within the same country. Many studies prove that psychological stress can induce a flare in the disease manifestation. The prevalence of metabolic comorbidities is found to be more with psoriatics than the control population. Psoriasis and comorbidities adversely affect each other which could be a reason for the changing trend in the comorbidities as well.

REFERENCES

1. Mansouri Y, Goldenberg G. New systemic therapies for psoriasis. Cutis. 2015;95(3):155-60.
2. Basko-Plluska JL, Petronic-Rosic V. Psoriasis: epidemiology, natural history, and differential diagnosis. Psoriasis: Targets and Therapy. 2012;2:67-76.
3. Naldi L. Epidemiology of psoriasis. Curr Drug Targets Inflamm Allergy. 2004;3:121-8.
4. Raychaudhuri SP, Farber EM. The prevalence of psoriasis in the world. J Eur Acad Dermatol Venereol. 2001;15:16-7.
5. Bell LM, Sedlack R, Beard CM, Perry HO, Michet CJ, Kurland LT. Incidence of psoriasis in Rochester, Minn, 1980-1983. Arch Dermatol. 1991;8:1184-7.
6. Huerta C, Rivero E, Garcia Rodriguez LA. Incidence and risk factors for psoriasis in the general population. Arch Dermatol. 2007;143(12):1559-65.
7. Christophers E. Psoriais-epidemiology and clinical spectrum. Clin Exp Dermatol. 2001;26:314-20.
8. Gelfand JM, Stern RS, Nijsten T, Feldman SR, Thomas J, Kist J, et al. The prevalence of psoriasis in African Americans: results from a population-based study. J Am Acad Dermatol. 2005;52(1):23-6.
9. Kurd SK, Gelfand JM. The prevalence of previously diagnosed and undiagnosed psoriasis in US adults: results from NHANES 2003–2004. J Am Acad Dermatol. 2009;60:218-24.
10. Raychaudhuri SP, Gross J. A comparative study of pediatric onset psoriasis with adult onset psoriasis. Pediatr Dermatol. 2000;17:174-8.
11. Dogra S, Yadav S. Psoriasis in India: Prevalence and pattern. Indian J Dermatol Venereol Leprol. 2013;76:595-601.
12. Sharma V, Orchards D. Paediatric psoriasis. Paediatrics and Child Health 2011;21(3):126-31.
13. Sticherling M, Augusti M, Boehncke WH, Christophers E, Domm S, Gollnick H, et al. Therapy of psoriasis in childhood and adolescence–a German expert consensus. J Dtsch Dermatol Ges. 2011;9(10):815-23.
14. Augustin M, Glaeske G, Radtke MA, Christophers E, Reich K, Schäfer I. Epidemiology and comorbidity of psoriasis in children. Br J Dermatol. 2010;162:633-6.
15. Swanbeck G, Inerot A, Martinsson T, Wahlström J, Enerbäck C, Enlund F, et al. Age at onset and different types of psoriasis. Br J Dermatol.1995;133:768-73.
16. Farber EM, Mullen RH, Jacobs AH, Nall L. Infantile psoriasis: a follow-up study. Pediatr Dermatol. 1986;3:237-43.
17. Fotiadou C, Lazaridou E, Ioannides D. Management of psoriasis in adolescence. Adolesc Health Med Ther. 2014;5:25-34.
18. Kumar B, Jain R, Sandhu K, Kaur I, Handa S. Epidemiology of childhood psoriasis: a study of 419 patients from northern India. Int J Dermatol. 2004;43:654-8.
19. Farber EM, Nall ML, Watson W. Natural history of psoriasis in 61 twin pairs. Arch Dermatol. 1974;109:207-11.
20. Elder J, Nair R, Guo S, Henseler T, Christophers E, Voorhees J. The genetics of psoriasis. Arch Dermatol. 1994;130:216-24.
21. Elder JT, Nair RP, Henseler T, Jenisch S, Stuart P, Chia N. The genetics of psoriasis 2001: the odyssey continues. Arch Dermatol. 2001;137:1447-54.
22. Valdimarsson H. The genetic basis of psoriasis. Clin Dermatol. 2007;25(6):563-7.
23. Rahman P, Elder JT. Genetic epidemiology of psoriasis and psoriatic arthritis. Ann Rheum Dis. 2005;64(Suppl 2):ii37-9.
24. Trembath R, Clough RL, Rosbotham JL, Jones AB, Camp RD, Frodsham A, et al. Identification of a major susceptibility locus on chromosome 6p and evidence for further disease loci revealed by a two stage genome-wide search in psoriasis. Hum Mol Genet. 1997;6:813-20.
25. Richardson SK, Gelfand J. Update on the natural history and systemic treatment of psoriasis. Adv Dermatol. 2008;24:171-96.
26. Chen YF, Chang J. PTPN22 C1858T and the risk of psoriasis: a meta-analysis. Mol Bio Rep. 2012;39:7861-70.
27. Naldi L, Chatenoud L, Linder D, Belloni Fortina A, Peserico A, Virgili AR, et al. Cigarette smoking, body mass index, and stressful life events as risk factors for psoriasis: results from an Italian case-control study. J Invest Dermatol. 2005;125:61-7.
28. Setty AR, Curhan G, Choi HK. Obesity, wait circumference, weight change, and the risk of psoriasis in women: Nurses' Health Study II. Arch Intern Med. 2007;167(15):1670-5.
29. Schafer T. Epidemiology oof psoriasis. Review and the German perspective Dermatology. 2006;212(4):327-37.
30. Poikolainen K, Reunala T, Karvonen J, Lauharanta J, Karkkainen P. Alcohol intake: a risk factor for psoriasis in young and middle-aged men? British Med J. 1990;300:780-3.
31. Naldi L, Peli L, Parazzini F. Association of early-stage psoriasis with smoking and male alcohol consumption: evidence from an Italian case-control study. Arch Dermatol. 1999;135:1479-84.

32. Higgins EM, du Vivier AW. Alcohol and the skin. Alcohol Alcohol. 1992;27:595-602.
33. Naldi L, Peli L, Parazzini F, Carrel CF, Psoriasis Study Group of the Italian Group for Epidemiological Research in Dermatology. Family history of psoriasis, stressful life event, and recent infectious diseases are risk factors for a first episode of acute guttate psoriasis: results of a case-control study. J Am Acad Dermatol. 2001;44:433-8.
34. Zhao G, Feng X, Na A, Yongqiang J, Cai Q, Kong J, et al. Acute guttate psoriasis patients have positive streptococcus hemolyticus throat cultures and elevated antistreptococcal M6 protein titers. J Dermatol. 2005;32:91-6.
35. Tsankov N, Irena A, Kasandjieva J. Drug-induced psoriasis: recognition and management. Am J Clin Dermatol. 2000;1:159-65.
36. Lionel F, Baker B. Triggering psoriasis: the role of infections and medications. Clin Dermatol. 2007;25:606-15.
37. Richards HL, Ray DW, Kirby B, Mason D, Plant D, Main CJ, et al. Response of the hypothalamic-pituitary-adrenal axis to psychosocial stress in patients with psoriasis. Br J Dermatol. 2005;153:1114-20.

CHAPTER 3

Etiopathogenesis

INTRODUCTION

Psoriasis is a systemic, immune-mediated disorder, characterized by inflammatory skin and joint manifestations. The exact etiopathogenesis of psoriasis has not been completely elucidated. Although psoriasis was first recognized as a distinct disease as early as 1808 by Willan, its pathogenic mechanisms have eluded investigators for decades.[1] This chapter will briefly see the various etiological and precipitating factors, pathology, and a succinct discussion on the pathogenesis of psoriasis.

Lack of a generally accepted animal model to study and prove the pathogenic factor in psoriasis, poses a major difficulty in elucidating the exact cause of the disease and its predictable course. Most of the hypothesis put forth depends much on the clinical studies and translational science done in patients with this disease. T lymphocytes play a key role as inducers of the disease phenotype. The pathogenic contribution of this cell type has now been tested through clinical studies of more than a dozen immune modifying biological agents in patients with psoriasis. The important role played by many inflammatory cytokines, infiltrating leukocytes, resident skin cells, and other chemokines prove the disease pathogenesis to be a complex process. Rather than viewing psoriasis as a disease caused by a single-cell type or a single inflammatory cytokine, it is probably best to conceptualize disease pathogenesis as linked to many interactive responses impacted by genetic, genomic, and immune contributions triggered by various environmental factors. Rapid progress has been made toward dissecting cellular and molecular pathways of inflammation that contribute to disease pathogenesis.[2]

- Cutaneous lymphocyte antigen (CLA)
- Immature dendritic cell (iDC)
- Interferon (IFN)
- Interleukin (IL)
- Lymphocyte function associated antigen-1
- Mature dendritic cell
- Major histocompatibility complex (MHC)
- Nuclear factor κB
- Natural killer T cells
- Plasmacytoid dendritic cell
- Psoriatic arthritis (PsA)
- Rheumatoid arthritis (RA)

- Signal transducer and activator of transcription (STAT)
- Tumor necrosis factor (TNF)
- T cell receptor (TCR)
- Target of rapamycin (TOR)
- Psoriasis susceptibility locus 2 (PSORS2)
- T cells
- Dendritic cells
- Gene expression or genomics
- Psoriasis genes or genetics.

It would be apt to consider psoriasis as the most prevalent autoimmune disease caused by inappropriate activation of the cellular immune system.

The disease is defined by a series of linked cellular changes in the skin that can be broadly categorized as:
- Hyperplasia of epidermal keratinocytes
- Vascular hyperplasia and ectasia and
- Cellular infiltration (T lymphocytes, neutrophils, and other types of leukocytes) in affected skin.

Psoriatic skin serves as a long-term reservoir of pathogenic immune cells. Growth and expansion of skin homing memory T cells can also occur exclusively within the skin. Psoriatic skin can potentially function as a surrogate of formal lymphoid tissue, at least for expansion of already differentiated skin homing T cells. It is worth remembering that psoriasis is a disease of the interfollicular epidermis, and it does not significantly alter the growth of follicular epithelia or the normal hair growth cycle. In people with psoriasis what are the factors causing T cells to malfunction is not due to a single factor. Genes that are linked to the development of psoriasis seem to play a major role. Other environmental factors also play a significant role in the disease manifestation or perpetuation.

This section will deal with the factors involved in the pathogenesis of psoriasis under the following headings:
- Etiology and precipitating factors
- Pathology
- Pathogenesis
- Immunopathogenesis
- Biomarkers.

ETIOLOGICAL OR PRECIPITATING FACTORS

Psoriasis typically starts or worsens because of a trigger that is identifiable in majority of the patients. The probable factors responsible for the disease are given in the Box 3.1 below:

Genetic Factors

Psoriasis is associated with complex genetic susceptibility. Knowledge on the genetic basis of psoriasis highlights genetic susceptibility factors that play a crucial role in regulation of immunity, epidermal proliferation, and skin barrier formation. Genetic susceptibility factors affecting both the immune system and epidermis could predispose to disease.

Although psoriasis has a multifactorial etiology, it is strongly influenced by genetic factors. Psoriasis affects people of all ages, with a strong tendency for disease onset in early adulthood in patients who develop psoriasis due to genetic transmission.[3]

BOX 3.1: Etiological or precipitating factors of psoriasis

- Genetic
- Trauma
- Infection
- Drugs
- Sunlight
- Metabolic factors
- Pregnancy and hormones
- Alcohol and smoking
- Stress
- Obesity

Major gene for psoriasis susceptibility is thought mainly to be located on chromosome 6, the site of human leukocyte antigen (HLA) class I (associated with early-onset disease) and II (late-onset disease) antigens which are thought to produce differing subtypes of the disease. Individuals with the Cw0602 allele are four times more likely to develop guttate psoriasis. A series of genes have been isolated in which mutations have been associated with psoriatic disease, including interleukin (IL)12-B9 (1p31.3), IL-13 (5q31.1), IL-23R (1p31.3), HLA-BW6, psoriasis susceptibility locus 6 (PSORS6), single transducer and activator of transcription 2 gene (STAT2/IL-23A) (12q13.2), tumor necrosis factor α-induced protein 3 gene (TNFA-IP3) (6q23.3), and interacting protein 1 gene TNIP1 (5q33.1). These genes play a role in helper T type 2 (Th2) cell and Th17 cell activity which have been noted in psoriatic lesions.[4,5] Several attempts have been made to detect psoriasis susceptibility loci by linkage studies. Up to now, at least 12 loci are known (PSORS1-12).[6] A strong association exists in early-onset psoriasis for the HLA-Cw6 allele.[7] Although psoriasis has a multifactorial etiology, it is strongly influenced by genetic factors proven by the observation that, when compared with the general population, a higher incidence of the disease has been identified among first-degree and second-degree relatives of psoriasis. The risk of psoriasis is greater in monozygotic twins than in dizygotic twins, confirming the genetic basis of the disease. The concordance of monozygotic twins both suffering from psoriasis has been reported to be approximately 70% and the sibling recurrence risk is estimated to range between 4 and 11. Late cornified envelope genes (LCE3C and LCE3B), is a common genetic factor for susceptibility to psoriasis in different populations.[8] In the susceptible genetic background, precipitating factors are more important in pediatric than in adult-onset psoriasis. They largely include trauma, infections, drugs, sunlight, metabolic causes, alcohol, smoking, stress, and obesity. Streptococcal pharyngitis or perianal streptococcal dermatitis typically provokes guttate psoriasis. Infection with human immunodeficiency virus (HIV) can induce or exacerbate psoriasis.

As early as 1995, Krueger et al. proposed a "framework hypothesis" stating that "there is an aberration throughout the skin of patients with psoriasis that is modified to disease expression by circulating factors" and that the primary skin defect could reside in the epidermis (keratinocyte) or dermis (fibroblast) and an altered gene could be a regulator of cytokines or growth factors.[9]

A major genetic determinant of psoriasis, designated PSORS1, resides in the major histocompatibility complex (MHC) on chromosome 6p21, tightly linked to HLA-Cw6, which is the most frequently detected allele in psoriasis.

The major locus strongly associated with psoriasis is PSORS1 on chromosome 6p21, spanning approximately 300 kb of the MHC class I region. In addition to PSORS1, linkage analyses and association studies have highlighted psoriasis loci on several other chromosomes outside of the MHC region. The loci of the susceptibility region and the molecules differentially regulated in psoriasis are given in Table 3.1.[6]

The pathogenesis of psoriasis involves a complicated interaction between genetic, immunological, and environmental components. Recent genome-wide association studies have identified a variety of genetic components involving both the immune system and the epidermis that affect psoriasis pathogenesis. Several genetic factors and pathways shared with autoimmune and inflammatory (immune-mediated) diseases

TABLE 3.1: Loci of the susceptibility region and the molecules differentially regulated in psoriasis

Susceptibility region	Locus	Molecules differentially regulated in psoriasis
PSORS1	6p21.3	HLA-Cw6, TNF, corneodesmosin, MHC class I
PSORS2	17q25	TIMP-2, SLC9A3R1, NAT9, RAPTOR
PSORS3	4q	VDBP, RRH
PSORS4	1q21	EDC, S100A7, S100A8, S100A9, LCE3B, LCE3C, Loricrin
PSORS5	3q21	Transferrin, SLC12A8
PSORS6	19p13	JunB, SGTA
PSORS7	1p	IL-23R
PSORS8	16q	NOD2
PSORS9	4q31–4q34	ND
PSORS10	18p11.23	ND
PSORS11	5q31.1–5q33.1	IL-12p40
PSORS12	20q13	ZNF313 (also termed RNF114)

EDC, epidermal differentiation complex; IL, interleukin; LCE, late cornified envelope protein; NAT, N-acetyltransferase; ND, not described; NOD, nucleotide-binding oligomerization domain; OMIM, online mendelian inheritance in man; PSORS, psoriasis susceptibility region; IL-23R, IL-23 receptor; RAPTOR, regulatory associated protein of mammalian target of rapamycin; RNF, RING finger protein; RRH, retinal pigment epithelium-derived rhodopsin homolog; SGTA, small glutamine-rich tetratricopeptide repeat-containing protein-α; SLC, solute carrier; TIMP, tissue inhibitor of metalloproteinases; TNF, tumor necrosis factor; VDBP, vitamin D-binding protein; ZNF, zinc finger protein; HLA, human leukocyte antigen; MHC, major histocompatibility complex.

highlight a common mechanism in different diseases. However, a substantial proportion of the involved genetic factors have yet to be identified. It is difficult to clarify how these genetic factors and pathways intersect and contribute to inflammation, proliferation, and altered differentiation in psoriasis.[10]

Based on the HLA association, Henseler and Christophers proposed that there are two types of psoriasis: a familial, early age of onset (<40 years) form, frequently associated with HLA-Cw6, DR7, B13, and B57; and a nonfamilial, later age at onset form that is associated with HLA-Cw2 and B27.[11] However, variable observation in the recent studies by Trembath et al. and others suggest a chief role for additional genes and/or environmental triggers.[12]

Patients with psoriasis also have different clinical features depending on whether they are HLA-Cw6 positive or negative. Besides having a lower age of onset, HLA-Cw*0602 positive patients have more extensive plaques on their arms, legs, and trunk, more severe disease, higher incidence of Koebner's phenomenon, reported more often that their psoriasis got worse during or after throat infections and frequently had a favorable response to sunlight. In contrast, dystrophic nail changes and (PsA) are more common in the Cw6-negative patients.[13]

It was also identified that chromosome 1q21, 17q25, and 20p the putative loci for atopic dermatitis are closely coincident with regions known to contain psoriasis susceptibility genes.[14] It was also found that there was a stronger association with TNF-α and D6S273 than with HLA-C.

Psoriasis and associated PsA are complex genetic diseases with environmental and genetic components. The identification of multiple loci for psoriasis susceptibility indicates that psoriasis and PsA are genetically heterogeneous. Dystrophic nail changes and PsA are more common in the Cw6-negative patients. An association of B27 with PsA is seen, especially in individuals with spinal disease. Genetic modifiers, such as caspase recruitment domain-containing protein 15 (CARD15), that play roles in the skin and synovium may predispose to PsA and it is hypothesized that CARD15 is a PsA gene that is independent of HLA-Cw*0602.

The risk of transmission of atopic disease from an affected mother is approximately four times higher than from an affected father. Similar parent-of-origin effects have been noted in psoriasis and PsA. However, in the two cases examined the disease appeared to be more likely to be inherited through the father, if he was affected.[15]

Trauma

A wide range of injurious local stimuli, in any form including physical, chemical, electrical, surgical, infective and inflammatory insults, has been recognized to elicit psoriatic lesions, which is clinically observed as Koebner's phenomenon.

In a cross-sectional survey, the prevalence of photosensitive psoriasis was 5.5%. Skin type I, familial history of photosensitivity, advanced age, and psoriasis affecting the hands were all significantly associated with photosensitivity.[16]

Infection

It is clearly demonstrated that bacterial, fungal, and viral infections seem to have significant role in inducing or modifying the disease manifestation. The important infective agents involved in the etiopathogenesis of psoriasis are mentioned in Box 3.2.

> **BOX 3.2: Role of infection in psoriasis**
> - Bacterial: Streptococcus
> - Fungal: Malassezia
> - Viral: HIV
>
> HIV, human immunodeficiency virus.

In children, streptococcal throat infection is strongly associated with guttate psoriasis. There is also evidence that streptococcal infection may be an important factor in chronic plaque psoriasis. It is interesting to note that episodes of guttate psoriasis are much more common in individuals with a family history of plaque psoriasis. The role of streptococcal infections in the etiology of psoriasis is known for many years. Recent evidences indicate that streptococcus induce Th1, Th17, Th22 response, epidermal activation and hyperplasia through the interaction with circulating skin-homing memory T cells and epidermal cells of psoriatic patients. In a study conducted by Ferran M et al. where activation of circulating psoriatic cutaneous lymphocyte-associated antigen, (CLA) + memory T cells cultured together with epidermal cells occurred only when streptococcal throat extracts were added, thereby demonstrating the direct involvement of streptococcal infection in pathological mechanisms of psoriasis, such as IL-17 production and epidermal cell activation. According to the study, an *in vitro* system partially recapitulates the initiation of a psoriatic lesion. Individuals with lesions elicited by streptococcal infection may have circulating CLA+ memory T cells that specifically recognize streptococcal antigen and home to the skin. These activated T cells, in cooperation with the epidermal cells, elicit massive cytokine milieu consisting of several cytokines implicated in this disease, such as IFN-γ, IL-22, IL-17, and inducible protein

(IP)-10. These components might have an important role in the initiation and triggering of a psoriatic lesion.[7]

Although no strong association of Malassezia species was formed with psoriatic lesion in general, the fungi may play a role in exacerbation of scalp psoriasis.

Psoriasis typically worsens after an individual has been infected with HIV. However, psoriasis often becomes less active in advanced HIV infection. The association between HIV infection and psoriatic arthropathy is not yet fully explained. However, the role of T cell seems to be an important factor.

The pathogenesis of psoriasis in patients with HIV is considered a medical paradox that revolves around three main quandaries. First, this T-cell-mediated disease manages to flourish in an environment of decreasing T-cell counts. Second, although various therapies targeting T lymphocytes are effective in psoriasis, the condition worsens with decreasing CD4 T-cell counts in patients with HIV. Third, HIV is characterized by a strong Th2 cytokine profile and psoriasis is characterized by a strong Th1 secretion pattern. The recognition of HIV-1 proteins and subsequent activation of T lymphocytes could trigger or maintain psoriatic lesions, as this locus has been proven to play an important role in susceptibility by increasing relative risk of developing psoriasis by 14–24 times.[18] The association between HIV infection and psoriatic arthropathy is not yet fully explained. However, the role of T cell seems to be an important factor in both HIV and psoriasis.

Drugs

Drugs can affect the diathesis of psoriasis by several ways including:
- Precipitation of psoriasis de-novo in predisposed and nonpredisposed individuals
- Exacerbation of pre-existing psoriatic lesions
- Induction of lesions in clinically normal skin in patients with psoriasis, and
- Development of treatment-resistant psoriasis.

The clinical presentation of drug-provoked psoriasis spans the spectrum of generalized plaque psoriasis, palmoplantar pustulosis, and erythroderma. Drug-provoked psoriasis can be divided into two categories. The first category, drug-induced psoriasis and the second, drug-aggravated psoriasis. The two categories of psoriasis are depicted in Flowchart 3.1. In the first type, discontinuation of the causative drug stops the further progression of the disease.

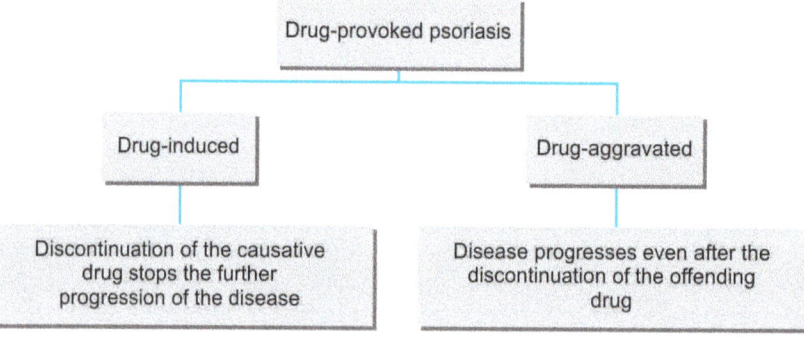

Flowchart 3.1: Drug-provoked psoriasis

TABLE 3.2: The differentiating features of drug-provoked psoriasis

Features	Drug-induced psoriasis	Drug-aggravated psoriasis
Past history of psoriasis	Need not be present	Usually present
Genetic predisposition	Need not be present	Usually present
Clinical presentation	Mostly as pustular lesions	Pustules less frequent
Nail involvement	Less frequent	May be present
Arthritis	Less frequent	May be present
Histology	Munro microabscess, vascular changes-sparse	Classical of psoriasis vulgaris
Discontinuation of drug	Stops progression of psoriasis	Psoriasis continues to progress
Response to treatment	Usually good	Resistant to treatment

Whereas, in the second category the disease progresses even after the discontinuation of the offending drug. True drug-induced psoriasis tends to occur in a de-novo fashion in patients with no family or previous history of psoriasis. The clinical presentation of these lesions may often mimic the pustular variant of psoriasis, often with no nail involvement or associated arthritis. Furthermore, there is an absence of munro's microabscesses, few macrophages and sparse vascular changes noted histologically. Drug-aggravated psoriasis exhibits a propensity to occur in patients with a history of psoriasis or with a genetic predisposition for the disease. Patients can have exacerbation of pre-existing psoriatic lesions or develop new lesions in previously uninvolved skin. Histological examination reveals features that are more characteristic of psoriasis vulgaris.[19] The differentiating features of drug-provoked psoriasis are given in Table 3.2.

Drugs play an important role in the onset or exacerbation of psoriasis. Lithium salts, antimalarial agents, β-adrenergic blocking agents, nonsteroidal anti-inflammatory drugs (NSAIDs), angiotensin-converting enzyme inhibitors and the sudden withdrawal of corticosteroids are the most common drugs precipitating or exacerbating psoriasis.

BOX 3.3: Drugs exacerbating psoriasis

- Antimalarials
- β-blockers
- Bupropion
- Calcium channel blockers
- Captopril
- Fluoxetine
- Glyburide
- Granulocyte colony-stimulating factor
- Interferon
- Interleukins
- Lipid-lowering drugs
- Lithium
- Penicillin
- Terbinafine

The list of drugs exacerbating psoriasis is given in Box 3.3.

The possible mechanisms by which common drugs like β-blockers, lithium, tetracyclines and NSAID induce or aggravate psoriasis are explained below.[20]

β-blockers

Several theories have been proposed regarding the pathogenesis of β-blocker-induced psoriasis. These include a delayed-type hypersensitivity reaction, immunological mechanisms including impaired lymphocyte transformation, or alterations in the cyclic adenosine monophosphate (cAMP) pathway. cAMP is an intracellular messenger that is responsible for the stimulation of proteins for cellular differentiation and inhibition of proliferation. The most reliable proposition is that, blockade of epidermal β2 receptors leads to a decrease in intraepidermal cAMP causing keratinocyte hyperproliferation. Biopsy specimens from eruptions caused by β1 blockers (metoprolol and atenolol) are characterized by excessive degranulation of neutrophils in the dermis. Nonselective β-blockers (propranolol, nadolol, and sotalol) were marked by excessive release of proteolytic enzymes from macrophages. Both groups of β-blockers exhibit excessive release of enzymes by lymphocytes, neutrophils, and macrophages, and it is believed that this event is responsible for the presence of hyperproliferation and psoriasis form change. Psoriasiform eruption of both drug-induced and drug-aggravated psoriasis from β-blocker therapy usually appear at 1–18 months after initiation of therapy. Re-exposure with oral challenge results in recurrence within a few days.

Psoriasiform eruptions from β-blockers are not true representations of psoriasis, β-blocker-provoked psoriasis improves upon discontinuation of medication, but usually does not completely resolve. With regard to β-blocker-induced, de-novo pustular psoriasis, the duration seemed to be much shorter. Reasons for these variations may be due to genetic, environmental, or racial backgrounds. It was found that the cumulative drug exposure to β-blockers is not a substantial risk factor for development of psoriasiform lesions.

Lithium

Psoriasiform eruptions are the most common cutaneous side effects, reported to occur in 3.4–45% of patients treated with lithium. Lithium causes depletion of inositol monophosphatase resulting in alterations in calcium homeostasis and serotonergic function. Inositol is an intracellular second messenger. Lithium inhibits the enzyme inositol monophosphatase, necessary for the recycling of inositol. The inhibition of the intracellular release of calcium appears to be the mechanism in which lithium provokes the development of a psoriasiform eruption. The support for the "inositol depletion hypothesis" comes from the clinical observation that inositol supplementation can reverse the exacerbation of lithium-provoked psoriasis. In addition, studies have shown that lithium increases the production of IL-2, TNF-α, and interferon-γ (IFN-γ) in psoriatic keratinocytes in the lesions. Lithium also increases intracellular tyrosine phosphorylation in psoriatic T cells but not in control T cells, with a possible implication to psoriasis lesion development. Main events in the pathogenesis of lithium-provoked psoriasis are given in Box 3.4.

There may be inherent factors that influence the induction or aggravation of psoriasis with lithium. When plaque-type psoriasis develops with lithium therapy, it may take longer to resolve compared to pustular psoriasis. It has been suggested that exacerbation of pre-existing psoriasis with lithium is more common than induction of new psoriatic lesions.

BOX 3.4: Pathogenesis of lithium-provoked psoriasis

- Intracellular depletion of inositol and calcium
- Increased production of IL-2, TNF-α, and IFN γ in psoriatic keratinocytes
- Increased intracellular tyrosine phosphorylation in psoriatic T cells

IL-2, interleukin-2; TNF-α, tumor necrosis factor-α; IFN-γ, interferon-γ.

Tetracyclines

Tetracyclines may theoretically provoke psoriasis through reduction of intracellular cAMP and by the interaction with arachidonic acid and its metabolites. It has been theorized that tetracyclines accumulate in higher concentrations in psoriatic lesions compared to uninvolved skin. Some tetracyclines may cause photosensitization, which may result in psoriasis, in predisposed patients who may experience exacerbation through the Koebner's phenomenon secondary to phototoxicity.

NSAIDs

Nonsteroidal anti-inflammatory drugs inhibit the metabolism of arachidonic acid by the cyclooxygenase (COX) pathway leading to accumulation of leukotrienes, which has been postulated to aggravate psoriasis or exacerbate arthritis. Nevertheless, in some patients, exacerbation of psoriasis and arthritis may coincidently occur simultaneously with the use of NSAIDs.

Sunlight

Though sunlight is beneficial to psoriasis, in some persons sunlight can exacerbate psoriasis. Females are more prone for photoexaggeration of psoriasis. It is also found that photoexaggerated psoriasis is associated with HLA-Cw6 and early-onset disease. However, in a cross-sectional survey, conducted by Ros et al., the prevalence of photosensitive psoriasis was found to be 5.5% where it was observed that skin type I, familial history of photosensitivity, advanced age, and psoriasis affecting the hands were all significantly associated with photosensitivity.[16]

Metabolic Factors

Hypocalcemia is known to precipitate psoriasis and can worsen pustular psoriasis. Hypocalcemia occurs in patients with psoriasis vulgaris, pustular psoriasis of von Zumbusch, and impetigo herpetiformis. It was observed that in pustular psoriasis of von Zumbusch precipitated by hypocalcemia, the exacerbation was due not to abnormal circulating levels of parathyroid hormone or vitamin D metabolites but to hypocalcemia. In most cases, hypocalcemia is caused by accompanying hypoalbuminemia, yet reductions in ionized serum calcium concentrations due to hypoparathyroidism or malabsorption have been reported. Stewart et al., reported the case of a patient with surgical hypoparathyroidism in which hypocalcemia precipitated typical pustular psoriasis of von Zumbusch. The psoriasis lesions rapidly cleared on two occasions when the patient's serum calcium was corrected by therapy with oral calcium and vitamin D or its analogs, and reappeared when treatment was discontinued.[21] According to Goldman, psoriasis, like gout, may be, at least partly, a result of disorder of urine metabolism and monosodium orate crystals may be responsible for the cell proliferation that is characteristic of psoriatic plaques.[22] Hyperuricemia is a common finding in psoriatic patients. Correction of hypocalcemia might be clinically useful for the global treatment of patients.[23] After analysis of 1,146 psoriasis patients, high incidence of asymptomatic hyperuricemia (18.8%) and elevated average levels of uric acid in these patients' blood were confirmed (346.8 ± 2.4 µmol/L). More severe forms of uric acid dysbolism lead to aggravated skin affections (psoriatic erythroderma, oxidative psoriasis), arthritis, occur in patients with familial predisposition to psoriasis. Advanced psoriasis patients are at risk to develop apparent gout.[24]

Pregnancy and Hormones

Pregnancy has dual effect on psoriasis. As most of them feel better, the disease can worsen in some. Impetigo herpetiformis (IH) is a form of pustular psoriasis which occurs only during pregnancy and recurs with every pregnancy. Though IH is considered as a distinct entity as it does not occur in nonpregnant women, the classical histology is that of pustular psoriasis. How pregnancy induces IH is not well proved. The main theories proposed include elevated levels of progesterone during third trimester, hypocalcemia and lower amounts of skin-derived antileukoprotienase activity probably contributing to the formation of epidermal pustule.[25]

Modulation of psoriasis severity by estradiol, during pregnancy, menstruation and menopause has been investigated previously. The correlation between sex hormones and psoriasis area severity index (PASI) has recently been studied in male psoriasis patients. Serum levels of testosterone and estradiol were significantly different between male patients with psoriasis and healthy controls. Testosterone was significantly increased in control patients and estradiol was significantly increased among male psoriatic patients. A significant inverse correlation was found between estradiol and PASI. However, the exact role of sex hormones in the pathogenesis of psoriasis in men has not been demonstrated.[26]

Alcohol or Smoking

Alcohol though is not known to induce psoriasis; it is well documented to exacerbate pre-existing disease in many. Excess drinking can also be a consequence of the disease that leads to treatment resistance and reduced therapeutic compliance. Abstinence has been reported to induce remission. Pietrzak A et al., have screened unreported excessive alcohol intake in psoriatics and are of the view that the knowledge of individual's drinking pattern may be of substantial importance for managing the disease.[27]

Smoking seems to be associated with development of palmoplantar pustular psoriasis. Smoking has shown to have a positive association with insulin resistance in psoriatics. Therefore, cutting back on smoking which is known to exacerbate psoriasis and cause cardiovascular disease may also help improve insulin resistance.[28] Thereby, abstinence from alcohol and smoking can both control psoriasis and reduce the adverse effects of metabolic comorbidities which are likely to develop in patients with psoriasis.

Stress

It is suggested that psoriasis is a stress-related disease and can be exacerbated by perceived stress. The exact mechanism by which psychological distress exacerbates or triggers psoriasis is poorly understood. May be that psychological stress has the potential to regulate the immune response, and there is emerging evidence that abnormal neuroendocrine responses to stress can contribute to the pathogenesis of psoriasis. Stress in the form of pathological worry has a deleterious effect not only on the disease course but also on response to therapy. The role of stress and psychological aspects are dealt in Chapter 12.

It was observed that serum neurotensin (NT) was increased in psoriasis patients, while lesional skin neurotensin and neurotensin receptor (NTR)–1 gene expression was decreased, as compared to controls. Neurotensin-induced vascular endothelial growth factor (VEGF) release from mast cells and was augmented by IL-33. Suggesting that, NT may play a role in the pathogenesis of the disease and its worsening with stress, at least through activation of skin mast cells.[29]

Obesity

Obesity is considered as a risk factor for psoriasis and can increase the severity of psoriasis.[30] Children with obesity and overweight get more adipose tissue. Onset or worsening of psoriasis with weight gain and/or improvement with weight loss is observed. The adipose tissue is a vigorous endocrine organ capable of secreting multiple pro-inflammatory adipocytokines, such as IL-6, IL-1, TNF-α11 and adiponectin which play an important role in the pathogenesis of psoriasis.

Expression of the disease much depends on the capacity of the epidermis to express the same. This is a complex process, linked to interaction of cells of the epidermis, dermis, immune system and humoral elements. The inherent phenotype has a capacity of the keratinocyte for hyperproliferation and altered differentiation, both of which are genetically controlled. A genetic aberration can, therefore, trigger the cascade of inflammatory events in the evolution of the disease.

PATHOLOGY AND PATHOGENESIS

From a histological point of view, psoriasis is a dynamic dermatosis that changes during the evolution of an individual lesion. Psoriasis vulgaris is a disease of the interfollicular epidermis, and it does not significantly alter the growth of follicular epithelia or the normal hair growth cycle.[2]

Lesions are usually diagnostic only in early stages or near the margin of advancing plaques. Hyperkeratosis, parakeratosis, Munro's microabscesses, spongiform pustule of Kogoj, diminished or absent granular layer, regular acanthosis, papillomatosis, tortuosity and dilatation of papillary capillaries, and chronic inflammation in the upper dermis are the common features seen in psoriasis. However, Munro's microabscesses and Kogoj's micropustules are diagnostic clues of psoriasis, but they are not always present in all cases at all stages. Not all features are demonstrable in a given section at a given point of time even in the same patient. According to some, the appearance of mononuclear leukocytes in the papillary dermis and polymorphonuclear leukocytes (neutrophils) in the stratum corneum are considered the defining features of psoriasis histopathology.[31] Many histological features of psoriasis features can be found in various types of eczemas and other dermatoses.[32] Depending on type, site, and stage of the disease histological features tend to differ (Figs 3.1 to 11). The histology in erythrodermic psoriasis will not show all the classical findings in all cases. Psoriasis

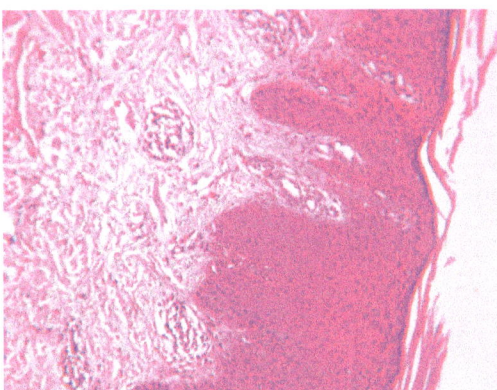

Fig. 3.1: Classical picture showing hyperkeratosis, parakeratosis, thin granular layer, and regular acanthosis

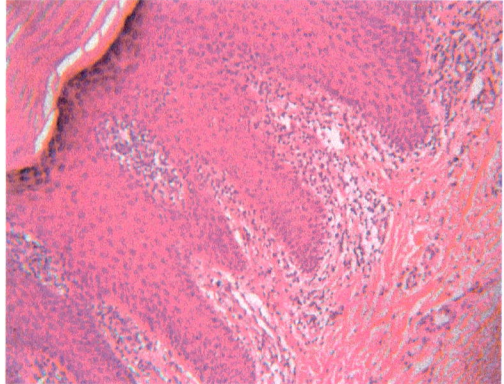

Fig. 3.2: Early papule showing papillae with squirting neutrophils

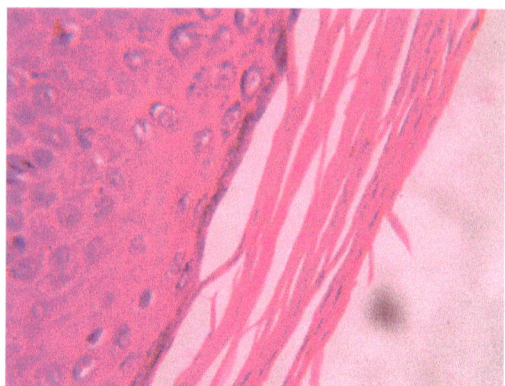

Fig. 3.5: High power view showing hyperkeratosis and parakeratosis with attenuated granular layer

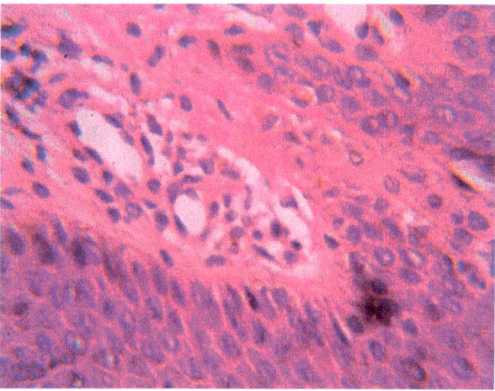

Fig. 3.3: Dilated tortuous capillary under high power

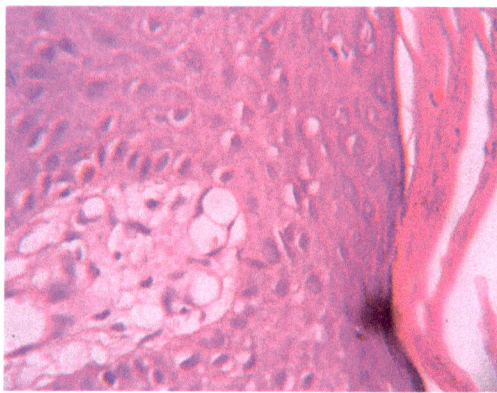

Fig. 3.6: High power view of formation of Munro's microabscess

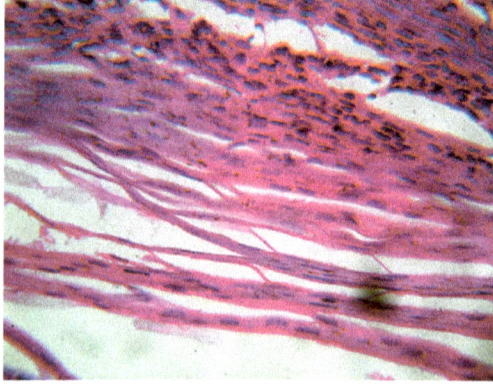

Fig. 3.4: High power view showing hyperkeratosis and parakeratosis of a plaque on the sole

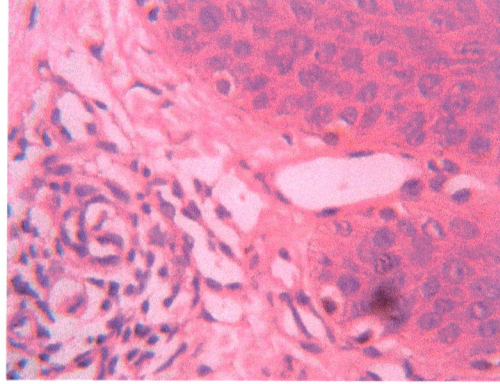

Fig. 3.7: High power view of spongiform pustule

Etiopathogenesis

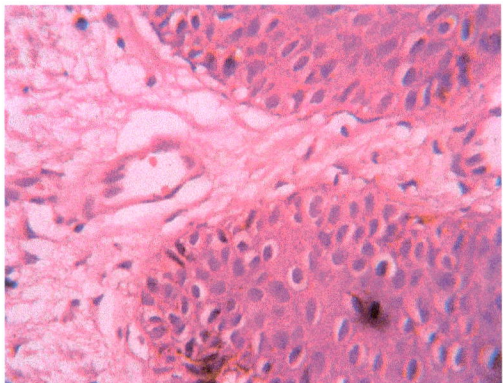

Fig. 3.8: High power view of the dilated papillary capillary

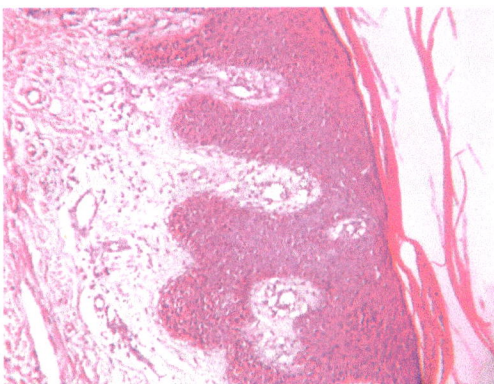

Fig. 3.11: Reduction in epidermal thickening and formation of granular layer after treatment

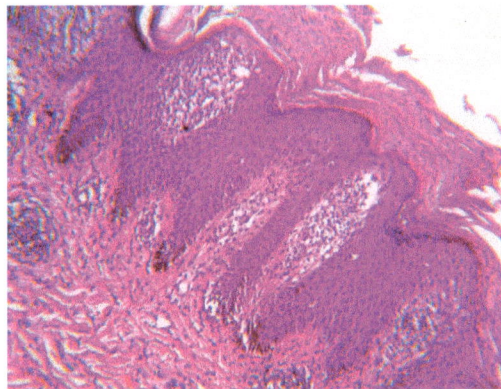

Fig. 3.9: Psoriasis of the palm showing massive hyperkeratosis, parakeratosis, suprapapillary thinning of epidermis, regular acanthosis, dilated papillary capillary with neutrophils

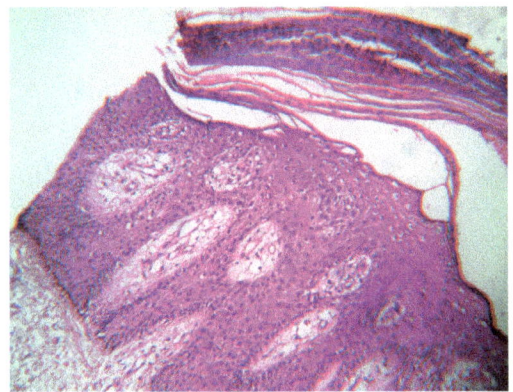

Fig. 3.10: Psoriasis of the sole with gross hyperkeratosis and psoriasis form acanthosis

contributes to nearly a third of erythroderma in neonates and infants where histological diagnosis can be delayed up to 11th month of life. The etiological diagnosis of erythroderma in infants is often a challenge. Keratinocyte proliferation and vascular changes are important microscopic findings in the early evolution of psoriasis. In infants, the most consistent feature of congenital erythrodermic psoriasis is regular acanthosis and dilatation of papillary capillaries with neutrophil squirting in to the epidermis. Munro's microabscess and spongiform pustule of Kogoj are not mandatory for the diagnosis of infantile erythrodermic psoriasis.[33] The mean accuracy of the histopathological diagnoses was less than 55%, even in adult erythroderma.[34]

The main components of psoriatic histology include changes in the:
- Keratinocytes
- Cellular component
- Vasculature, and
- Neural structure.

Acanthosis is probably due to an increase in the number of cycling cells rather than reduction in the cell cycle time. There is approximately seven fold increase in the number of such proliferating cells.[4] The epidermal growth or differentiation program in psoriasis is largely regenerative hyperplasia, a type of hyperplasia programmed in keratinocytes as an injury–repair response pathway. The immune trigger may relate to direct damage to keratinocytes produced by leukocyte trafficking in the epidermis and/or a response to inflammation related cytokines.[35]

According to some, the inflammatory infiltrate appears to be the central reason for the entire pathogenesis of psoriasis. It was observed that increased numbers of T lymphocytes are a highly consistent finding in psoriasis biopsies. With immune histochemical staining, T lymphocytes are found interspersed between keratinocytes throughout the epidermis and in somewhat larger quantities in the dermis. Dendritic cells form another major class of leukocytes that is found in increased abundance in psoriatic skin lesions. Langerhans cells, considered as one type of immature dendritic cell, are resident in normal epidermis and also can be found in psoriasis lesions, sometimes in increased abundance.[36] There is induction of selectin and upregulation of intracellular adhesion molecule-1 that leads to accumulation of skin-homing T lymphocytes within lesional skin. The above pathogenic mechanisms perhaps are best reflected in the histology as very early changes of psoriasis. Abnormal regulation of T cells coupled with interaction between keratinocytes and complex cytokine network is involved in the pathogenesis of the disease. Human skin mast cells are previously recognized as IL-22 producers. It is now established that skin mast cells express IL-17. Thus mast cells might play an important role in the physiopathology of psoriasis a well as atopic dermatitis.[37]

With regard to vascular changes, there is dilatation and elongation of capillary loops with increase in endothelium of superficial microvasculature. These findings, point toward the importance of angiogenesis in the pathogenesis of psoriasis. It is interesting to note that the epidermal keratinocytes are the primary source of angiogenic activity. They produce soluble mediators including VEGF having angiogenic activity which is overexpressed in psoriatic epidermis. Many studies point to a primary role for the immune system in the pathogenesis of psoriasis. However, it cannot be ruled out that vascular change precedes the immune response. Some patients with erythrodermic or severe plaque psoriasis have evidence of systemic capillary leak, such as proteinuria. In such patients, circulating VEGF is detectable and correlates with proteinuria, a well-known complication of erythroderma. Dermal capillaries in addition to vascular growth, contribute to the inflammatory process. There is dilatation and elongation of vertical dermal capillary loops in lesional skin and a four fold increase in endothelium of superficial but not deep microvasculature, indicating that these changes are confined to the upper plexus. There is localization of endothelial proliferation and microvascular expansion in active plaque psoriasis. These vascular changes may point toward the importance of angiogenesis, in the pathogenesis of psoriasis.

It was observed that serum NT was increased in psoriasis patients, while lesional skin NT and NTR-1 gene expression was decreased, as compared to controls. The above findings suggest that NT may play a role in the pathogenesis of psoriasis and its worsening with stress, through activation of skin mast cells.[29]

There is marked proliferation of cutaneous nerves and increased levels of neuropeptides have been detected in lesional psoriatic skin, potentially contributing to the development of psoriasis.[34]

Histology

Histological confirmation of psoriasis is not always mandatory as most of the cases are clinically diagnosed even in children. However, early skin biopsy is helpful in the diagnosis of neonatal and infantile erythroderma where the etiology of erythroderma can be made and timely diagnosis will help manage the child better. Histology does help in adults to rule out other causes of erythroderma. It also helps differentiate atopic dermatitis from psoriasis in both children and adults. However, there are instances where both diseases can coexist (Fig. 3.12).[33] Though recruitment of T cells into the skin and their effector responses are the key features in the pathogenesis of atopic dermatitis and psoriasis, the clinical presentation depends on the localization of the subset of immune cells in to inflamed skin which further mediate their clinical difference. Histologically, psoriasis plaques show hyperkeratosis, parakeratosis, and marked acanthosis. There will be mixed dermal infiltrate, including CD4+ T cells, dendritic cells, macrophages, and mast cells. Dermis shows dilated tortuous papillary blood vessels. Whereas, spongiosis is the predominant feature in atopic dermatitis, intraepidermal neutrophil collection and angiogenesis in the dermis are characteristic features of psoriasis.

Following are the diagnostic histologic features of various types of psoriasis:

Psoriasis Vulgaris

A classical psoriatic papule or plaque shows hyperkeratosis, parakeratosis, hypogranulosis, and neutrophil collection in the stratum corneum, (Fig. 3.13) regular elongation of rete with marked acanthosis and clubbing of the base of the rete. Dermis shows dilated and tortuous capillaries. These changes are variable depending on the stage of the lesion biopsied.

Histology of early papule is characterized by mounds of parakeratosis and few neutrophils in stratum corneum. There will be focal loss of granular layer and slight epidermal hyperplasia. Keratinocytes may reveal increased number of mitotic figures. One can also see slight spongiosis and exocytosis. Perivascular infiltrate consisting of lymphocytes and neutrophils are present in the upper dermis (Fig. 3.14).

Histopathological features of well-developed plaque shows characteristic findings. Stratum corneum shows confluent parakeratosis with collection of neutrophils

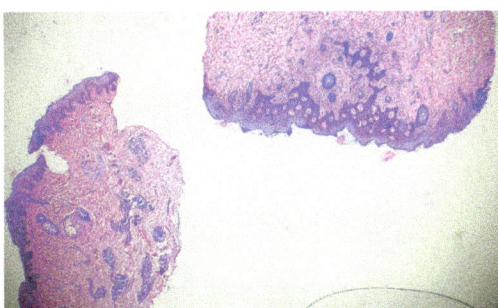

Fig. 3.12: Child with erythroderma showing features of both psoriasis (chest) and eczema (leg) at the same time

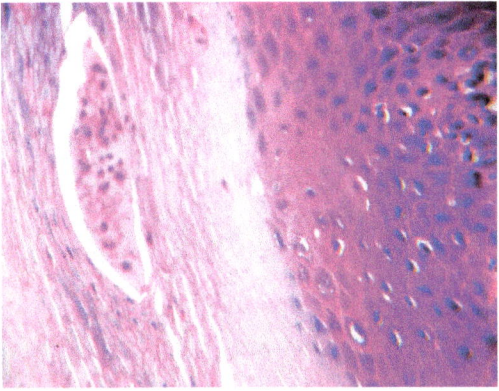

Fig. 3.13: Intracorneal neutrophil collection X400

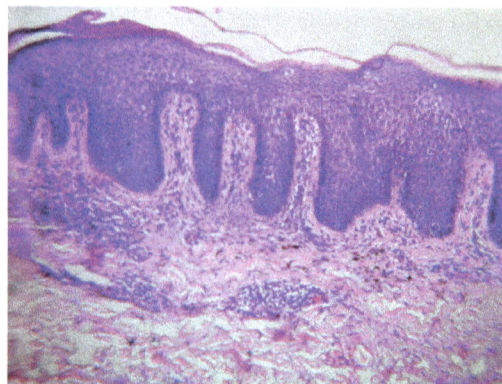

Fig. 3.14: Early papule showing parakeratosis, focal loss of granular layer, spongiosis, and epidermal hyperplasia

which may also be seen in the upper malpighian layer, the spongiform pustule of Kogoj. The upper portion of epidermis may reveal keratinocytes with pale cytoplasm. There will be hypogranulosis and prominent psoriasiform epidermal hyperplasia with regular elongation of rete ridges, sparing the epidermis over the dermal papilla seen as suprapapillary thinning. Exocytosis of lymphocytes may be observed in the lower epidermis. The basal cell layer often shows focal increase in mitotic figures. Dermal papillae are thinned out elongated and contain fibrillary collagen. The papillary capillaries appear dilated and tortuous. Upper dermal vessels may show perivascular infiltrate composed of lymphohistiocytes and neutrophils.

Histology of late stage of plaque psoriasis is characterized compact orthokeratosis instead of parakeratosis. The main histological feature includes acanthosis and elongation of rete. There is conspicuous bulbous enlargement of the tips of the bases which can show bridging of the rete ridges. The suprapapillary plate is thinned. The dermal papillae show dilated tortuous capillaries.

It is conspicuos that dilated capillaries and keratinocyte proliferation are the consistant features in all stages of psoriasis.

Guttate Psoriasis

Histological features of guttate psoriasis include that of early lesions of psoriasis vulgaris (Fig. 3.15).

Erythrodermic Psoriasis

Biopsy from skin of an erythrodermic patient generally displays less characteristic features of psoriasis. In the early stages, stratum corneum may not show hyperkeratosis, and the parakeratosis may be scant. In some patients, the stratum corneum may be absent. However, typical histology of psoriasis may be seen in some individuals with erythroderma. Parakeratosis, neutrophil infiltrate in the stratum corneum, epidermal hyperplasia with spongiosis with slight exocytosis and dilated papillary capillaries along with dermal infiltrate are seen.

Pustular Psoriasis

Histopathology of pustular psoriasis shows features similar to that of psoriasis but with less marked epidermal hyperplasia. Characteristic findings of pustular psoriasis include collection of neutrophils in the upper

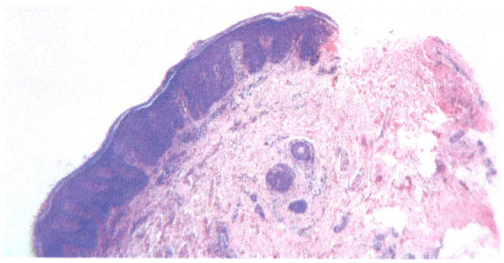

Fig. 3.15: Guttate psoriasis in a child showing features of early psoriasis

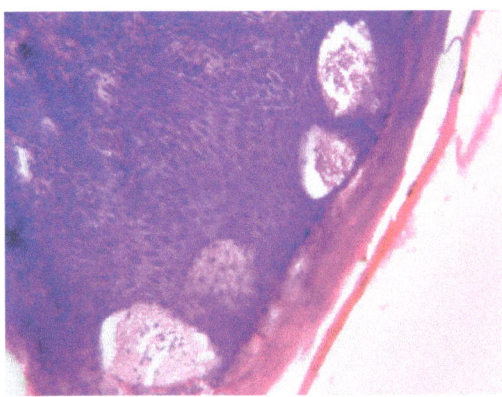

Fig. 3.16: Classical spongiform pustule of Kogoj of pustular psoriasis

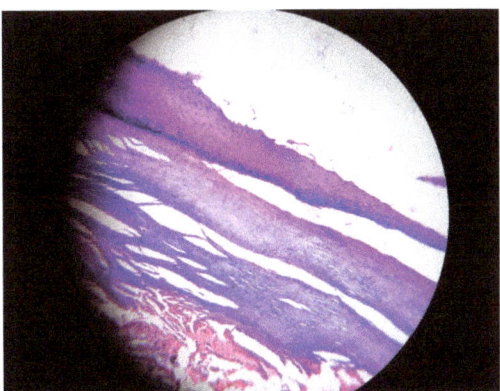

Fig. 3.17: Nail psoriasis showing hyperkeratosis, parakeratosis, and few neutrophils

epidermis. Presence of pockets of neutrophils within the stratum corneum gives rise to intracorneal pustules. Neutrophils collections are also seen below the stratum corneum, giving rise to the subcorneal pustule. Neutrophil with a sponge like array in the upper half of epidermis results in spongiform pustule of Kogoj. Discrete collection of neutrophils in the spinous zone gives rise to the Munro's microabscesses (Fig. 3.16).

Histological findings of pustular psoriasis closely resemble that of Reiter's syndrome.

Nail Psoriasis

Histopathology of nail psoriasis varies according to the clinical focus of the disease. Presence of neutrophils in the nail bed epithelium is the most important finding to make a diagnosis of nail psoriasis. Other histopathological findings include: hyperkeratosis with parakeratosis, serum exudates, focal hypergranulosis, and nail bed epithelium hyperplasia (Fig. 3.17).

Palmoplantar Psoriasis

Psoriasis and eczematous dermatitis of the skin of palms and soles share similar histologic features. Vertically situated multiple foci of parakeratosis, alternating with orthokeratosis, were found to be the only statistically significant feature seen in psoriasis that was not seen in eczema. Multiple foci of parakeratosis, loss of granular layer at least in focal areas, presence of neutrophils at the summits of parakeratosis, presence of neutrophils and/or plasma in the parakeratosis foci, psoriasiform epidermal hyperplasia, spongiosis restricted to the lower parts of the epidermis, dyskeratotic cells, thinning of suprapapillary plate, edema of the papillary dermis, presence of tortuous and dilated capillaries in the papillary dermis, and extravasated erythrocytes were found to be more common in palmoplantar psoriasis compared with eczematous dermatitis; but none of them was statistically significant. It was observed that spongiotic vesicles were seen in most of the patients with psoriasis. Many features of palmoplantar psoriasis overlap with those of eczematous dermatitis. The differential diagnosis of nonpustular psoriasis affecting palmoplantar skin might be troublesome because of the anatomic properties of this region. Presence of multiple parakeratosis foci, placed vertically, alternating with orthohyperkeratosis, could

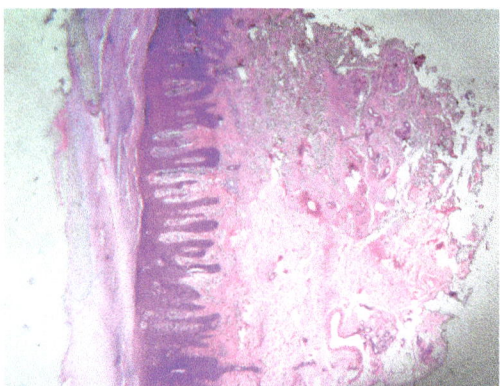

Fig. 3.18: Massive hyperkeratosis seen in psoriasis of the palm

be considered in favor of palmoplantar psoriasis (Fig. 3.18).[32]

Resolving or Treated Psoriasis

There is progressive reduction of neutrophils within the stratum corneum in psoriatic plaques resolving due to treatment. This histological finding is followed by reduction in the amount of parakeratosis. The granular layer starts regenerating. The epidermal changes like acanthosis will take time to resolve. In such cases if there had not been a pretreatment biopsy to compare, histopathologic clue of the disease that may remain is the persistence of papillary dermal capillary dilatation and tortuosity.

Histology of eczema can mimic that of psoriasis. In psoriasiform eczema, there will be more of spongiosis. Absence of Munro's microabscess and spongiform pustule will exclude psoriasis. Dilated tortuous papillary capillaries are not feature of eczema. Late lesions of psoriatic plaque histologically resemble lichen simplex chronicus. In a given patient with psoriasis, overlap with lichen planus and atopic dermatitis are not uncommon. Pustular psoriasis mimics Reiter's syndrome histologically.

Pathogenesis of Psoriasis as a Multisystem Disease

Current evidence prove that psoriasis is no longer a disease of the skin and joints alone, but a disease that can have an impact on other systems and hence, dermatologists should consider the disease as a possible multisystem disease and warn the patients for the prospective negative effects of their disease.

Role of Oxidative Stress and Enzymes in Psoriasis

Oxidative-free radicals and apoptosis have been linked to chronic skin diseases. Higher levels of oxidative radicals and the release of mitochondrial cytochrome C may have a role in the pathogenesis of psoriasis. In a study when patients were subjected for tests, to detect the levels of serum malondialdehyde (MDA), nitric oxide (NO), superoxide dismutase (SOD), catalase (CAT), total antioxidant status (TAS), and serum cytochrome C concentrations, Gabr and Al-Ghadir made the following observations:

- Increase in the levels of MDA and NO; and decrease in SOD, CAT, and TAS levels in all patients with different degrees of psoriasis
- Positive correlation of PASI with the increase in MDA and NO and negative correlation with decreased SOD, CAT, and TAS levels
- Significant increase in cytochrome C level among psoriasis patients which showed negative correlation to MDA and NO levels in mild and positive correlation with moderate and severe groups.

The release of mitochondrial cytochrome C indicates the induction of apoptosis, mediated via oxidative stress which ultimately plays an important role in the pathogenesis of psoriasis.[38]

Etiopathogenesis

Hashemi et al., have shown that serum adenosine deaminase activity and trypsin inhibitory capacity were increased in psoriatic patients. In parallel, serum total antioxidant activity was decreased in these patients.[39] It has been determined that the activity of the prolidase enzyme increases due to the increased collagen turnover in psoriasis patients. Increased serum oxidant levels and oxidative stress indices values may play a role in the pathogenesis of psoriasis.[40]

Psoriasis and atherosclerosis also share common enzymatic sources of reactive oxygen species (ROS), and these ROS influence several cellular signaling pathways implicated in the pathogenesis of both diseases.[41] High plasma overexpression of osteopontin (OPN) and low plasma Selenium (Se) levels are predictable factors for occurrence of psoriasis. However, further studies examining the effects of Se supplementations on the levels of plasma OPN, together with their effects on psoriasis outcome and cardiovascular risk factors in these patients, are needed.[42] It has been determined that the activity of the prolidase enzyme increases due to the increased collagen turnover in psoriasis patients. Increased serum oxidant levels and oxidative stress indices values may play a role in the pathogenesis of psoriasis.[40]

IMMUNOPATHOGENESIS

Psoriasis is now recognized as the most prevalent autoimmune disease caused by inappropriate activation of the cellular immune system. The disease is defined by a series of linked cellular changes in the skin namely, hyperplasia of epidermal keratinocytes; vascular hyperplasia and ectasia; and infiltration of T lymphocytes, neutrophils and other types of leukocyte in affected skin. Substantial evidences implicate both innate and acquired immunity in the disease pathogenesis. Dendritic and T cells play major role in the immunopathogenesis of psoriasis, wherein dendritic and T helper (Th17, Th1) cells secrete varying cytokines that further increase and recruit leukocyte activation and ultimately causing the systemic inflammation. Simple version of immunopathogenesis of psoriasis in the skin is depicted below (Fig. 3.19).

The normal cycle of maturation of keratinocytes is 28–30 days. In psoriasis, this is accelerated to 3–4 days. The immune system has been strongly implicated in the pathogenesis of psoriasis since it resembles a T cell-mediated autoimmune disease. During lesion formation, inflammation precedes epidermal hyperproliferation and increased numbers of T cells have been demonstrated in the uninvolved skin of psoriatics. T cells isolated from involved psoriatic skin may also enhance keratinocyte proliferation. Both CD4+ and CD8+ T cells in active skin lesions are strongly polarized as Th1 cells (Th1 and Tc1, respectively) and there is also a significant increase in circulating type 1 T cells in most patients. Psoriasis serves as the clearest (polar) example of a type 1-deviated skin disease.[1]

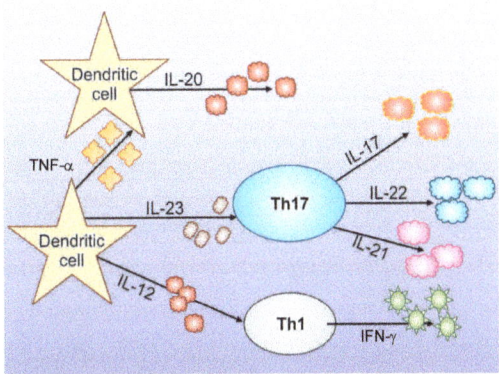

TNF, tumor necrosis factor; Th, T helper; IL, interleukin; IFN, interferon.

Fig. 3.19: Immunopathogenesis of psoriasis in skin

Rapid progress has been made toward dissecting cellular and molecular pathways of inflammation that contribute to disease pathogenesis that encompasses, genetic basis; cellular basis and epidermal proliferation; angiogenesis and vascular changes; immunologic basis and immunologic events including an immunogenetic spin off which determines the clinical manifestation and outcome.

The presence of innate immune cells and their products in psoriatic skin plaques suggests a role for innate immunity in this disease. In addition, the innate immune system can direct the development of pathogenic Th cells in psoriasis.[43]

Several studies have demonstrated that both involved and uninvolved skin, from psoriatic individuals differs from the skin of normal subjects in several ways. The following observations made in psoriatic skin may provide an insight to the pathogenesis of the disease:

- Keratinocyte stem cells (β1 integrin$^+$ K1/K10$^-$) in the uninvolved skin of psoriatic subjects are inherently hyperresponsive to proliferation signals mediated by T cell lymphokines
- Keratinocytes from both involved and uninvolved psoriatic skin are 100 times less sensitive to growth inhibition by 1, 25-dihydroxyvitamin D3 than normal keratinocytes
- Psoriatic keratinocytes show abnormal patterns of integrin α2β1, α3β1, α5β1, and α6β4 expression. Aberrant integrin expression by keratinocytes can have dramatic results as is seen in transgenic mice for integrin β1
- Overexpression of platelet-derived growth factor (PDGF), transforming growth factor-α (TGF-α), IL-6, IL-8, IFN-γ, and monocyte chemoattractant protein-1 (MCP-1) are seen in lesional skin and PDGF is over expressed in uninvolved skin. PDGF induces IL-6 and MCP-1, whereas TGF-α induces IL-8 and MCP-1. TGF-α and IL-8 have been shown to stimulate keratinocyte proliferation
- Fibroblasts from psoriatic skin but not normal skin can induce hyper proliferation of normal keratinocytes. Fibroblasts from uninvolved psoriatic skin proliferate faster than normal fibroblasts in the presence of normal human serum and proliferate to an even greater extent in the presence of serum from psoriatic patients
- The expression of insulin-like growth factor-1 and epidermal growth factor is increased in psoriatic lesional skin
- Fibroblasts from lesional and nonlesional psoriatic skin produce increased amounts of IL-8 compared with fibroblasts from normal skin. The important cellular changes observed in psoriatic skin are tabled in Box 3.5.

Psoriatic skin, therefore, appears to be sensitized toward disease which may be triggered by exogenous or endogenous factors.[11]

One of the most compelling susceptibility factors for psoriasis is the presence of

> **BOX 3.5: Changes observed in psoriatic skin**
>
> - Hyper-responsiveness of keratinocyte stem cells to proliferation signals
> - Decreased sensitivity of keratinocytes to growth inhibition
> - Aberrant integrin expression by keratinocytes
> - Overexpression of PDGF, TGF-α, IL-6, IL-8, IFN-γ and MCP-1
> - Hyperproliferation of fibroblasts
> - Increased production of IL-8 by fibroblast
> - Increased expression of IGF-1 and EGF
>
> PDGF, platelet-derived growth factor; TGF, transforming growth factor; MCP-1, monocyte chemoattractant protein-1; IL-6, interleukin-6; IFN, interferon; IGF, insulin-like growth factor; EGF, epidermal growth factor.

HLA-Cw*0602. Other susceptibility loci for psoriasis reside on chromosomes 1q21, 3q21, 4q, 7p, 8, 11, 16q, 17q, and 20p. It is postulated that alternative pathways of leukocyte activation would converge to activate type 1 inflammatory genes which, in turn, regulate end stage inflammation in skin and the appearance of the psoriasis phenotype.[2]

The immunologic evolution of psoriasis can be studied in three phases: (i) the sensitization phase, (ii) the silent phase, and (iii) the effector phase.[44]

In the first phase, specific effector Th17 and Th1 cells evolve from naïve T cells under the influence of dendritic cells in secondary lymphatic organs, such as the lymph nodes or tonsils. This sensitization phase is followed by the second phase which remains silent for a variable period of time, without any clinical manifestation. As long as the sensitization phase is not associated with an infection or other triggering factor, it is clinically unnoticeable and not characterized by any skin alterations. This is followed by a silent phase of variable duration. In the presence of precipitating or triggering factor like infection or trauma, the third phase namely the effector phase begins with the skin infiltration of various immune cells monocytes or macrophages, various subpopulations of dendritic cells, subpopulations of T cells, and neutrophilic granulocytes.

It has been demonstrated that epidermal keratinocytes are the primary source of angiogenic activity. The expression of P- and E-selectin in dermal blood vessels makes it easier for the infiltration to occur. Immigration of these immune cells activates local tissue macrophages, dendritic cells, and mast cells which liberate their products. Aberrant production of IL-8 and thrombospondin-1 by psoriatic keratinocytes mediates angiogenesis.

As this phase continues, biology of the keratinocytes changes resulting in increased proliferation and altered terminal differentiation. While most studies suggest a primary role for the immune system in psoriasis pathogenesis, it has been argued that vascular change precedes the immune response. Investigations of the active edge of plaque psoriasis showed vascular proliferation to precede changes in epidermal keratin. In the absence of adequate control of inflammation, in the form of treatment, skin lesions persist leading to other consequences.

The sequence of the immunologic events that are theorized to occur in psoriasis would be:[45]
- Antigenic stimuli contribute to the activation of plasmacytoid dendritic cells and other innate immune cells in the skin
- Proinflammatory cytokines produced by innate immune cells, including IFN-α, stimulate the activation of myeloid dendritic cells in the skin
- Myeloid dendritic cells produce cytokines, such as IL-23 and IL-12 that stimulate the attraction, activation and differentiation of T cells
- Recruited T cells produce cytokines that stimulate keratinocytes to proliferate and produce pro-inflammatory antimicrobial peptides and cytokines
- Cytokines produced by immune cells and keratinocytes perpetuate the inflammatory process via participation in positive feedback loops.

The formation of the pustules in IH could be related to imbalance of the skin elastase and its inhibitors as a result of low levels of skin-derived antileukoproteinase (SKALP).

Keratinocytes of patients with atopic dermatitis and psoriasis show an intrinsically abnormal and different chemokines production profile and favor the recruitment of distinct leukocyte subsets into the skin.

However, in spite of their differences, both atopic dermatitis and psoriasis share epidermal hyperplasia, aberrant immunity, and skin barrier anomalies. Genetic studies of both psoriasis and atopic dermatitis suggest that defects affecting cells of the skin need to be as seriously considered as defects in adaptive immunity. The epidermal differentiation complex has been implicated in both atopic dermatitis and psoriasis. It transcribes within terminally differentiating keratinocytes and contains many genes that may modify immune processes in the epithelium. The colocalization of atopic dermatitis to psoriasis loci indicates that atopic dermatitis is influenced by genes that modulate dermal responses independently from atopic mechanisms. What spins off the immune system and decides on the pathogenesis, clinical presentation in a genetically prone individual, needs further elucidation.[46]

Immunopathogenesis of Psoriasis Involving Joints

Inflammatory arthritis is a joint disease characterized by leukocyte invasion and synoviocyte activation followed by cartilage and bone destruction. Variable etiologies contribute to the pathogenesis of joint involvement in PsA. Bone erosion, observed in PsA is solely dependent on osteoclast activation as these cells possess the cellular and molecular machinery required to perform the bone-resorbing function. The extent of bone-resorption correlates with an increase of synovial fluid mononuclear cells and synovial macrophage in the synovial inflammatory infiltrate. The bone resorbing phenotype depends on the osteoclast precursor infiltration into the joint and their activation and differentiation to osteoclasts.[47]

The spondyloarthropathies are a group of rheumatic diseases that are associated with inflammation at anatomically distal sites, particularly the tendon-bone attachments (entheses) and the aortic root. Serum concentrations of IL-23 are elevated and polymorphisms in the IL-23 receptor are associated with ankyosing spondylitis. However, it remains unclear whether IL-23 acts locally at the entheses or distally on circulating cell populations. It has been shown that IL-23 is essential in enthesitis and acts on previously unidentified IL-23 receptor retinoic acid-receptor (RAR)-related orphan receptor and entheseal resident T cells. The presence of these entheseal resident cells and their production of IL-22, which activates signal transducer and activator of transcription 3-dependent osteoblast-mediated bone remodeling, explains why dysregulation of IL-23 results in inflammation at this precise anatomical site.[48]

Synovial tissue in PsA is characterized by a sublining infiltrate with T cells and B cells, vascular proliferation and a relatively thin lining layer of proliferating intimal synoviocytes. Indeed, studies would suggest that the synovitis in PsA can be distinguished from rheumatoid arthritis, with quantitative differences in the features of the tissue, although there are no unique pathological hallmarks in either disease. Local cytokines IL-17, IL-6, and IL-23 further increase inflammation in joint and entheseal complex. Localized inflammation leads to activation of osteoclasts and erosion formation. The presence of novel resident entheseal T cells expressing related orphan receptor respond to IL-23 activation and further secrete IL-22 and enhance IL-6. IL-22 may activate further inflammation.[49]

The events of immune pathogenesis of PsA are depicted in the Fig. 3.20.

Etiopathogenesis

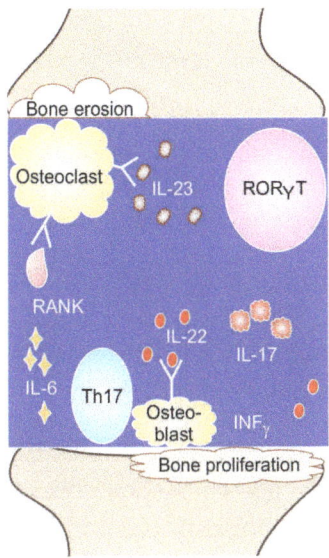

ROR, related orphan receptor; RANK, receptor activator of nuclear factor kappa B; IL, interleukin; IFN, interferon; Th, T helper.

Fig. 3.20: Immunopathogenesis of psoriasis in joint

BIOMARKERS

Ever since research has tried to pin down the exact cause for psoriasis, the need for a marker to predict the chances of the disease in any individual and also the chances of comorbidities in an affected individual has been the target. Various genetic, cellular, and biochemical markers have been discovered in association with psoriasis. It is also scientifically proved that few of these are shared between other associated conditions as well.

Genetic Markers

The HLA region (specifically the version of the HLA-C gene called HLA-Cw0602) was the first genetic marker to be associated with psoriasis.[50] Linkage analysis studies have identified twelve chromosomal loci associated with psoriasis, named PSORS1 to PSORS12. The major psoriasis genetic determinant is PORS1, located within the major MHC on chromosome 6p which probably accounts for 35–50% of the heritability of the disease. Psoriasis has a strong genetic component; a child with two affected parents has a 50% chance of developing the disease; siblings have a three to six fold risk. But the genes responsible for psoriasis have not yet been completely understood.

There is an association between psoriasis and various HLA markers: HLA-B13, B16, B17, B37, Cw6, and DR7 are associated with skin disease; HLA-B27, B38, B39, DR4, and DR7 are associated with skin plus joint disease; the relative risk is 9–15 times normal for HLA-Cw6. There is linkage disequilibrium for HLAs Cw6, B13, and Bw57 as well as an early onset in type I psoriasis, frequently showing positive family history. Whereas, type II psoriasis manifesting at a later age, is more frequently associated with Cw2 and B27 than normal.

Cellular Markers

Keratins can be used as biomarkers of psoriasis severity. Immunostaining with anti-K16, anti-K6, anti-K1, and anti-K10 antibodies reflects abnormal hyperproliferation and differentiation of keratinocytes, whereas K1 and K10, representing markers of terminal differentiation of keratinocytes are down regulated in psoriatic skin lesions. Keratins (K16 and K17) have been identified as markers of keratinocyte hyperproliferation in psoriasis *in vivo* and *in vitro*. At least six markers of abnormal keratinocyte differentiation have been found, and all have implications in the pathogenesis of the disease. These include aberrations of keratinocyte transglutaminase type I, SKALP, migration inhibitory factor-related protein-8, involucrin, filaggrin, and keratin expression.[51]

Serum and Inflammatory Biomarkers

Higher levels of C-reactive protein (CRP) have been demonstrated in patients with psoriasis compared with controls showing a significant correlation to disease severity. VEGF levels were found to be increased and to correlate with disease severity. Indeed, circulating levels of VEGF were higher during active psoriasis and in the presence of PsA, and were lowered during disease remission. Adiponectin, leptin, ghrelin, resistin, inflammatory cytokines (IL- 6, 8, 17, 18, 23, 1β; TNFs, plasminogen activator inhibitor 1), uric acid, CRP and lipid abnormalities are other biomarkers found to be altered in psoriasis. Many other molecules have been proposed as biomarkers of cutaneous psoriasis, including metalloproteinase-1 (a marker of tissue damage), transforming growth factor-β1, and tissue inhibitor of metalloproteinase-1. Expression of toll-like receptor 4 has been found in guttate psoriasis, spectrum of psoriasis that is known to be precipitated by bacterial infection.

Markers of Comorbidity

From the genetic point of view, patients with the cutaneous form of psoriasis and those with PsA share the majority of the predisposing gene variants, in particular, an association with HLA-Cw6. Other class I antigens are also associated with PsA, including HLA-B13, HLA-B57, HLA-B39, and HLA-Cw7. Basal IL-1β, IL-6, and IL-22 levels in synovial fluid were correlated with CRP levels and these cytokines were significantly reduced after this therapy. Other markers that have been detected in the circulation of patients with PsA reflect cartilage destruction and bone remodeling. These include metalloproteinase-3, osteoprotegerin, and the ratio between C-propeptide of type II collagen and collagen fragment neoepitopes (CPII: C2C). The serum level of the receptor activator of nuclear factor kappa-B ligand (RANKL) reflects the extent of bone erosion and has been proposed as a predictive marker of progressive joint damage. Circulating osteoclast precursors in patients with PsA have also been proposed as cellular biomarkers of disease severity because of their correlation with bone erosion. Leptin and resistin could be investigated further as candidate biomarkers for prediction of development of insulin resistance and atherosclerosis in patients with psoriatic disease.

Biomarkers not only provide insights into the mechanisms involved in the pathogenesis of the disease but also help to some extent in the distinction between the different clinical variants of the disease, assessment of disease activity and severity, and prediction of the outcome of a therapeutic intervention. Biomarkers could also allow the selection of patient-tailored therapy to maximize the beneficial effect. A field of great importance is the use of biomarkers for prediction of development of comorbidities, such as arthritis, cardiovascular disease, and metabolic syndrome. In a study done by Hermans using the biomarkers like CRP, human soluble CD40 ligand (sCD40L), oxidized low-density lipoprotein (ox-LDL), human matrix Gla-protein (MGP), and fetuin-A, it was observed that CRP ($p <0.0001$), sCD40L ($p<0.0001$) and MGP ($p <0.0001$) were elevated in the patient cohort. Fetuin-A showed decreased serum levels in patients with psoriasis ($p<0.0001$), whereas ox-LDL did not show any significant difference.[52]

According to Boehncke S et al., sex hormone–binding globulin (SHBG) performed well as a sensitive biomarker for insulin resistance and systemic inflammation in psoriatic patients. Its improvement, as well as the reduction of resistin serum levels, most likely reflects a state of reduced cardiovascular risk in patients undergoing effective continuous systemic therapy. Long-term safety data will help to assess whether this effect translates into reduced cardiovascular mortality.[53]

Thorslund K et al., investigated to find if the increased expression of serotonin transport protein in psoriasis correlated with the severity of disease, chronic stress, and depression who suggest that the serotonergic system may be involved in the chronic inflammation evident in psoriatic skin who add that by modulating the levels of serotonin transporter protein, there might be a therapeutic possibility for reducing chronic inflammation in psoriasis.[54] Salama et al., evaluated the role of psoriasin, koebnerisin, IL-12, and IL-23 in the pathogenesis of psoriasis and their relations to PASI and obesity and opine that psoriasin is the first biomarker to confirm the link between obesity with psoriasis. It was also noted that the risk of development of psoriasis was directly related to higher body mass index.[55]

CONCLUSION

Genetic factors, trauma—both physical and emotional play a major role in the etiology of the disease. Infections caused by bacteria, fungi, and virus and a wide range of drugs can worsen psoriasis. Metabolic factors, pregnancy and hormones, alcohol and smoking do play an important role in determining the exacerbation of the disease. Obesity has been documented to be an individual risk factor associated with psoriasis that can lead to many adverse sequelae on its own and through a state of insulin resistance.

Better understanding of the pathology and immunopathogenesis has paved way to the discovery of many drugs including biologics. The application of biomarkers will help us to study and understand individual patient better, thereby making the choice of therapy easier. Advances in the scientific research with a better understanding of the etiopathogenesis will hopefully keep the disease under control and reduce the complications in future.

REFERENCES

1. Bowcock AM, Cookson WO. The genetics of psoriasis, psoriatic arthritis and atopic dermatitis. Hum Mol Genet. 2004;13(suppl 1):R43-55.
2. Krueger JG, Bowcock A. Psoriasis pathophysiology: current concepts of pathogenesis. Ann Rheum Dis. 2005;64(Suppl II):ii30-6.
3. Lebwohl M. Psoriasis. Lancet. 2003;361:1197-204.
4. Lowes MA, Kikuchi T, Fuentes-Duculan J, Cardinale I, Zaba LC, Haider AS, et al. Psoriasis vulgaris lesions contain discrete populations of Th1 and Th17 T cells. J Invest Dermatol. 2008;128:1207-11.
5. Hüffmeier U, Lascorz J, Becker T, Schürmeier-Horst F, Magener A, Ekici AB, et al. Characterization of (PSORS6) in patients with early onset psoriasis and evidence for interaction with PSOR1. J Med Genet. 2009;46(11):736-44.
6. Wagner EF1, Schonthaler HB, Guinea-Viniegra J, Tschachler E. Psoriasis: what we have learned from mouse models. Nat Rev Rheumatol. 2010;6:704-14.
7. Henseler T. The genetics of psoriasis. J Am Acad Dermatol. 1997;37:S1-11.
8. Riveira-Munoz E, He SM, Escaramís G, Stuart PE, Hüffmeier U, Lee C, et al. Meta-analysis confirms the LCE3C_LCE3B deletion as a risk factor for psoriasis in several ethnic groups and finds interaction with HLA-Cw6. J Invest Dermatol. 2011;131(5):1105-9.
9. Kadunce DP, Krueger JG. Pathogenesis of psoriasis. Current concepts. Dermatol Clin. 1995;13:723-37.
10. Liangdan Sun, Xuejun Zhang. The immunological and genetic aspects in Psoriasis. Berlin, Heidelberg: Springer 2014. Vol. 1. p. 3.
11. Bhalerao J, Bowcock AM. The genetics of psoriasis: a complex disorder of the skin and immune system. Hum Mol Genet. 1998;7(10):1537-45.
12. Trembath RC, Clough RL, Rosbotham JL, Jones AB, Camp RD, Frodsham A, et al. Identification of a major susceptibility locus on chromosome 6p and evidence for

further disease loci revealed by a two stage genome-wide search in psoriasis. Hum Mol Genet. 1997;6:813-20.
13. Guedjonsson JE, Karason A, Antonsdottir AA, Runarsdottir EH, Gulcher JR, Stefansson K, et al. HLA-Cw6-positive and HLA-Cw6-negative patients with Psoriasis vulgaris have distinct clinical features. J Invest Dermatol. 2002;118:360-5.
14. Capon F, Novelli G, Semprini S, Clementi M, Nudo M, Vultaggio P, et al. Searching for psoriasis susceptibility genes in Italy: genome scan and evidence for a new locus on chromosome 1. J Invest Dermatol. 1999;112:32-5.
15. Karason A, Gudjonsson JE, Upmanyu R, Antonsdottir AA, Hauksson VB, Runasdottir EH, et al. A susceptibility gene for psoriatic arthritis maps to chromosome 16q: evidence for imprinting. Am J Hum Genet. 2003;72;125-31.
16. Ros AM, Eklund G, Odont D. Photosensitive psoriasis. An epidemiologic study. J Am Acad Dermatol. 1987;17:752-8.
17. Ferran M, Galván AB, Rincón C, Romeu ER, Sacrista M, Barboza E, et al. Streptococcus induces circulating (CLA+) memory T-cell-dependent epidermal cell activation in psoriasis. J Invest Dermatol. 2013;133:999-1007.
18. Patel RV, Weinberg JM. Psoriasis in the patient with human immunodeficiency virus, part 1: review of pathogenesis. Cutis. 2008;82:117-22.
19. Kim GK, Del Rosso JQ. Drug-provoked psoriasis: Is it drug induced or drug aggravated?: understanding pathophysiology and clinical relevance. J Clin Aesthet Dermatol. 2010;3(1):32-8.
20. Katz M, Seidenbaum M, Weinrauch L. Penicillin-induced generalized pustular psoriasis. J Am Acad Dermatol. 1987;17:918-20.
21. Stewart AF, Battaglini-Sabetta J, Millstone L. Hypocalcemia-induced pustular psoriasis of von Zumbusch. New experience with an old syndrome. Ann Intern Med. 1984;100(5):677-80.
22. Goldman M. Uric acid in the etiology of psor iasis. Am J Dermatopathol. 1981;3(4):397-404.
23. Gisondi P, Targher G, Cagalli A, Girolomoni G. Hyper-uricemia in patients with chronic plaque psoriasis. J Am Acad Dermatol. 2014;70(1):127-30.
24. Golov KG, Ivanov OL, Balkarov IM, Novoselov VS. Clinical significance of hyperuricemia in psoriasis. Klin Med (Mosk). 1994;72(3):34-6.
25. Roth MM, Feier V, Cristodor P, Moguelet P. Impetigo herpetiformis with postpartum flare-up: a case report. Acta Dermatovenerol Alp Pannonica Adriat. 2009;18:77-82.
26. Cemil BC, Cengiz FP, Atas H, Ozturk G, Canpolat F. Sex hormones in male psoriasis patients and their correlation with the psoriasis area and severity index. J Dermatol. 2015;42(5):500-3.
27. Pietrzak A. Psoriasis and unreported excessive alcohol intake a simple screening approach. J Euro Acad Dermatol Venereol. 2011;25:1265-68.
28. Pereira RR, Amladi ST, Varthakavi PK. A study of the prevalence of diabetes, insulin resistance, lipid abnormalities, and cardiovascular risk factors in patients with chronic plaque psoriasis. Indian J Dermatol. 2011;56(5):520-6.
29. Vasiadi M, Therianou A. Alysandratos KD, Katsarou-Katsari A, Petrakopoulou T, Theoharides A, et al. Serum neurotensin (NT) is increased in psoriasis and NT induces VEGF release from human mast cells. Br J Dermatol. 2012;166(6):1349-52.
30. Takahashi H, Tsuji H, Takahashi I, Hashimoto Y, Ishida-Yamamoto A, Iizuka H. Plasma adiponectin and leptin levels in Japanese patients with psoriasis. Br J Dermatol. 2008;159:1207-8.
31. Mobini N, Toussaint S, Kamino H. Papulosquamous disorders. In: Elder DE, Elenitsas R, Johnson BL, Murphy GF, Xu X (Eds). Lever's Histopathology of Skin, 10th edition. New York: Lippincott Williams & Wilkins Co; pp. 169-203.
32. Aydin O, Engin B, Oğuz O, Ilvan S, Demirkesen C. Non-pustular palmoplantar psoriasis: is histologic differentiation from eczematous dermatitis possible? J Cutan Pathol. 2008;35(2):169-73.
33. Parimalam K, Thomas J, Dineshkumar D. Histology of infantile erythrodermic psoriasis–a study of eight cases. E-Journal of the Indian Society of Teledermatology. 2012;6:28-33.
34. Chiricozzi A, Chimenti S. Effective topical agents and emerging perspectives in the treatment of psoriasis. Expert Rev Dermatol. 2012;7:283-93.
35. Tominaga K, Yoshimoto T, Torigoe K, Kurimoto M, Matsui K, Hada T, et al. IL-12 synergizes with IL-18 or IL-1beta for IFN-gamma production from human T cells. Int Immunol. 2000;12:151-60.
36. McGregor JM, Barker JN, Ross EL, MacDonald DM. Epidermal dendritic cells in psoriasis possess a phenotype associated with antigen presentation: in situ expression of beta 2-integrins. J Am Acad Dermatol. 1992;27:383-8.
37. Mashiko S, Bouguermouh S, Rubio M, Baba N, Bissonnette R, Sarfati M. Human mast cells are major IL-22 producers in patients with psoriasis and atopic dermatitis. J Allergy Clin Immunol. 2015; pii:S0091-6749(15)00175-X.
38. Gabr SA, Al-Ghadir AH. Role of cellular oxidative stress and cytochrome c in the pathogenesis of psoriasis. Arch Dermatol Res. 2012;304:451-7.
39. Hashemi M, Mehrabifar H, Daliri M, Ghavami S. Adenosine deaminase activity, trypsin inhibitory capacity and total antioxidant capacity in psoriasis. J Eur Acad Dermatol Venereol. 2010;24:329-34.
40. Sürücü HA, Aksoy N, Ozgöztas O, Sezen H, Yesilova , Turan E. Prolidase activity in chronic plaque psoriasis patients. Postepy Dermatol Alergol. 2015;2:82-7.

41. Armstrong AP, April W, Voyles SV, Armstrong EJ, Fuller EN, Rutledge JCJ. Angiogenesis and oxidative stress: Common mechanisms linking psoriasis with atherosclerosis. J Dermatol Science. 2011;63:1-9.
42. Kadry D, Rashed L. Plasma and tissue osteopontin in relation to plasma selenium in patients with psoriasis. J Euro Acad Dermatol and Venereol. 2012;26(1):66-70.
43. Sweeney CM, Tobin AM, Kirby B. Innate immunity in the pathogenesis of psoriasis. Arch Dermatol Res. 2011;303(10):691-705.
44. Sabat R, Philipp S, Höflich C, Kreutzer S, Wallace E, Asadullah K, et al. Immunopathogenesis of psoriasis. Exp Dermatol. 2007;16:779-98.
45. Nestle FO, Kaplan DH, Barker J. Psoriasis. N Eng J Medicine. 2009:361-496.
46. Parimalam K, Thomas J. Congenital erythrodermic psoriasis with atopic dermatitis: an example of immunogenetic spinoff. Indian J Pathol Microbiol. 2013;56:72-3
47. Adamopoulos IE. Autoimmune or Autoinflammatory? Bad to the Bone. Int J Clin Rheumatol. 2015;10(1):5-7.
48. Sherlock JP, Joyce-Shaikh B, Turner SP, Chao CC, Sathe M, Grein J, et al. IL-23 induces spondyloarthropathy by acting on ROR–gt +CD3 +CD4 –CD8- entheseal resident T cells. Nat Med. 2012;18(7):1069-76.
49. Huynh D, Kavanaugh A. Psoriatic arthritis: current therapy and future approaches. Rheumatology (Oxford). 2015;54(1):20-28.
50. Walter H, Brachtel R, Eckes L, Hilling M. Psoriasis vulgaris and genetic markers. Hum Genet. 1977;37:169-81.
51. Molteni S, Reali E. Biomarkers in the pathogenesis, diagnosis, and treatment of psoriasis. Psoriasis: Targets and Therapy. 2012;2:55-66.
52. Hermans MM, Brandenburg V, Ketteler M, Kooman JP, van der Sande FM, Boeschoten EW, et al. Association of serum fetuin-A levels with mortality in dialysis patients. Kidney Int. 2007;72(2):202-7.
53. Boehncke S, Salgo R, Garbaraviciene J, Beschmann H, Ackermann H, Boehncke WH, et al. Changes in the sex hormone profile of male patients with moderate-to-severe plaque-type psoriasis under systemic therapy: results of a prospective longitudinal pilot study. Arch Dermatol Res. 2011;303(6):417-24.
54. Thorslund K, Amatya B, Dufva AE, Nordlind K. The expression of serotonin transporter protein correlates with the severity of psoriasis and chronic stress Arch Dermatol Res. 2013;305(2):99-104.
55. Salama RH, Al-Shobaili HA, Al-Robaee AA, Alzolibani AA. Psoriasin: A novel marker linked obesity with psoriasis. Dis Markers. 2013;34(1):33-9.

CHAPTER 4

Clinical Aspects

INTRODUCTION

Over 125 million people worldwide, approximately 2-3% of the total population has psoriasis. Studies show that between 10% and 30% of people with psoriasis also develop psoriatic arthritis (PsA). Psoriasis in children is not uncommon. About one out of three people with psoriasis report having a relative with psoriasis. If one parent has psoriasis, a child has about a 10% chance of having psoriasis. If both parents have psoriasis, a child has approximately a 50% chance of developing the disease. A positive family history, precipitating trigger factors, and age of onset can to some extent predict the prognosis of the disease in children. A positive family history has been reported in 23.4-71% of children with psoriasis.[1,2] Identical twins have more chances of manifesting psoriasis than fraternal twins.[3] Clinical features of psoriasis are variable from patient to patient.

This portion of the topic will be dealt under the following headings:
- History and evaluation
- Clinical variants
- Associations
- PsA.

HISTORY AND EVALUATION

It is an art to elicit history and evaluate a patient with any disease, more so with a disease like psoriasis, which is now considered as a systemic disorder with psychological implications and lot of associated comorbidities. Thorough knowledge about the disease will help elicit proper history which will aid in early diagnosis and appropriate treatment. It is of utmost importance to spend time with the patient while eliciting history. This will help to develop a good patient doctor rapport which has got a long way to go in effective control of the disease. Winning the patient's confidence is the first step in getting good patient compliance. The following aspects should be necessarily concentrated upon while evaluating the patient:
- Symptoms
- Age of onset
- Triggering and exacerbating factors

- Signals of psoriasis
- Grading
- Associations.

Symptoms of Psoriasis

Psoriasis is usually an asymptomatic disease. Itching is very variable in psoriasis, ranging from complete absence to severe pruritus in a minority of patients. Intense itching may give a clue to the unstable course of the disease. The degree of itching may reflect the emotional state of the patient and, if severe, may be a symptom of anxiety or depression. Itching is also a sign of unstable psoriasis. Pain is a frequent complaint in patients having palmoplantar pustulosis (PPP) and keratoderma with fissures due to psoriasis. Pain is also a common feature in severe nail psoriasis. Pustular and erythrodermic patterns are more usually accompanied by sensations of burning or tightness. Joint pain may indicate PsA. Severe hair loss is seen in erythrodermic psoriasis. Psoriasis of the scalp does not cause hair loss except in conditions, like tinea amiantacea.

Age of Onset

Variations exist between studies regarding the age of onset of psoriasis. The first manifestation of psoriasis may occur at any age from birth to old age, females tending to present the disease earlier than males. The mean age of onset for the first presentation of psoriasis can range from 15–20 years of age, with a second peak occurring at 55–60 years.[4] Peak age of onset in childhood psoriasis is between 8 years and 12 years.[5] Family history of psoriasis predicts early disease.[6] The disease duration may vary from a few weeks to a whole lifetime. The course is unpredictable and the variations are numerous. Psoriasis type I and type II, are distinguished by a bimodal age of onset (Figs 4.1A and B). Type 1 begins on or before the age of 40 years; type II begins after the age of 40 years. Type I disease accounts for more than 75% of the cases. Elderly-onset patients have shown a lower incidence of family history, with a milder psoriasis area and severity index (PASI) score. The proportion of guttate and generalized pustular psoriasis (GPP) type was lower, and the involvement of knee and trunk was found to be low in elderly-onset psoriasis. Whereas, proportion of erythrodermic psoriasis and scalp involvement was found to be more in the elderly-onset group.

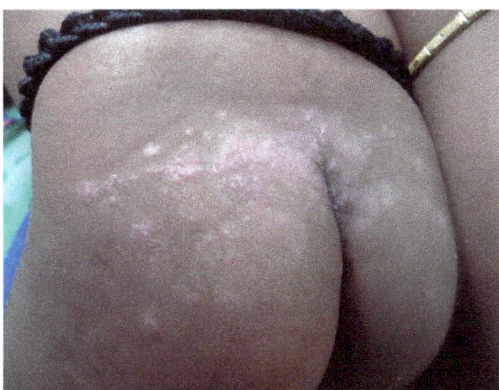

Fig. 4.1A: Type I psoriasis with onset in childhood

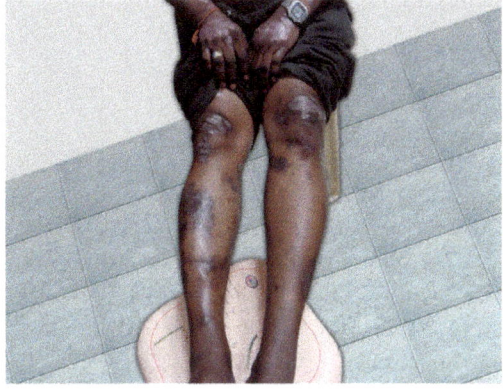

Fig. 4.1B: Type II psoriasis having onset during adult life

Triggering and Exacerbating Factors

Precipitating factors are more important in pediatric, than in adult-onset psoriasis. They largely include trauma, infections, drugs, and stress. The appearance of psoriatic lesions in uninvolved skin at sites of former trauma is known as isomorphic response or Koebner's phenomenon. Various types of trauma may elicit a psoriatic papule in previously uninvolved skin. The Koebner's reaction usually occurs 7–14 days after injury. Koebner's reaction can be seen in nearly three-fourth of patients with psoriasis. If psoriasis occurs at one site of injury, it does so at all sites of injury demonstrating an all-or-none phenomenon. This is of significance in situations like road traffic accidents. Clearing of existing psoriasis following injury is termed the reverse Koebner reaction. Koebner's and reverse Koebner reactions are mutually exclusive. The Koebner reaction is observed more frequently in actively spreading, severe psoriasis. It appears to be a marker for a subgroup of patients with a tendency to early-onset of the disease. Koebner's phenomenon may also indicate possibility of early relapse after various forms of therapy.

Any form of trauma including physical, chemical, thermal, surgical or inflammatory trauma can result in exacerbation of psoriasis. Streptococcal pharyngitis or perianal streptococcal dermatitis typically provokes guttate psoriasis and childhood pustular psoriasis can be elicited by the streptococcal antigen.[7,8] Infection with human immunodeficiency virus (HIV) can induce or exacerbate psoriasis.[9] Whereas, the use of β-blocking agents and lithium is a well-known trigger of psoriasis in adult patients [Figs 4.1C(a to d)]. Use of antimalarials and withdrawal of oral or topical corticosteroids play a more important role in rebound or induction of childhood psoriasis.[10-12] In addition, several studies emphasize the influence of psychological and psychosomatic factors like stress or lack of social support in the course of psoriasis.[13] Inflammatory focus was the most frequent trigger factor observed by Barisic-Drusko and Rucevic.[14] One must understand that gradation exists among psoriatic patients and in the same individual over time, ranging from apparently healthy, with minor signs to overt clinical manifestations. Environmental risk factors triggering psoriasis are categorized in Box 4.1.

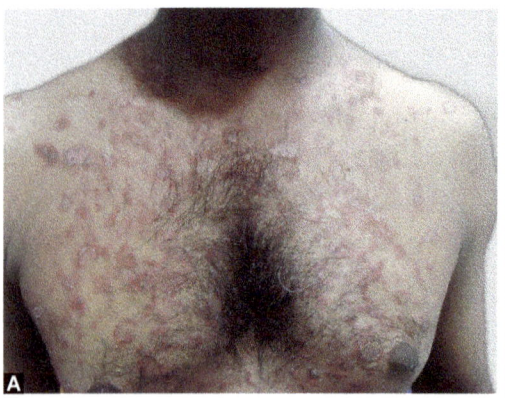 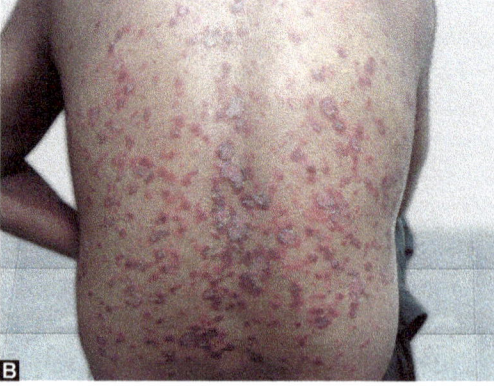

Figs 4.1C(A and B): Man who's psoriasis got exacerbated with β-blocker

Clinical Aspects

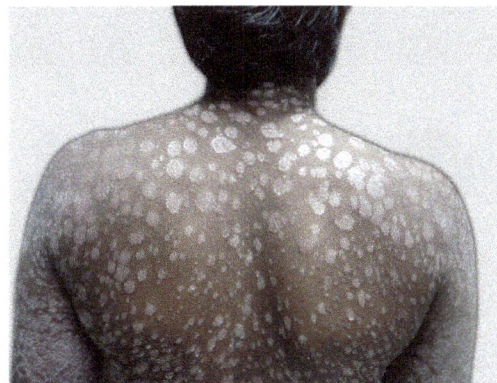

Fig. 4.1C(C): Psoriasis triggered by β-blocker in an adult

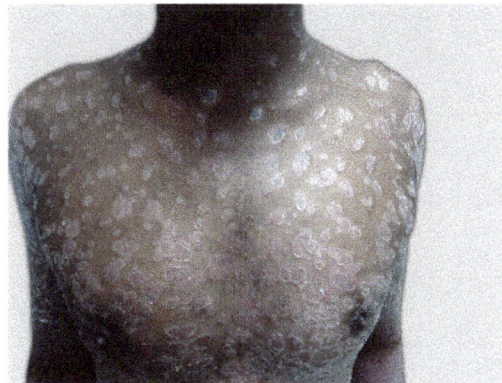

Fig. 4.1C(D): Psoriasis triggered by β-blocker in an adult. Note the varying stages, guttate papules, plaques, and lichenoid hue

Signals of Psoriasis

Even before development of classical papule or plaque of psoriasis, patients may present with any one of the following subtle symptoms which should not be brushed aside.
- Worsening of a pre-existing erythematous plaque
- Sudden onset of pustules
- Recent infection, especially streptococcal sore throat or tonsillitis
- Pain in an asymptomatic plaque in the vicinity of affected joint
- Pruritus (sometimes in guttate psoriasis)

BOX 4.1: Environmental risk factors triggering psoriasis
- Trauma:
  - Physical
  - Chemical
  - Electrical
  - Surgical
  - Infective and inflammatory insults
- Infection:
  - Concurrent streptococcal infection, particularly of the throat
  - HIV infection
- Drugs:
  - Lithium salts
  - Antimalarials
  - β-adrenergic blockers
  - NSAIDs
  - ACE inhibitors
  - Withdrawal of corticosteroids.
- Sunlight
- Metabolic factors
- Hormonal–estrogens
- Hypocalcemia
- Psychogenic factors
- Stress
- Alcohol and smoking
- AIDS

NSAIDs, nonsteroidal anti-inflammatory drugs; ACE, angiotensin converting enzyme inhibitors HIV, human immunodeficiency virus; AIDS, acquired immunodeficiency syndrome.

- Dystrophic nails
- Long-term rash with recent presentation of joint pain
- Joint pain without any visible skin findings.

The so called minor signs usually considered as "stigmata" of psoriasis are easily missed out and the diagnosis is delayed if not looked for (Figs 4.1D to M).[15] The clinical features that help as the signals of psoriasis are given in Box 4.2.

The most common skin manifestations are scaling erythematous macules, papules,

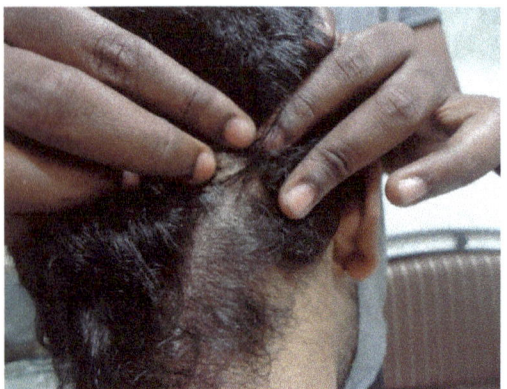

Fig. 4.1D: Severe seborrhoeic dermatitis in a college student, an indicator of psoriasis

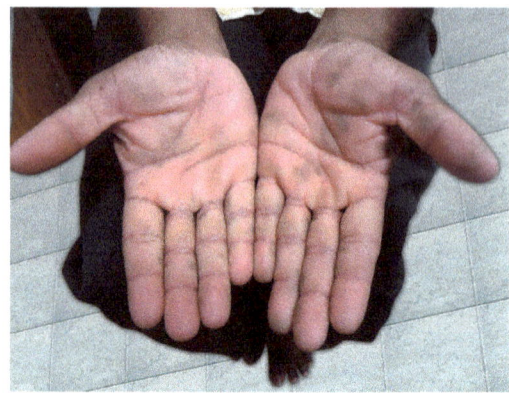

Fig. 4.1G: Keratolysis punctata like lesions on the palms: an early sign of psoriasis

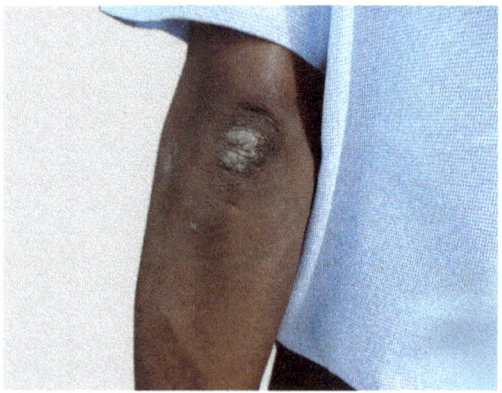

Fig. 4.1E: Hyperkeratotic nonscaly plaque on the elbow of a man: a signal of psoriasis

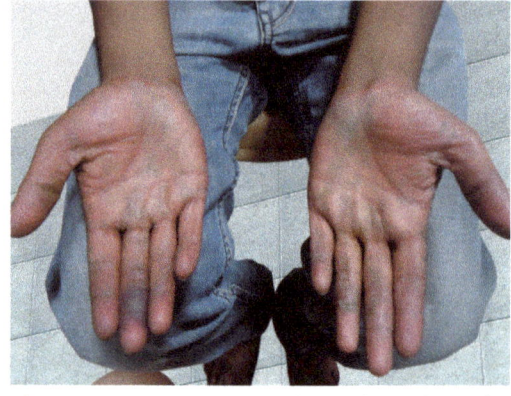

Fig. 4.1H: Eczematous patch on the palms of a young man signaling psoriasis. He also had severe dandruff

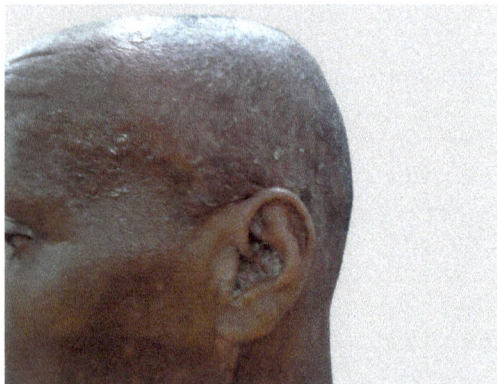

Fig. 4.1F: Psoriasis can be missed in patients presenting with recalcitrant otitis externa

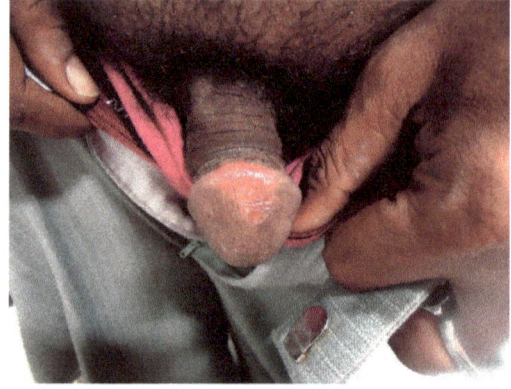

Fig. 4.1I: Sharply marginated erythema of the penile skin should arouse suspicion of psoriasis

Clinical Aspects

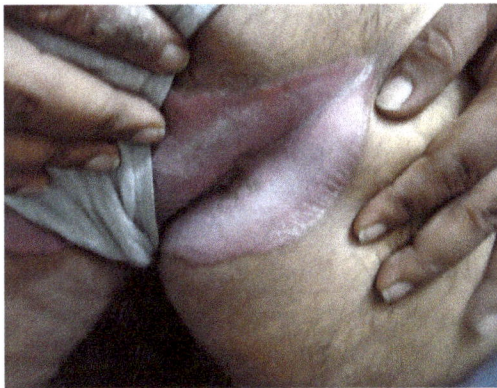

Fig. 4.1J: Intertrigo with sharply marginated erythema may be a sign of psoriasis

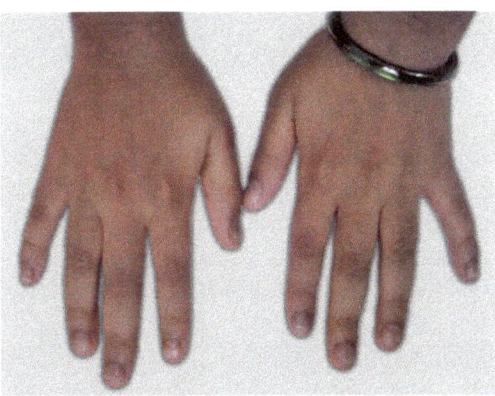

Fig. 4.1L: Nail pitting is a sign of psoriasis

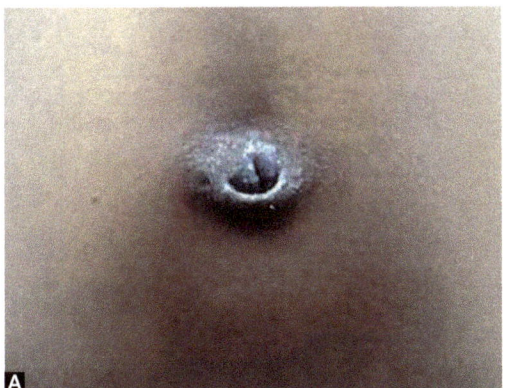

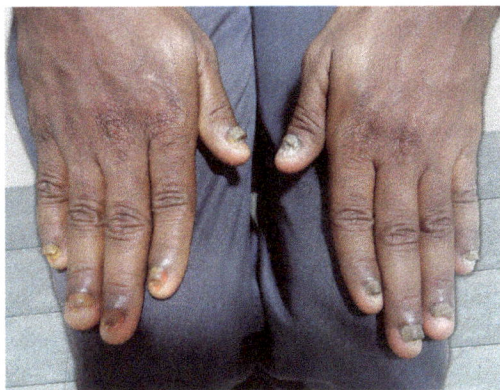

Fig. 4.1M: Subungual hyperkeratosis with onycholysis indicating psoriasis

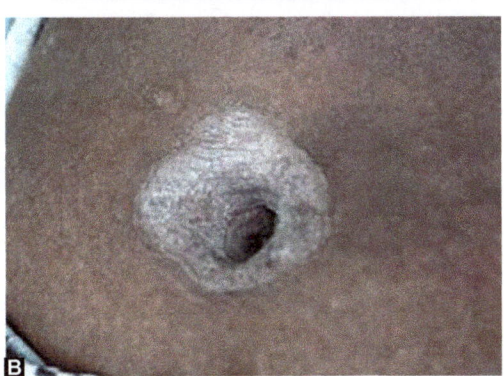

Fig. 4.1K(A and B): Periumbilical erythema and scaling may be a sign of flexural psoriasis which can be easily missed in colored skin

BOX 4.2: Signals of psoriasis

- Severe dandruff
- Hyperkeratotic nonscaly plaques on extensor surfaces
- Recalcitrant scaly otitis externa
- Keratolysis-like lesions of the palms and soles
- Eczematous patches on palms and soles
- Sharply marginated areas of erythema over the penile skin
- Intertrigo with sharp margination of erythema
- Nail pittings
- Subungual hyperkeratosis and onycholysis
- Sterile multiple paronychia

and plaques. Typically, the macules are seen first, and these progresses to maculo papules and ultimately to well-demarcated, noncoherent, silvery plaques overlying a glossy homogeneous erythema. The area of skin involvement varies with the form of psoriasis. The clinical types of psoriasis are more or less the same as in adults and children with some variation in the incidence and manifestations of different types.

Plaque type psoriasis, scalp psoriasis, guttate psoriasis, nail psoriasis, flexural psoriasis, napkin psoriasis, unstable psoriasis, pustular psoriasis are the types of psoriasis commonly encountered in children. Congenital psoriasis, congenital psoriatic erythroderma, and infantile psoriasis are rare forms of psoriasis seen in the first year of life. Erythrodermic psoriasis and PsA are less frequent when compared to adulthood psoriasis. Mucosal involvement has been rare in Indian children.[16] Psoriasis with its wide spectrum of presentation can now be considered as a disease manifesting from "womb to tomb".

The disease in children is more pruritic, and the lesions are relatively thinner, softer, and less scaly. The classical erythematous scaly papule or plaque will mostly give a clue to diagnosis.

The following features are pertinent and helpful in the clinical diagnosis of psoriasis (Figs 4.1N to Q):[17]

- The isomorphic response or Koebner phenomenon, which is occurrence of lesions in areas of trauma
- The Auspitz sign: pinpoint bleeding at the base of scale that has been removed
- Presence of nail pitting, which can aid in diagnosis of the disease
- Altered pigmentation with lesional clearance.

The first two findings are useful to assess the disease activity.

Grading

Severity grading for psoriasis is usually based on surface area and severity.

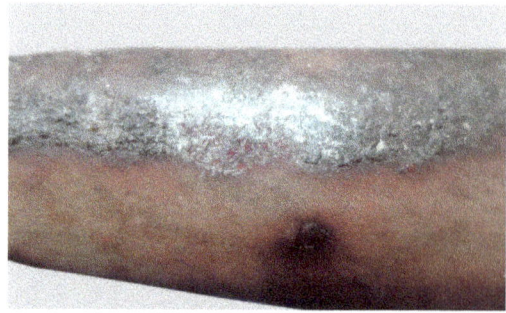

Fig. 4.1O: Large plaque of psoriasis showing silvery white scale. Note the pinpoint bleeding spots, the "Auspitz sign" indicating activity of the disease

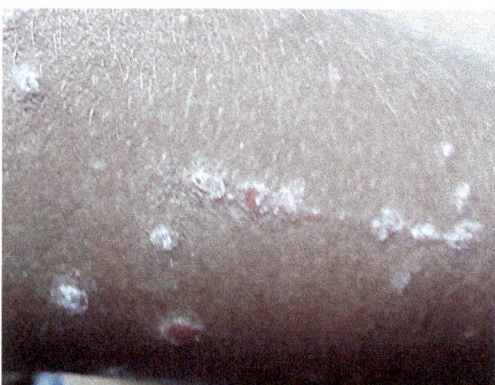

Fig. 4.1N: Isomorphic response in psoriasis. Note the Auspitz' sign as well

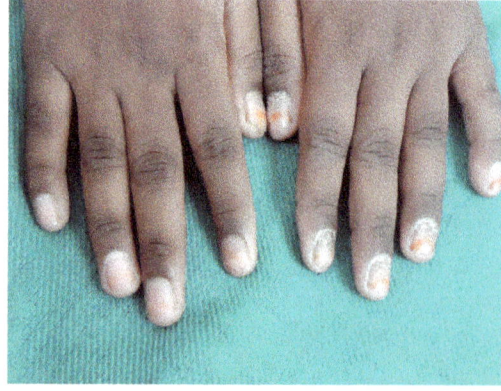

Fig. 4.1P: Nail pitting in a boy who later developed skin lesions of psoriasis

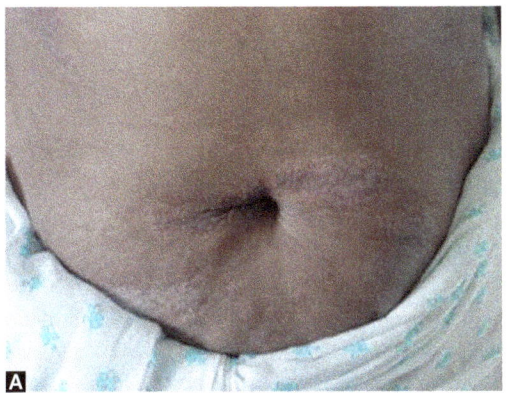 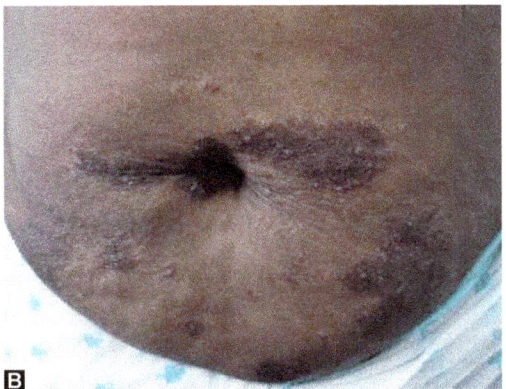

Fig. 4.1Q(A and B): Note the altered pigmentation in psoriatic plaque treated with ultraviolet B (UVB). Steroid treated plaques may show hypopigmentation

Psoriasis area and severity index is the most widely used tool for the measurement of severity of psoriasis. PASI combines the assessment of the severity of lesions and the area affected into a single score in the range 0 (no disease) to 72 (maximal disease). Within each area, the severity is estimated by three clinical signs: erythema (redness), induration (thickness), and desquamation (scaling). Severity parameters are measured on a scale of 0–4, from none to maximum.

The sum of all three severity parameters is then calculated for each section of skin, multiplied by the area score for that area and multiplied by weight of respective section (0.1 for head, 0.2 for arms, 0.3 for body, and 0.4 for legs). The calculation of precise PASI corrects the undesired inaccuracies of PASI in the lower body surface area (BSA) ranges and is a tool to use as an endpoint in trials aiming to detect differences in the lower ranges of BSA.

A simpler way to assess the severity would be mild, moderate, and severe which are represented as less than 3%, 3 to 10%, and more than 10% BSA, respectively.[18] Some define it as limited, less than 3% BSA, or, extensive, greater than 3% BSA. Whereas, in clinical trials, severe psoriasis is defined as, the presence of lesions involving more than 10% BSA. However, these calculations do not take into consideration the impact on the patient's quality of life.

Associations

A detailed history must be elicited to find all the known associations of psoriasis. It is important to elicit relevant findings about the other systems whenever systemic therapy or phototherapy in contemplated.

CLINICAL VARIANTS

Psoriasis is highly variable in morphology, distribution, and severity. Despite the classic presentation described, the morphology can range from small papules (guttate form) to generalized erythema and scaling (erythrodermic form). Skin can be affected without involvement of other structures like nail. In many patients, there can be involvement of more than one structure, skin, nail mucosa and joint. Psoriasis may be symptomatic with patients complaining of intense pruritus or burning. The disease in most patients is asymptomatic, localized or it can be widespread and disabling. Further,

BOX 4.3: Clinical spectrum of psoriasis

- Based on type of disease:
    - Plaque
    - Guttate
    - Linear
    - Follicular
    - Pustular
    - Erythrodermic
    - Unstable
- Based on site of involvement:
    - Scalp
    - Flexural
    - Palmoplantar
    - Mucosal
    - Ocular
    - Nail
- Based on disease manifestation:
    - Latent
    - Mild
    - Moderate
    - Moderate to severe
    - Severe
    - Guarded prognosis

psoriasis may have a variable course. It can present as chronic, stable plaques or may present acutely, with a rapid progression and widespread involvement. The different spectrums of psoriasis are outlined in Box 4.3.

The different types of psoriasis based on type of disease include plaque type, guttate psoriasis, linear psoriasis, follicular psoriasis, pustular psoriasis, erythrodermic psoriasis, and unstable psoriasis.

Based on Type of Disease

Plaque-type Psoriasis

Psoriasis vulgaris or plaque-type psoriasis is, by far, the most common clinical type of psoriasis both in children and adults accounting to as high as 80%. Classical plaque is characterized by erythema and silvery white scales. The color, a full rich red referred to as "salmon pink" is characteristic of psoriasis which is not seen in other close mimickers like eczema, seborrhoeic dermatitis or lichen simplex. However, the depth of color differs in too fair an individual and lost in too dark an individual. Scale in psoriasis can vary in thickness. The amount of scaling varies among patients and even at different sites on a given patient. In acute inflammatory or exanthematic psoriasis, scaling can be minimal and erythema may be the predominant clinical sign.[19] The common sites involved include, scalp, postauricular area, elbows, knees, umbilical region, and buttocks. The lesions may initially begin as erythematous macules (flat and <1 cm) or papules, extend peripherally, and coalesce to form plaques of one to several centimeters in diameter [Figs 4.2A(a to h)]. One can observe some degree of uniformity in the clinical appearance of plaques of psoriasis modified little by site size. While the scaling varies in degree, the hue remains consistent. The plaques are well-defined, with a sharply delineated edge. Annular and gyrate figures may be produced with central normal appearing skin by merger of these plaques. The plaques are always raised and hence

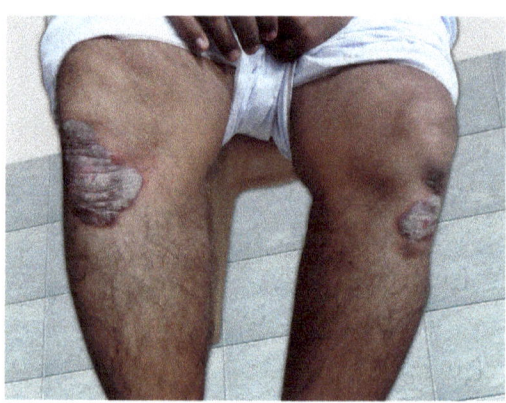

Fig. 4.2A(A): Plaque psoriasis showing Auspitz sign

Clinical Aspects

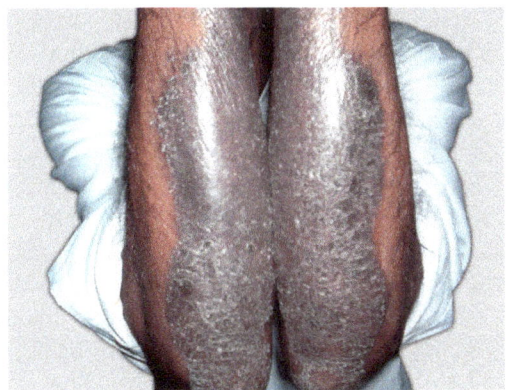

Fig. 4.2A(B): Persistence of plaque psoriasis due to constant friction acting as Koebnerization

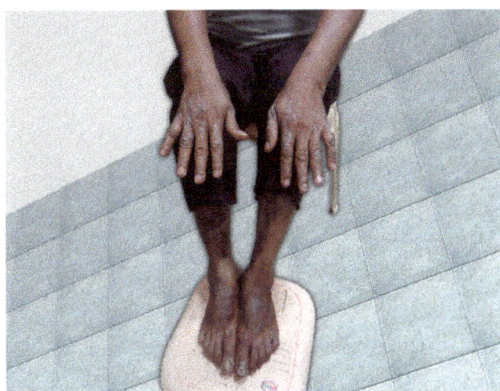

Fig. 4.2A(E): Plaque type psoriasis of the hands and feet

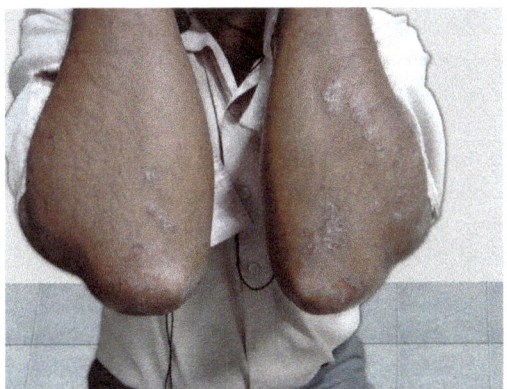

Fig. 4.2A(C): Plaque type psoriasis affecting the extensor surface

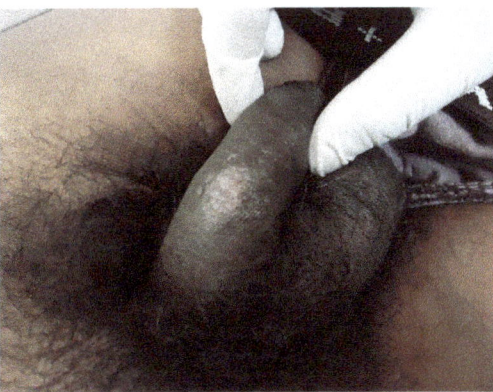

Fig. 4.2A(F): Rare site for plaque type psoriasis

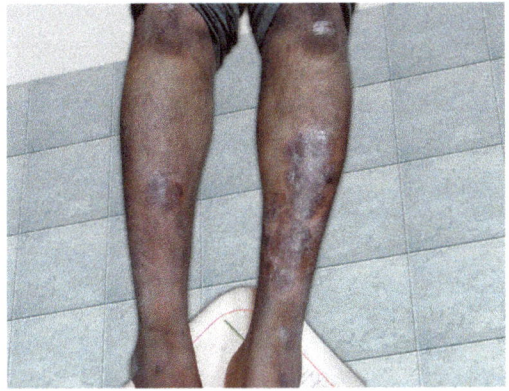

Fig. 4.2A(D): Psoriasis vulgaris affecting the shin

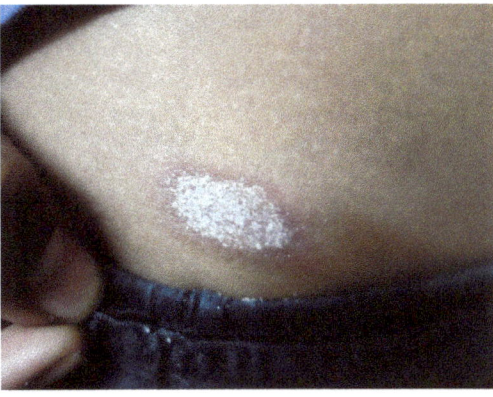

Fig. 4.2A(G): Classical silvery scale of psoriasis

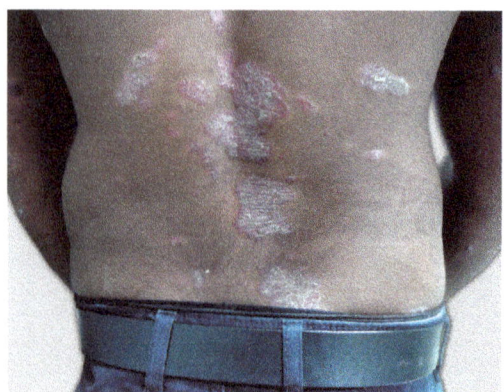

Fig. 4.2A(H): Salmon pink plaques with silvery white scales of psoriasis, showing uniform appearance

easily palpable due to epidermal thickening characteristic of the psoriatic process which helps in differentiating seborrheic dermatitis of the scalp. Treatment and washing may result in temporary loss of this palpability but only temporarily.

Plaques vary in size with diameter ranging from one to several centimeters. They can be round, oval or irregular in shape. Similarly, the number is also variable from single plaque to any number of lesions. Symmetry is invariably observed, if there are multiple plaques. Large plaques are commonly seen on the legs, forearms, and sacral region. Fissuring is a common manifestation seen over the plaques involving the palmoplantar skin and plaques occurring across the line of joint movement. A white blanching ring, known as Woronoff's ring, may be observed in the skin surrounding a psoriatic plaque, especially in resolving lesions.

Scalp is the most common initial site affected. Facial involvement in children is a frequent observation in majority of the reports, which varies from 18% to 46%.[20]

Presence of Koebner's' response (development of isomorphic skin lesion along the line of trauma) is an indicator of disease activity. Eczema can sometimes closely mimic psoriasis, when the scales are loose. Auspitz sign is the characteristic clinical finding that helps in the diagnosis of psoriatic papules and plaques and demonstration of Auspitz sign will help diagnosing psoriasis though it is not pathognomonic for psoriasis. It is always advisable to examine the hidden sites of psoriasis as they are sometimes the true signals. Bowen's disease and cutaneous T-cell lymphoma can mimic plaque type psoriasis and should be ruled out by pathological study in a chronic plaque of psoriasis that does not respond to treatment. The severity of plaque type psoriasis can be assessed using PASI score.

Rupioid, elephantine, and ostraceous psoriasis are special forms of plaque psoriasis characterized by gross hyperkeratosis. Rupioid psoriasis refers to limpet-like cone-shaped lesions while the term elephantine psoriasis is used to describe very persistent, thickly scaling, and large plaques. These are seen on the back, limbs, hips or elsewhere. Ring-like hyperkeratotic lesion with a concave surface, resembling an oyster shell is known as ostraceous psoriasis.

Guttate Psoriasis

Guttate (gutta meaning a droplet) psoriasis presents as small salmon-pink papules, 1–10 mm in diameter, predominately on the trunk [Figs 4.2B(a to c)]. These are usually distributed in a centripetal fashion although guttate lesions can also involve the head and limbs. The lesions may be scaly. Papules frequently appear suddenly, 2–3 weeks after an upper respiratory infection with group A β-hemolytic streptococci which can be the presenting episode of psoriasis in children and occasionally in adults. Guttate psoriasis has been reported to follow Kawasaki disease.[21] Guttate psoriasis accounts for 2% of the total cases of psoriasis. The number of lesions may range from five or 10 to over 100. In children, an acute episode of guttate psoriasis is usually self-limiting. Whereas, in adults, guttate flares may complicate course of chronic plaque disease. Although few studies have assessed the long-term prognosis of children with acute guttate psoriasis, nearly one-third of patients with guttate psoriasis eventually develop plaque type of psoriasis. Pityriasis rosea and early papule of lichen planus can be differentiated with evolution of the disease. There will be intense itching in lichen planus. However, patients with lichen planus prefer rubbing to scratching, where elicitation of Auspitz sign will be painful. Wickham's striae which are white crisscross beaded lines observed using a hand lens after applying mineral oil to the papule will differentiate lichen planus from psoriatic papule.

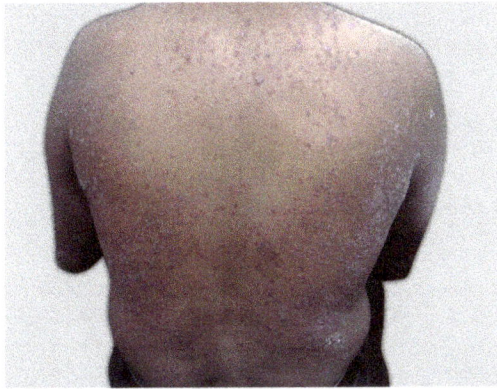

Fig. 4.2B(A): Guttate psoriasis in an adult

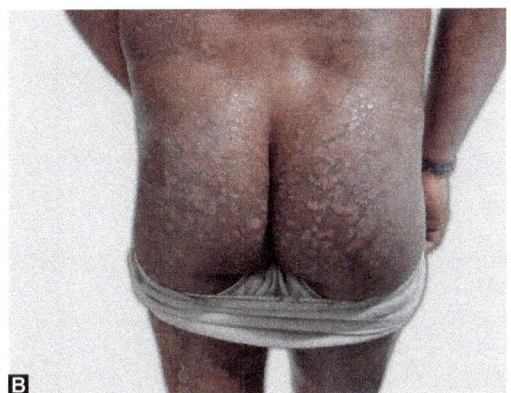

Linear Psoriasis

Erythematous scaly papules or plaques following the lines of Blaschko are features of this rare variant, linear psoriasis. Unlike inflammatory linear verrucous epidermal nevus (ILVEN), there is no or only mild pruritus (Fig. 4.2C). Presence of Koebner's phenomenon and demonstration of Auspitz sign will help clinical diagnosis which can be further confirmed with biopsy, the histology of which will show psoriasiform features.

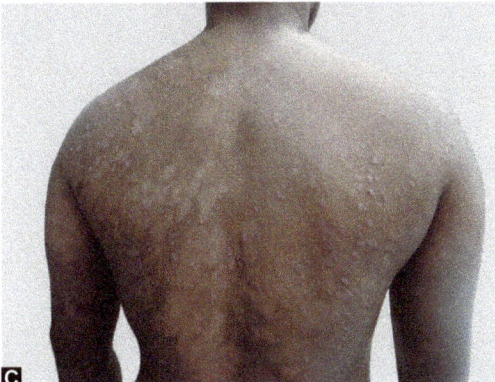

Figs 4.2B(B and C): Guttate lesions in adult evolving to psoriasis vulgaris

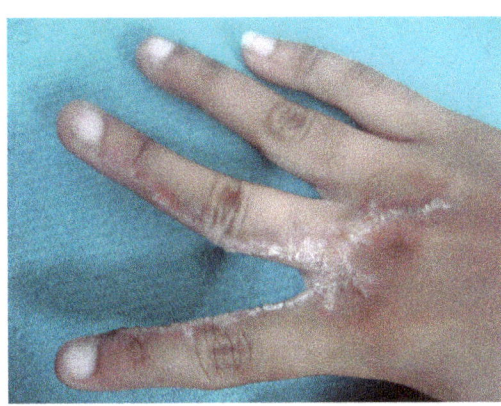

Fig. 4.2C: Linear psoriasis in an adult

Family history for psoriasis is often positive in patients with Blaschko's linear psoriasis.[22] ILVEN, a disease with linear morphology should be differentiated from linear psoriasis. There is lower expression of keratin 10 in psoriasis as compared to normal levels in ILVEN. Whereas, lower levels of cell surface expression markers of T-cell subsets, such as CD8, CD45RO, CD2, CD94, and CD161 are features of ILVEN.[23]

Follicular or Spinulosic Psoriasis

Follicular psoriasis is rare form of psoriasis, but is more frequent in children. It may be mistaken for pityriasis rubra pilaris which is characterized by rough follicular papules on an erythematous base, especially on the dorsal aspect of the fingers, and by large orange-red plaques with distinctive "islands of sparing". An orange-red waxy palmar and plantar keratoderma is also peculiar. Histologically, pityriasis rubra pilaris differs from that of psoriasis due to the presence of alternating parakeratosis and hyperkeratosis in both vertical and horizontal directions (spotty parakeratosis). Recurrent infundibulo folliculitis, a clinical feature of atopic dermatitis may clinically mimic follicular psoriasis due to scaly follicular lesions. Histologically, presence of spongiosis of the hair follicle will clinch the diagnosis of infundibulo folliculitis. Neutrophil infiltration of the stratum corneum, which is an important feature of psoriasis, is not seen in pityriasis rubra pilaris and follicular eczema.

Pustular Psoriasis

Pustular psoriasis presents as sterile pustules appearing locally or diffusely over the body [Figs 4.2D(a to l)]. Pustular psoriasis may cycle through erythema, pustules, then scaling. Pustular psoriasis can develop de novo or in a patient with psoriasis vulgaris. The clinical presentation can vary from a single plaque studded with pustule to the whole body showing pustules, sometimes in severe cases, lakes of pus. For easy clinical approach, pustular psoriasis can be classified as, localized or generalized. Localized pustular psoriasis predominantly involves the hands and feet, whereas GPP affects the entire body surface. GPP can evolve into erythroderma which is a dermatological emergency

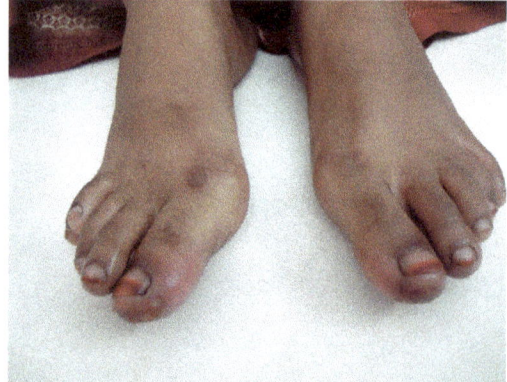

Fig. 4.2D(A): Localized pustular psoriasis of the feet

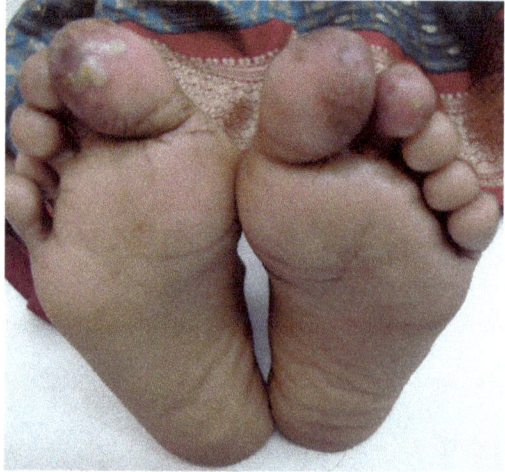

Fig. 4.2D(B): Note pustules with erythema and scaling early stage of acrodermatitis continua

Clinical Aspects

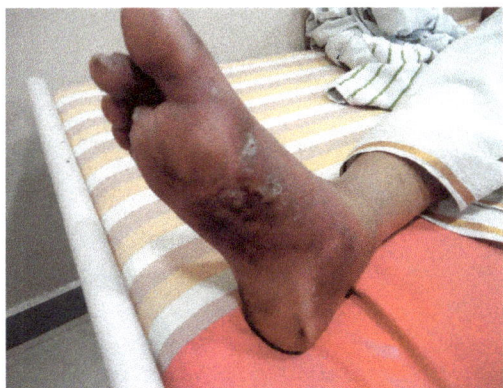

Fig. 4.2D(C): Localized pustular psoriasis of the sole

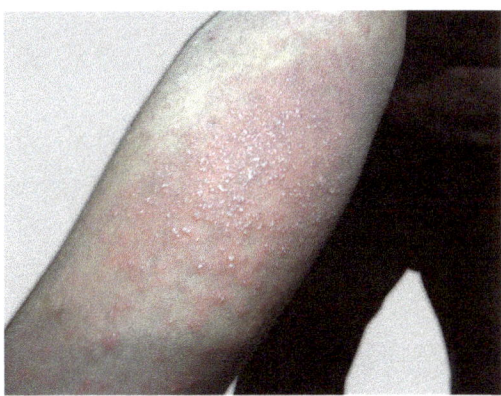

Fig. 4.2D(F): Pinpoint pustules in early pustular psoriasis

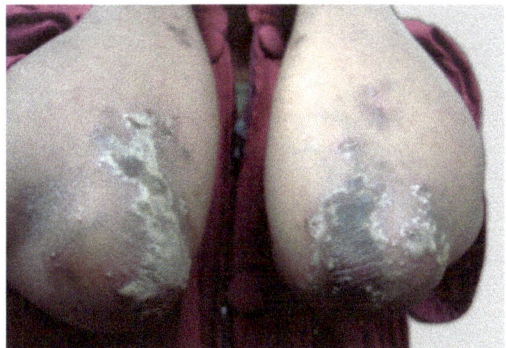

Fig. 4.2D(D): Localized form of pustular psoriasis in an adolescent boy who was having plaque type psoriasis

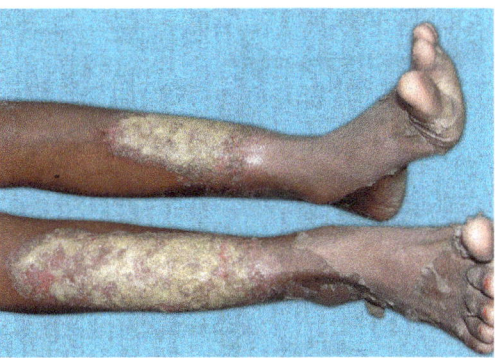

Fig. 4.2D(G): Superficial pustules after sudden withdrawal of systemic steroids

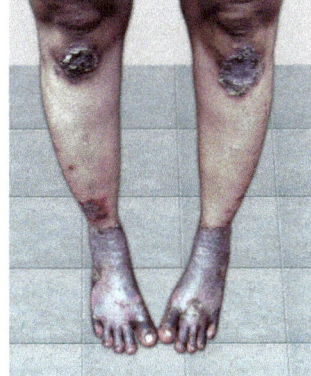

Fig. 4.2D(E): Localized form of generalized pustular psoriasis resolving after therapy and resuming the original plaque morphology

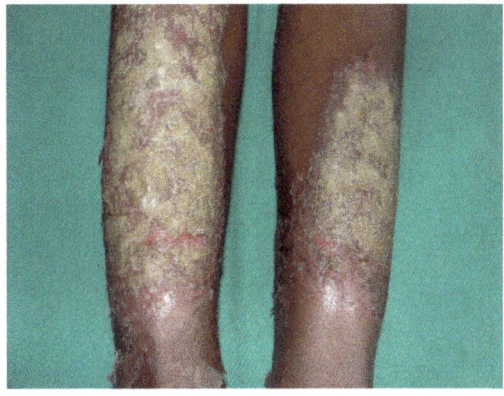

Fig. 4.2D(H): Lake of pus in acute generalized pustular psoriasis

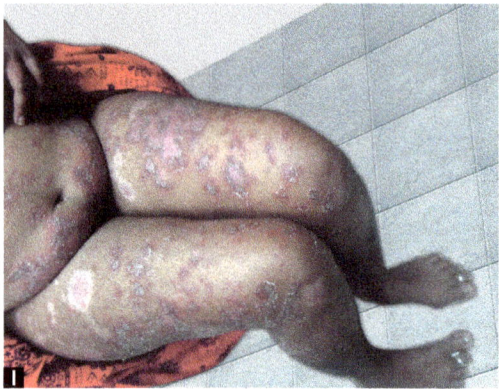
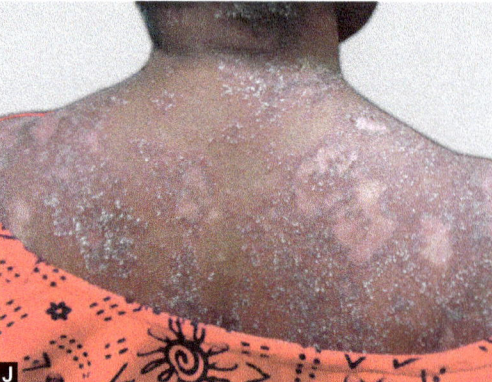

Figs 4.2D(I and J): Acute generalized pustular psoriasis of von Zumbusch

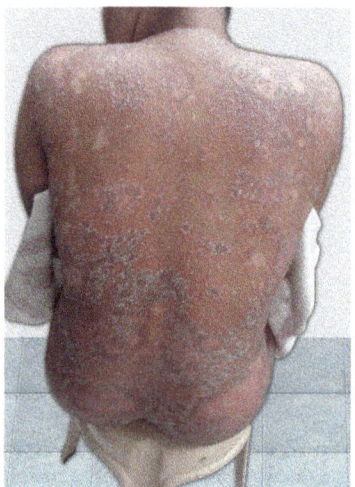
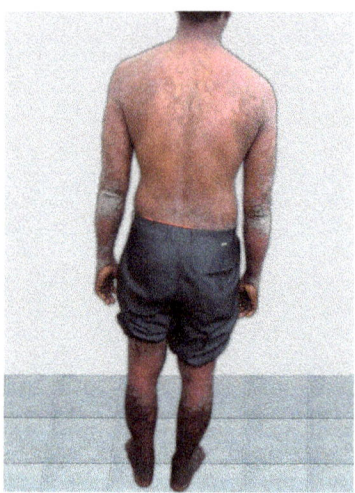

Fig. 4.2D(K): Generalized pustular psoriasis mimicking acute generalized exanthematous pustulosis

Fig. 4.2D(L): Generalized pustular psoriasis in a man with psoriasis vulgaris following steroid withdrawal

requiring inpatient care. Erythroderma due to GPP, if not properly managed can lead to multiorgan failure. Box 4.4 gives the types of pustular psoriasis.

Localized Pustular Psoriasis

Palmoplantar Pustulosis

The relationship of PPP to psoriasis vulgaris is controversial.[24,25] PPP was previously considered to be a localized form of pustular psoriasis, but about 10–20% of patients with

> **BOX 4.4: Types of pustular psoriasis**
> - Localized pustular psoriasis:
>   - Palmoplantar pustulosis
>   - Acrodermatitis continua of Hallopeau
> - Generalized pustular psoriasis (GPP):
>   - Acute GPP
>   - GPP of pregnancy
>   - Infantile and juvenile GPP
>   - Circinate, annular, linear GPP
>   - Localized form of GPP

PPP have psoriasis elsewhere. It is now known that they are distinct conditions with different genetic backgrounds.

Smoking has been shown as a probable provocative factor for PPP.[26] PPP is much more common in smokers. It is thought that activated nicotine receptors in the sweat glands induce an inflammatory process.[27]

Acrodermatitis Continua of Hallopeau

This form of localized pustular psoriasis often starts at the tip of the digit, the skin becoming red and scaly, and pustules develop subsequently. Vesiculo pustules are followed by a fringe of undermined epidermis with a red glazed skin. Nail bed may be involved, leading to nail dystrophy and even onycholysis. Bony changes can occur leading to osteolysis of the tuft of the distal phalanx. The free end of the digit may become wasted and tapered with disturbance in the vasculature. Acrodermatitis continua, though is a disease of children may also affect adults. Acrodermatitis continua of Hallopeau in adults may evolve into GPP. The tongue may become involved with fissuring or show features of geographic tongue also known as annulus migrans of pustular psoriasis. Tinea manuum is usually asymmetric in distribution and demonstration of the fungal element will help in establishing the diagnosis which is sometimes challenging. Contact dermatitis can be confirmed with a patch test. Parakeratosis pustulosa in children can mimic acrodermatitis continua. However, the occurrence of pustules is rare. There is predominant scaling along with nail dystrophy.[28] Histological examination will confirm psoriasis which will show neutrophilic microabscess.

Generalized Pustular Psoriasis

Generalized pustular psoriasis is an uncommon variant of psoriasis characterized by eruption of sterile pustules which can be acute, subacute or occasionally chronic. GPP can be considered as an extreme form of psoriasis in which all the main pathological features of the disease are accentuated. Its relationship to psoriasis vulgaris is clear, due to the following facts: patients with pustular psoriasis have family history of psoriasis. Some may have phases of ordinary psoriasis before or after the GPP, pustular psoriasis has a classical psoriatic histology. In addition, systemic drugs like methotrexate (MTX), etretinate, and cyclosporine A are effective in both psoriasis vulgaris and GPP.

Amongst the many predisposing factors, steroid withdrawal seems to be the most common cause of pustular eruption in psoriasis. Other factors contributing to the etiology of pustular psoriasis include infection, pregnancy, and hypocalcemia associated with hypoparathyroidism.

Provocation is most obvious in the acute forms of pustular psoriasis. The irritation caused by inadvertent use of coal tar and dithranol may provoke pustulation in patients with psoriasis. Intensive topical therapy with very potent corticosteroids under occlusion has also been implicated. It was also documented that withdrawal of cyclosporine therapy could induce GPP.[21,22] Chronic, previously stable acrodermatitis continua have been converted to GPP by high-dose oral prednisolone followed by sudden withdrawal. There are many drugs that can precipitate GPP which are listed in Box 4.5.

Acute Generalized Pustular Psoriasis (Von Zumbusch)

Two main groups have been distinguished. In the first, typical psoriasis of early-onset develops into pustular psoriasis after some years, often after a triggering factor. In the second, late-onset psoriasis undergoes spontaneous progression to the generalized pustular form.[29] The onset may be preceded by sensation of burning followed by dryness of the skin. An abrupt onset of high fever and severe malaise precedes development of generalized eruption of pinpoint pustules. Sheets of erythema and pustulation spread to involve previously unaffected skin, the flexures and genital regions being particularly involved. Different configurations like isolated pustules, lakes of pus, circinate lesions, plaques of erythema with pustular collarets or a generalized erythroderma can be seen. Waves of pustulation may succeed each other, and the pustules dry.

The nails become thickened or separated by subungual lakes of pus. The buccal mucosa and tongue may be involved. Geographic tongue and fissured tongue are the common oral manifestations.[30] Remission occurs within days or weeks. Exhaustion, toxicity or infections are the common causes of death in untreated cases. Remission is followed by erythroderma or return to the original state. Relapses are common. GPP should be differentiated from acute generalized exanthematous pustulosis (AGEP), which is difficult at times. Withdrawal of systemic or topical corticosteroids can precipitate or worsen acute generalized pustular psoriasis and these agents should be used with caution. The following features will help differentiating GPP and AGEP. Difference between GPP and AGEP are given in Table 4.1.

Childhood Pustular Psoriasis

Childhood pustular psoriasis is a rare disease which usually appears at 2-10 years of age constituting less than 1% of childhood

> **BOX 4.5: Drugs precipitating generalized pustular psoriasis**
>
> - Salicylates
> - Iodide
> - Lithium
> - Phenylbutazone
> - Oxyphenbutazone
> - Progesterone
> - Terbinafine
> - Amfebutamone
> - Withdrawal of steroid

TABLE 4.1: Differentiating features of generalized pustular psoriasis and acute generalized exanthematous pustulosis

Features	GPP	AGEP
History of psoriasis	Mostly present	Possible (if the patient is also a psoriatic)
History of drug intake	May be present	Must be present
History of arthritis	Common	Not relevant
Duration of fever	Longer	Shorter
Duration of pustules	Longer	Shorter
Onset	Anywhere may be over a psoriatic plaque	Intertriginous area or face
Distribution	More generalized	Predominantly in the folds
Oral mucosal involvement	Invariably present	Mild in up to 20%
Eosinophilia	Not significant	May be seen

Continued

Continued

Features	GPP	AGEP
Histology:		
• Subcorneal/intraepidermal pustules	+	+
• Acanthosis	+	−
• Keratinocyte necrosis	+	−
• Eosinophil exocytosis	−	+
• Papillomatosis	+	−
• Papillary dermal edema	−	+
• Papillary capillary dilatation	+	−
• Vasculitis	−	+
Altered liver enzymes	Invariably present, may be very high though transient	Mild elevation
Course	Tends to recur	Resolution on withdrawal of offending drug

GPP, generalized pustular psoriasis.

psoriasis.[31,32] A male preponderance is seen in GPP of childhood in contrast to GPP in adults.

A review of 1,262 cases of childhood psoriasis found a 0.6% rate of pustular variants. Four clinical patterns of pustular psoriasis have been described in children namely, GPP or von Zumbusch, annular pustular psoriasis, exanthematic pustular psoriasis, and localized pustular psoriasis. Annular form seems to be the most common presentation. They are not necessarily mutually exclusive and mixed variants are also possible.[33]

In children, GPP manifests as an acute, episodic, and potentially life-threatening form of psoriasis and classically presents as widespread sheets of sterile pustules on bright erythematous skin that resolves within 3–4 days, with recurrent waves of inflammation. The acute postulation is typically associated with fever and toxic changes.[34] Compared with the adult forms, the first manifestation of GPP in children is usually more severe, presenting with high fever accompanied by generalized pustules. Few of these cases eventually develop psoriasis vulgaris. The younger the age of onset, the more severe the patient's condition can be.

Pustular Psoriasis of Infancy

Nearly one-fourth of pustular psoriasis can have the onset during the first year of life. The disease may begin in the first few weeks of life and two cases of congenital GPP have been described.[35] Infantile cases are usually benign. Systemic symptoms are often absent and spontaneous remissions are known to occur. History suggestive of psoriasis in the form of an eruption diagnosed as seborrheic dermatitis, napkin dermatitis could be elicited in some infants. Rarely more severe forms with fever and toxicity occur. Infants with congenital erythroderma can have supervening pustular eruption.

Circinate, Annular, and Linear Forms of Pustular Psoriasis

Circinate type of pustular psoriasis appears as discrete areas of erythema, which become raised and edematous. Pustules appear at the edges of the round lesions, spread centrifugally, and may mimic erythema annulare centrifugum. The pustules dry out and leave a trail of scale as the lesion grows. Annular and other patterned lesions may be seen in acute GPP, but are more characteristic of the subacute or chronic forms of widespread pustular psoriasis. It may occur alone or as a phase in the evolution of GPP. Linear forms of pustular psoriasis are occasionally observed within the context of more generalized pustulosis.

Localized form of Pustular Psoriasis

These must be distinguished from PPP or acropustulosis. The term "psoriasis with pustules" is perhaps more appropriate. One or more plaques of psoriasis vulgaris may develop pustules especially after excessively irritant topical therapy.

Erythrodermic Psoriasis

Erythrodermic psoriasis is a particularly inflammatory form of psoriasis that often affects most of the body surface. It generally appears on people who have unstable plaque psoriasis, where lesions are not clearly defined. It is characterized by periodic, widespread, fiery redness of the skin. Histopathological confirmation to establish the cause of erythroderma as psoriasis is not always possible during the acute stages. When the patient presents with erythroderma for the first time without a definite history of psoriasis, one has to wait for the acute phase to settle to establish the diagnosis. Systemic steroids should be used with extreme caution in such cases.

There are two forms of erythrodermic psoriasis based on the onset. In the first form, chronic plaque evolves gradually into an exfoliative phase. In this type, one can see extensive plaque psoriasis involving the entire cutaneous surface, however, showing some areas of uninvolved skin. Here, the plaques retain the characteristics of the disease. In the second form, patients present suddenly with erythroderma which is marked by severe itching or burning as the case may be. It is frequently seen in unstable psoriasis, GPP and due to intolerance to topical treatment, or phototherapy. It can be precipitated by infections, hypocalcemia, antimalarials, tar, and classically by sudden withdrawal of corticosteroids. In this form of erythroderma, the characteristics of the disease are lost. Patient will be ill with erythema edema and scaling involving more than 80% of body surface.

Erythrodermic psoriasis presents as generalized erythema, pain, itching, and fine scaling.

It typically encompasses nearly the entire BSA [Figs 4.2E(a to k)]. It may be accompanied by fever, chills, hypothermia, and dehydration secondary to the large BSA involvement. Presence of psoriatic plaques in classic locations, nail changes characteristic of psoriasis, facial sparing, and inflammatory arthritis will help suspect psoriasis as the cause for erythroderma in a patient seen for the first time. Itching may be severe, when the other causes of erythroderma like eczematous dermatitis or Sezary syndrome, should be ruled out. Presence of

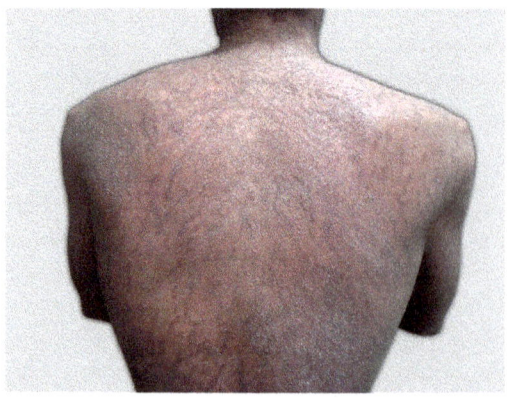

Fig. 4.2E(A): Erythrodermic psoriasis in a college student

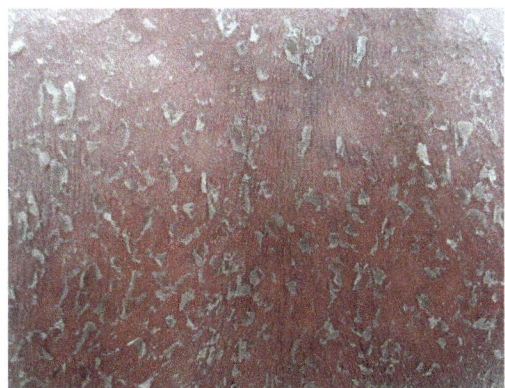

Fig. 4.2E(B): Note crimson red erythema of psoriatic erythroderma

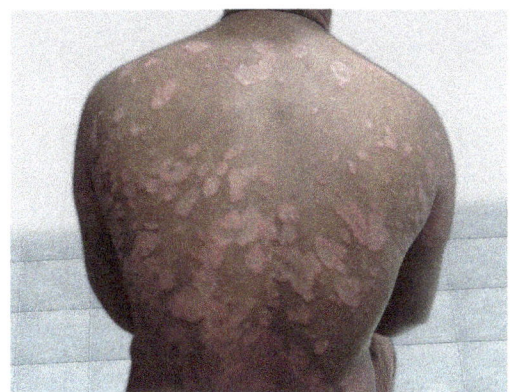

Fig. 4.2E(E): Psoriasis starting as guttate lesion progressing to plaque type and rapidly evolving to erythroderma: an unstable form of psoriasis

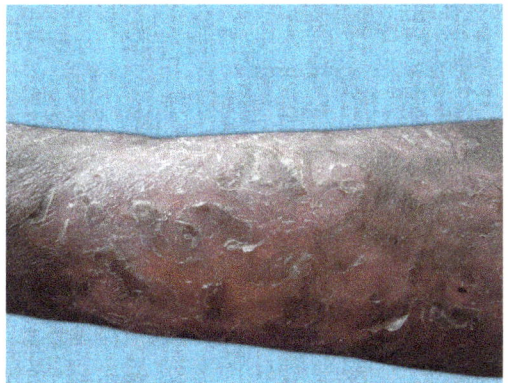

Fig. 4.2E(C): Closer view of scaling and erythema of erythrodermic psoriasis

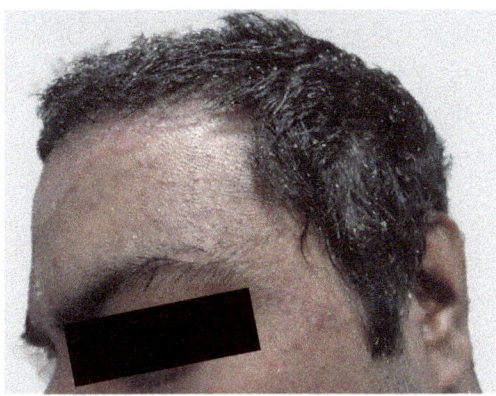

Fig. 4.2E(F): Note involvement of scalp in erythrodermic psoriasis

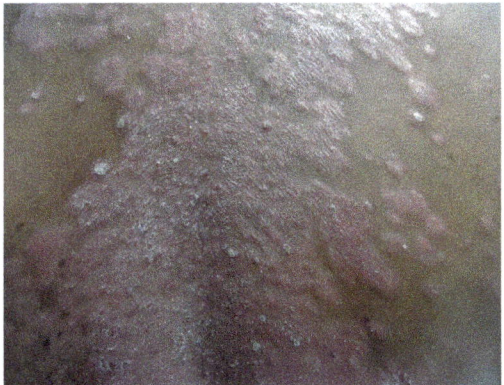

Fig. 4.2E(D): Plaque psoriasis evolving into erythroderma

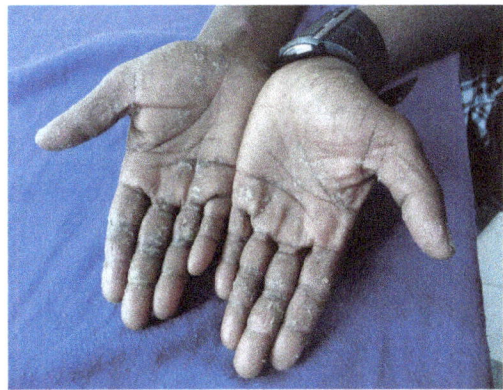

Fig. 4.2E(G): Involvement of palm in erythrodermic psoriasis

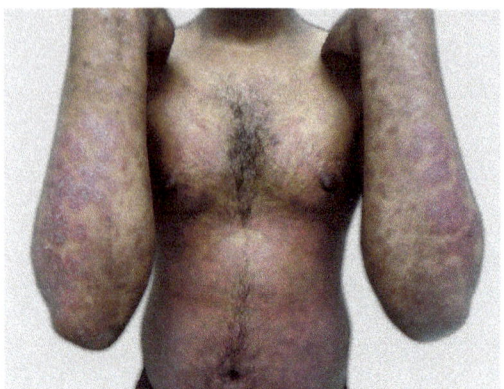

Fig. 4.2E(H): Large easily removable scales with intense erythema in erythrodermic psoriasis

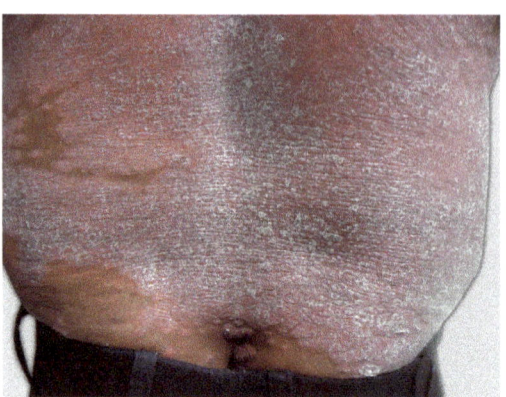

Fig. 4.2E(K): Erythrodermic psoriasis with guarded prognosis

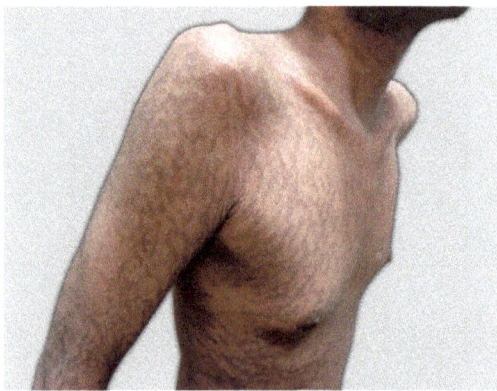

Fig. 4.2E(I): Erythrodermic psoriasis recalcitrant to treatment

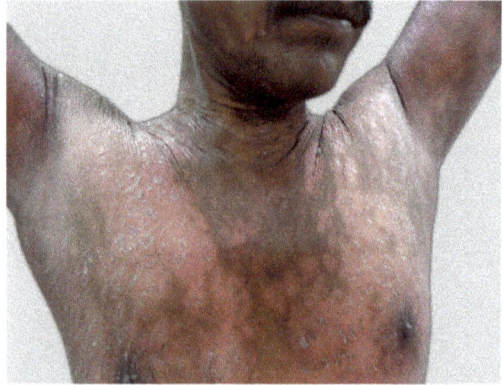

Fig. 4.2E(J): Psoriatic erythroderma with relative sparing of the face and sun exposed skin

lymphadenopathies is also a more common finding in both erythroderma and Sezary syndrome which has to be assessed properly.

Patients with severe pustular or erythrodermic psoriasis may require hospital admission for metabolic and pain management. Older patients with erythrodermic psoriasis may experience cardiac instability and hypotension due to massive vascular shunting in the skin.

Pedal edema, especially around the ankles, may also develop along with infection. Disruption in the thermoregulatory mechanism leads to shivering episodes. Infection, pneumonia, and congestive heart failure brought on by erythrodermic psoriasis can be life-threatening.

Erythrodermic Psoriasis in Children

Erythrodermic psoriasis is a rare clinical presentation in childhood psoriasis. It may arise from any type, commonly from the plaque type. It may arise from any type of psoriasis. Drugs, environmental, psychological, and metabolic factors can trigger the onset of erythrodermic form of the disease. This spectrum of psoriasis is characterized by generalized erythema, edema, desquamation, and systemic compromise. The child will present with fever, dehydration, malaise, and malnutrition. The overall presentation can range from mild-severe form. The erythrodermic form occurs in about 1.4% of psoriasis cases in children and adolescents. Over all, less than 3% of childhood psoriasis manifests with erythroderma.

Congenital Erythrodermic Psoriasis

Congenital psoriasis, meaning psoriasis present at birth or appearing during the neonatal period, is exceptional. Congenital occurrence of psoriasis, defined as the development of any of its clinical variants at birth or during very first days of life is considered very rare. In the recent times, psoriasis is emerging as the most common cause for erythroderma in infants. Clinicopathologic correlation is mandatory in confirming congenital erythroderma due to psoriasis.

Unstable Psoriasis

Unstable psoriasis is a dermatological emergency. People with stable chronic plaque psoriasis may suddenly progress to unstable psoriasis. It also involves forms like the erythrodermic form and the pustular form that can rapidly progress and cause dangerous sometimes fatal medical complications, even death. The erythema and scaling of the skin are often accompanied by severe itching and pain. Erythrodermic psoriasis is a particularly inflammatory form of psoriasis that often affects most of the body surface. When it appears on people who have unstable plaque psoriasis, where lesions are not clearly defined, it is characterized by periodic, widespread, fiery redness of the skin [Figs 4.2F(a to c)]. Such erythrodermic psoriasis "throws off" the body chemistry, causing protein and fluid loss that can lead to severe illness. Common triggers include infections, drugs, alcohol, and abrupt cessation of steroids. The course of disease is unpredictable and the condition is a medical emergency and will require inpatient multidisciplinary care. Intense pruritus and skip areas of normal skin may arouse a suspension of cutaneous lymphoma which has to be differentiated by histology [Fig. 4.2F(d)].

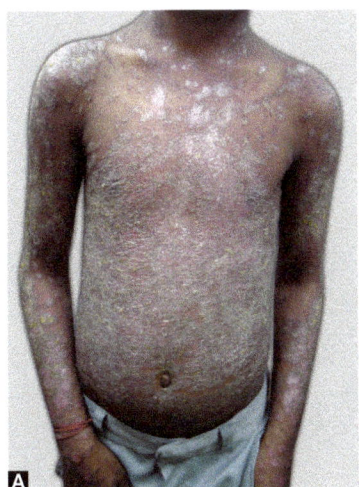 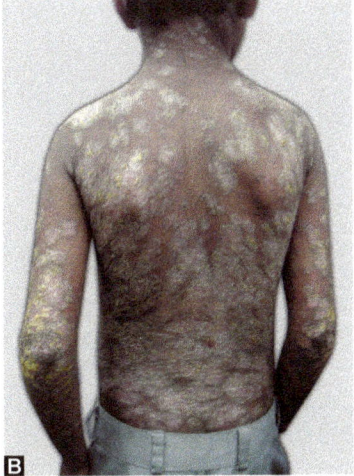

Figs 4.2F(A and B): Unstable psoriasis with severe itching

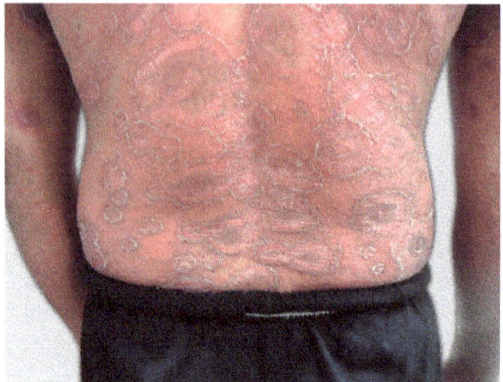

Fig. 4.2F(C): Unstable psoriasis. Note the fiery red erythema

erythema typically transgress the frontal hair line feature that helps in differentiating from seborrheic dermatitis. Circumscribed scaly plaques are sometimes the only presentation. There can be diffuse hair loss in those with erythrodermic psoriasis. The most common condition that can be confused with psoriasis is seborrheic dermatitis of the scalp. In psoriasis, the scales are silvery white and the plaque extends beyond the hair margin where as in seborrheic dermatitis, the scales are greasy and the patch is limited to the hair bearing area [Figs 4.2G(a to g)].

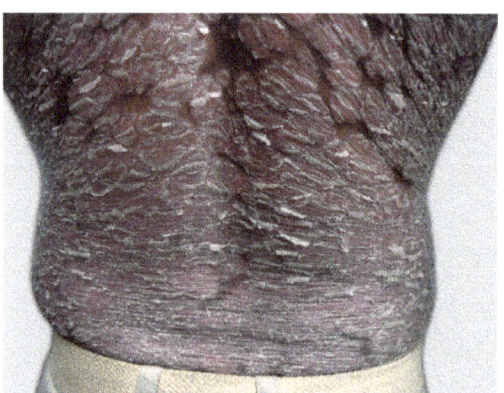

Fig. 4.2F(D): Intense pruritus and skip areas of normal skin of unstable psoriasis require detailed work up to rule out lymphoma

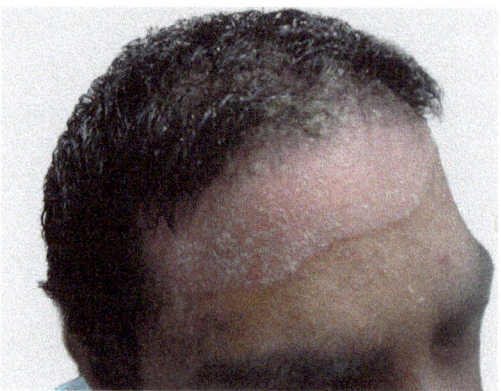

Fig. 4.2G(A): Scalp psoriasis showing psoriatic corona

Psoriasis According to Site of Involvement

Scalp Psoriasis

Scalp psoriasis affects approximately 50% of patients. Scalp is the most common site involved both in children and adults. Itching and hair loss are common symptoms though not a feature seen in all. Scalp can be involved either as an isolated site of affection or as part of plaque type psoriasis, pustular psoriasis and erythrodermic psoriasis. The scaling and

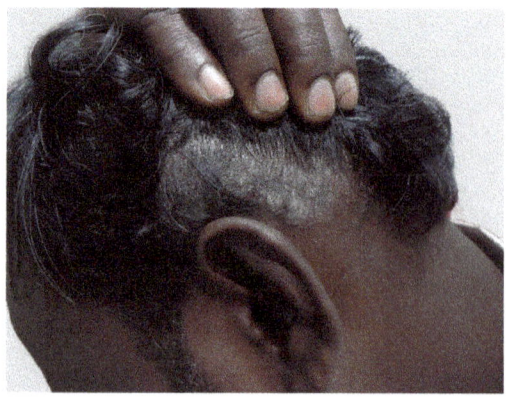

Fig. 4.2G(B): Scalp psoriasis showing Auspitz sign

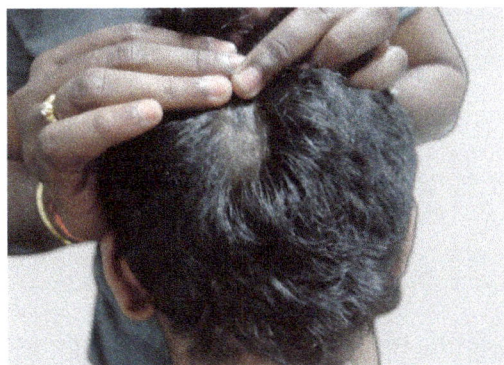

Fig. 4.2G(C): Scalp psoriasis which can be easily missed as seborrhoeic dermatitis in a hairy scalp, if thorough examination is not carried out.

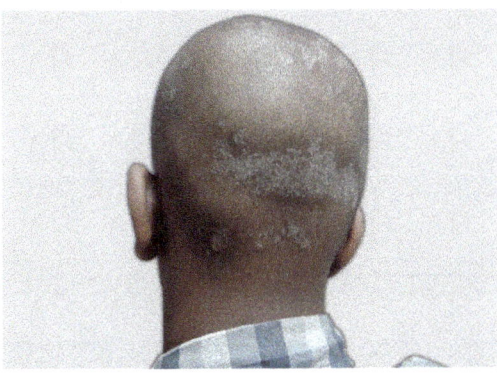

Fig. 4.2G(F): Posterior view of patient in psoriasis of the scalp mimicking seborrhoeic dermatitis. Note the silvery white dry scale as against greasy scales of seborrhoeic dermatitis

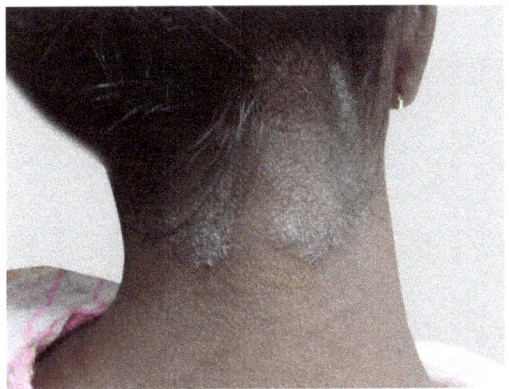

Fig. 4.2G(D): Scalp psoriasis mimicking Lichen simplex chronicus

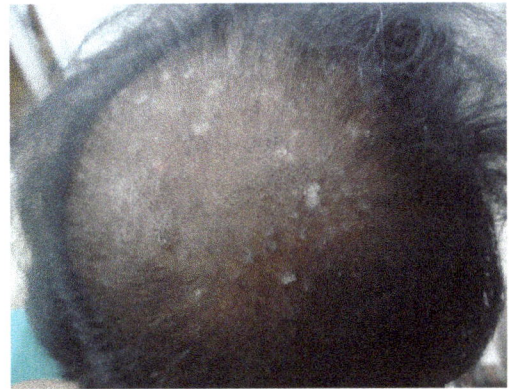

Fig. 4.2G(G): Scalp psoriasis showing scaly papules and Auspitz sign

Flexural Psoriasis or Inverse Psoriasis

This is a variant of psoriasis that spares the typical extensor surfaces and affects intertriginous (i.e., axillae, inguinal folds, infra mammary creases) areas with minimal scale. It is characterized by smooth, inflamed lesions without scaling, due to the moist nature of the area where this type of psoriasis is located [Figs 4.2H(a to d)].

Flexural psoriasis may occur as a primary disorder or as a Koebner phenomenon on top of infective or seborrheic intertriginous dermatoses. Failure to respond to antibacterial or antifungal preparations should

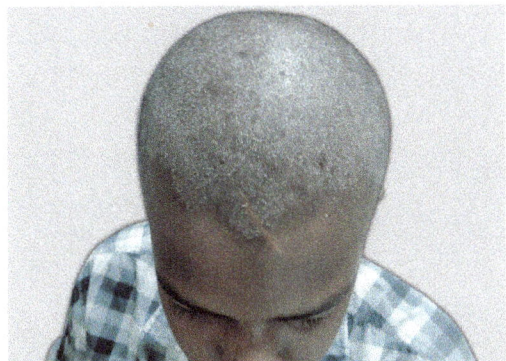

Fig. 4.2G(E): Psoriasis of the scalp mimicking seborrhoeic dermatitis. Note the silvery white dry scale as against greasy scales of seborrhoeic dermatitis

arouse suspicion of psoriatic etiology. Candidal intertrigo should be considered as a differential diagnosis and there can be candida overgrowth in flexural psoriasis [Fig. 4.2H(e)].

Psoriatic plaques of flexures are anhidrotic however, the effect of hyperhidrosis of the surrounding skin, maceration, and friction alter the appearance of the psoriasis, which still retains its characteristic color and well-defined borders. The surface has a glazed hue and fissuring at the depth of the fold is common, especially in the gluteal cleft.

Psoriasis of the retroauricular fold or the external auditory meatus should be differentiated from seborrheic dermatitis.

Flexural psoriasis was observed in nearly 10% of childhood psoriasis. Localization of

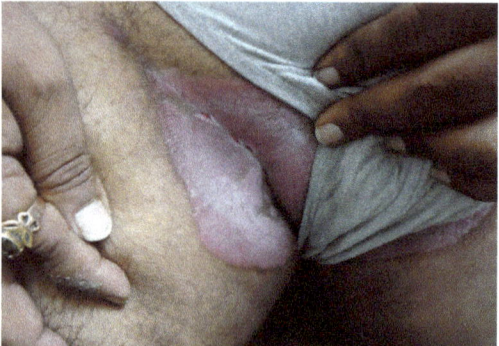

Fig. 4.2H(A): Note the sharply marginated erythema with deep fissures in flexural psoriasis; candidal infection should be ruled out

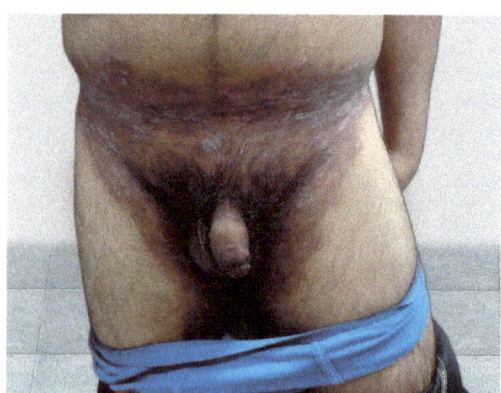

Fig. 4.2H(B): Flexural psoriasis: male

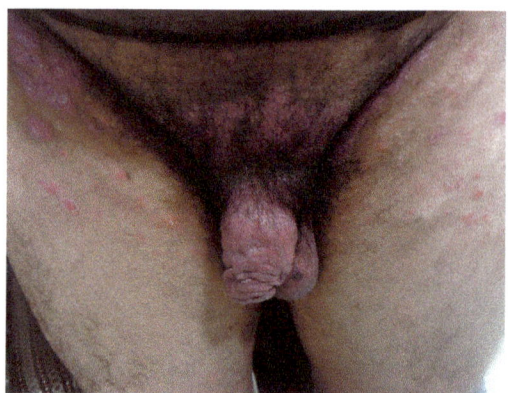

Fig. 4.2H(D): Flexural psoriasis with psoriasis vulgaris

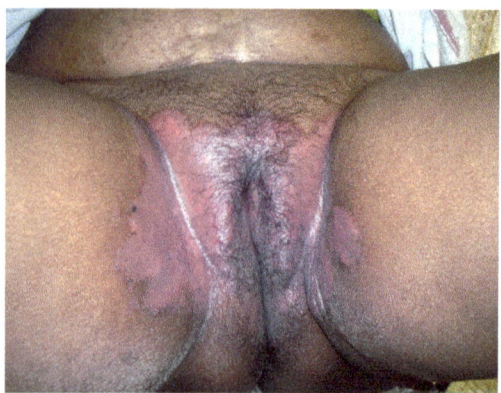

Fig. 4.2H(C): Flexural psoriasis: female

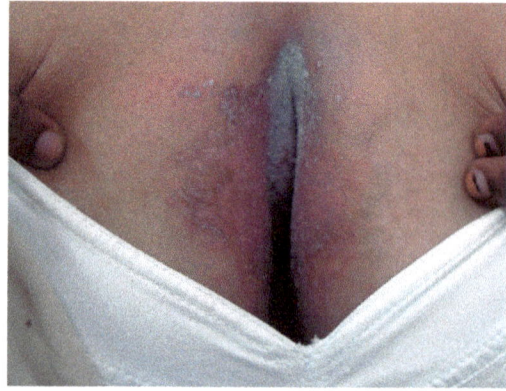

Fig. 4.2H(E): Flexural psoriasis with candidal intertrigo

erythematous, sometimes macerated, thick plaques to the folds of the skin, including axillae and groin can be associated with plaque type psoriasis in other sites. In infants, diaper dermatitis may be mistaken for psoriasis and vice versa. Dissemination with widespread eruption of erythemato-squamous lesions on the whole body may follow. In obese adults, flexural psoriasis of the groin and axilla is easily mistaken for candida intertrigo while both can coexist.

Palmoplantar Psoriasis

Psoriasis of the palms and soles can manifest in four different ways namely:
- Typical scaly, red patches similar to psoriasis elsewhere
- Thickening and scaling of the skin accompanied with the formation of deep, painful fissures on the palms and soles
- Generalized thickening and scaling of the palms and soles (keratoderma)
- Sheets of tiny yellow-brown pustules (PPP, already discussed).

Palmoplantar psoriasis tends to be a chronic recurrent condition. In many patients, PPP is a painful condition limiting day to day activities resulting in poor job performance. Psoriasis of the palm can mimic hand eczema and may often be difficult to distinguish as sometimes both may coexist or alternate. Well-defined edge at the wrist or forearm and absence of vesiculation are clues towards psoriatic etiology. In addition one can observe that skin over the knuckles frequently show a dull red thickening of the skin. Tinea pedis, eczema, syphilis, and keratoderma due to other causes are to be excluded before contemplating antimitotic agents as treatment [Figs 4.2I(a to m)]. In general, PPP occurs in people between 20 and 60 years old, affecting females more than males [Fig. 4.2I(o)].

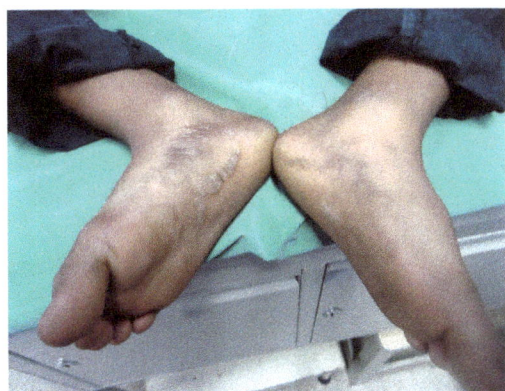

Fig. 4.2I(A): Early stage of plantar psoriasis

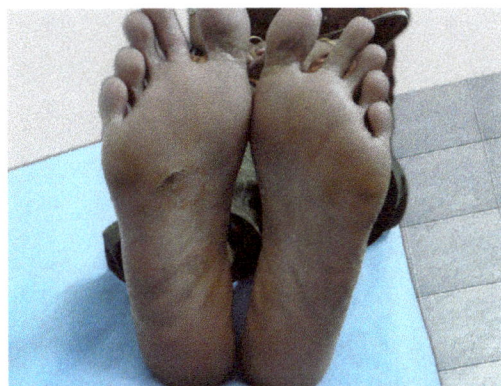

Fig. 4.2I(B): Plantar psoriasis

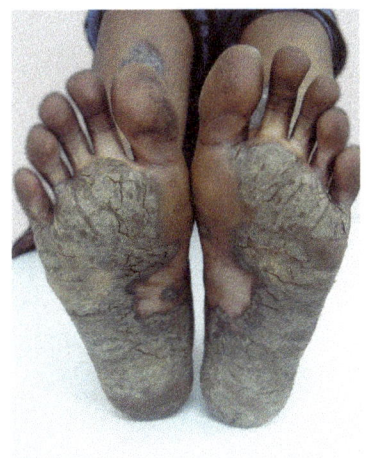

Fig. 4.2I(C): Plantar psoriasis severe form

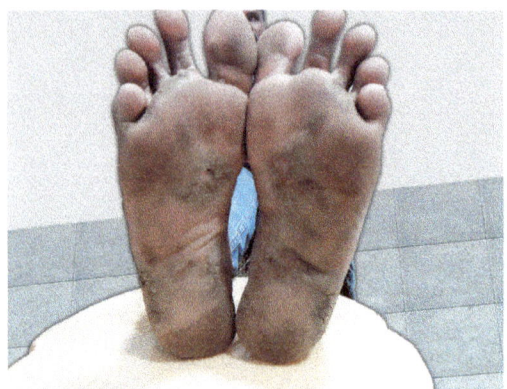

Fig. 4.21(D): Plantar psoriasis affecting the instep and the heel. This type will need systemic therapy even if there are no lesions elsewhere

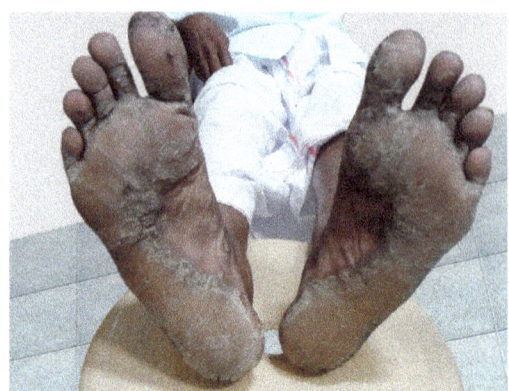

Fig. 4.21(G): Plantar psoriasis sparing the instep

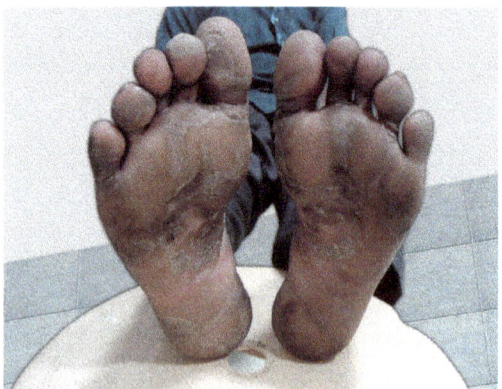

Fig. 4.21(E): Plantar psoriasis affecting the entire sole

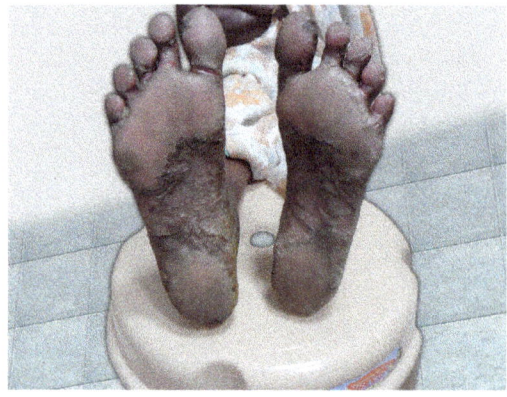

Fig. 4.21(H): Plantar psoriasis with clean deep fissures in an agricultural worker

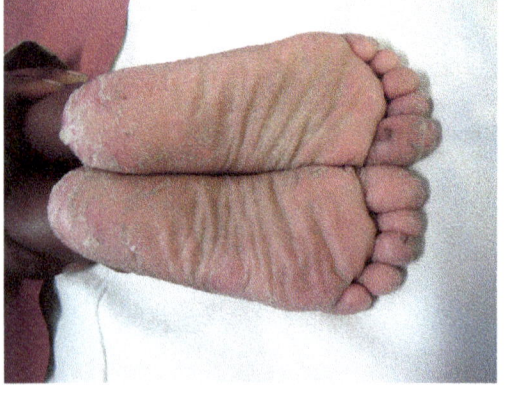

Fig. 4.21(F): Plantar psoriasis mimicking tinea pedis

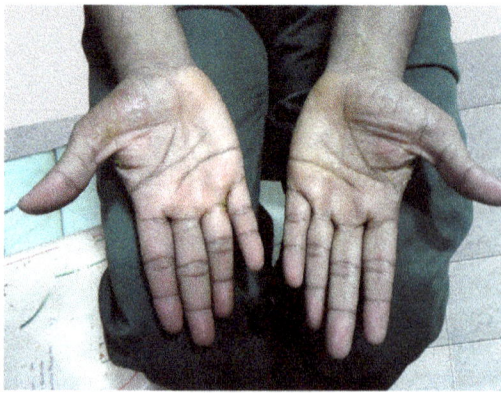

Fig. 4.21(I): Psoriasis of the palm: mild form

Clinical Aspects

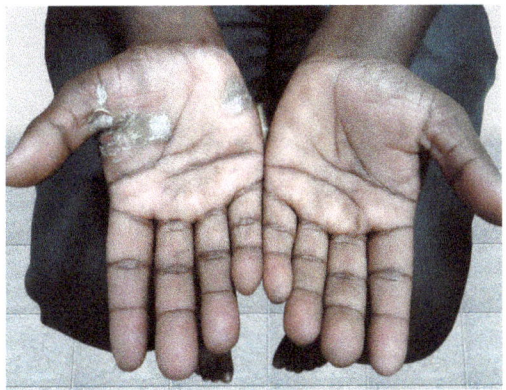

Fig. 4.2I(J): Psoriasis of the palm: classical plaque with fissuring and scaling

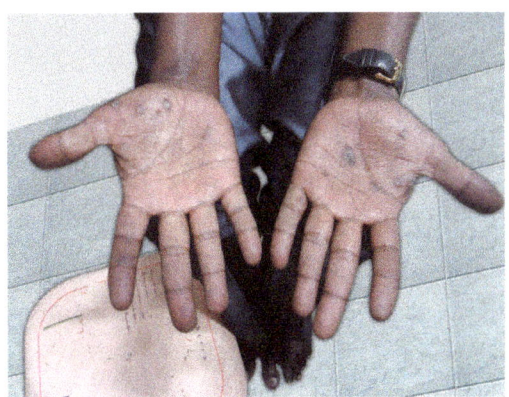

Fig. 4.2I(M): Psoriasis mimicking secondary syphilis

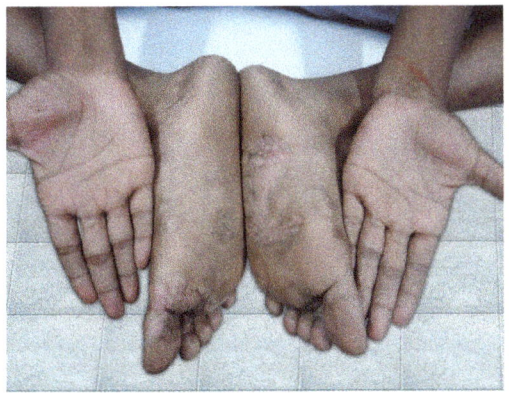

Fig. 4.2I(K): Psoriasis of the palms and soles

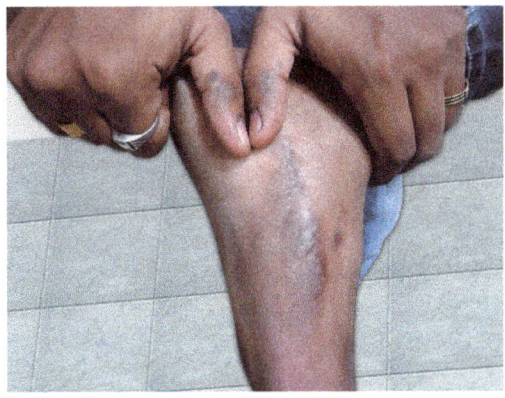

Fig. 4.2I(N): Psoriasis resembling eczema

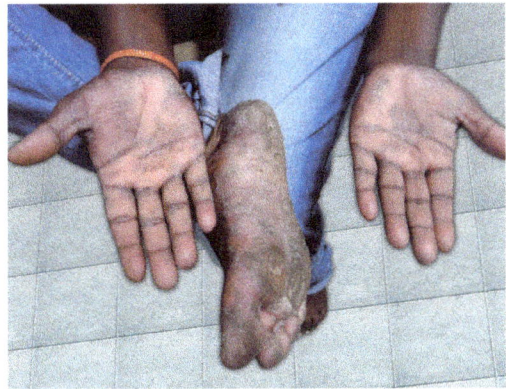

Fig. 4.2I(L): Psoriasis of the palms and soles severe form warranting photo or systemic therapy

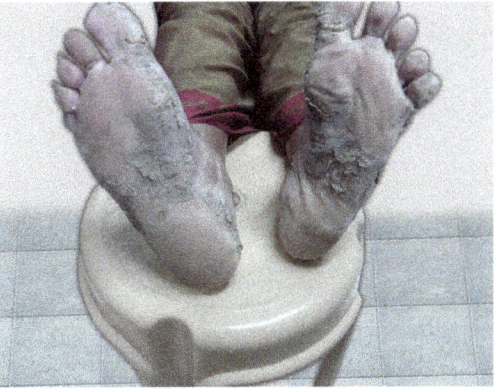

Fig. 4.2I(O): Thickening and scaling of the skin accompanied with the formation of deep, painful fissures on the soles

Plantar psoriasis, the one with highest discomfort, was observed in about 12.8 % of children with psoriasis in an Indian study.

Mucosal Psoriasis

Annular plaques on the tongue may be noted in patients with psoriasis. Geographic tongue is a common presentation of pustular psoriasis (Fig. 4.2J). Fissured tongue is yet another manifestation of pustular psoriasis. Erythema, ulcers, desquamative gingivitis, and pustules are other manifestation observed in psoriasis. Involvement of mucosa is seen in up to 7% of children.

Ocular Psoriasis

Ocular symptoms may occur in approximately 10% of psoriasis patients (Fig. 4.2K). Ocular involvement is more common in men than in women. It is rare to have involvement of the eye prior to skin involvement of psoriasis. The incidence of ocular psoriasis can vary widely, and may include ocular conditions, such as xerosis, symblepharon, trichiasis, blepharitis, conjunctivitis, uveitis, and iritis, as well as reported cases of secondary corneal involvement resulting in keratitis. Chronic uveitis has been found,[36] particularly in patients with PsA. Eye problems may be directly related to flare-ups around the eyes or due to the disease affecting the eye, which can also lead to problems within the eye itself that when left untreated can cause permanent vision loss. Psoriasis has early and extensive ocular involvement, sometimes earlier than joints.

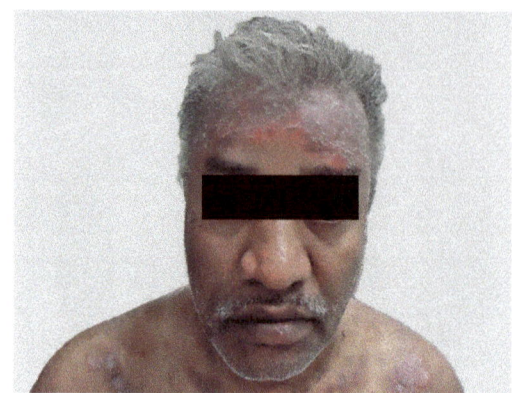

Fig. 4.2K: Ocular manifestation in unstable psoriasis

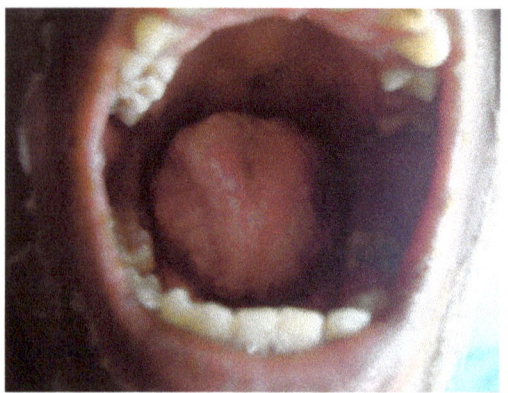

Fig. 4.2J: Geographic tongue as oral mucosal involvement in psoriasis

Nail Psoriasis[37]

The clinical findings associated with psoriatic nail disease correlate with the anatomical location of the nail unit that is affected by the disease.

Nail changes in psoriasis may be seen in up to 40% [Figs 4.2L(a to m)]. Nail pitting is the most common manifestation. Nail involvement can precede, coincide with, or succeed psoriasis and may even rarely appear isolated. Nail abnormalities are more frequent in PsA and in digital skin involvement. Psoriasis of the nails occurs in about three quarters of psoriatic patients with arthritis, but only in about one-third of those with skin lesions alone. Nail involvement is not an uncommon feature in psoriasis. While isolated nail involvement is seen in 5–10%

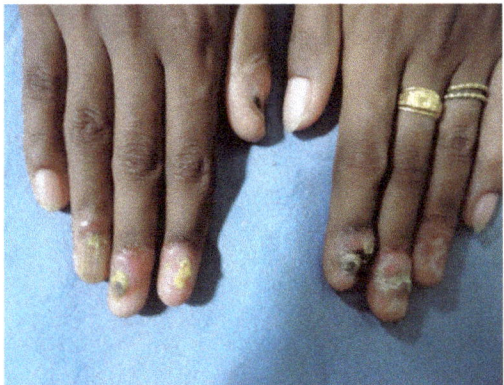

Fig. 4.2L(A): Nail involvement in psoriasis showing frequent changes: pitting, yellow discoloration, subungual keratosis and onycholysis

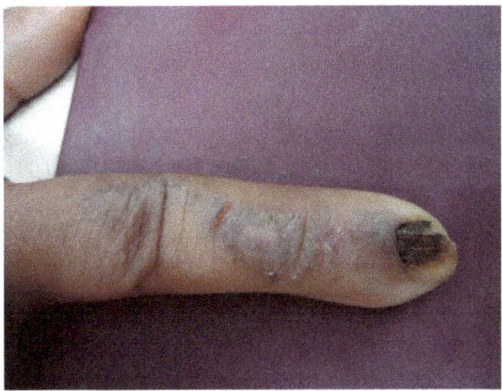

Fig. 4.2L(D): Nail dystrophy in psoriasis. Note the linear plaque that simulates lichen planus

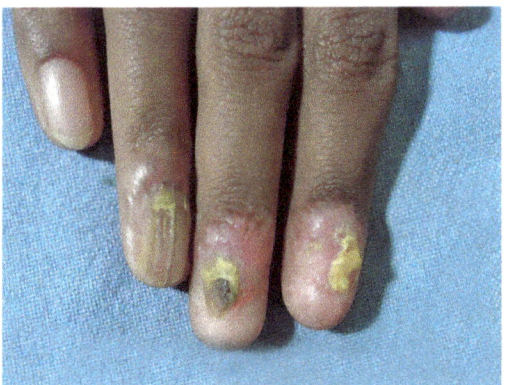

Fig. 4.2L(B): Note the yellowish discoloration and subungual hyperkeratosis and the normal little finger nail

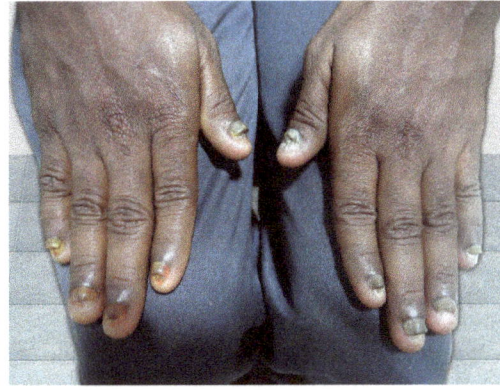

Fig. 4.2L(E): Psoriasis nail with onychomycosis

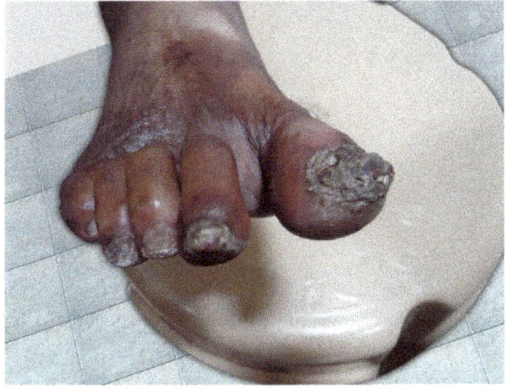

Fig. 4.2L(C): Severe involvement of nail in psoriasis

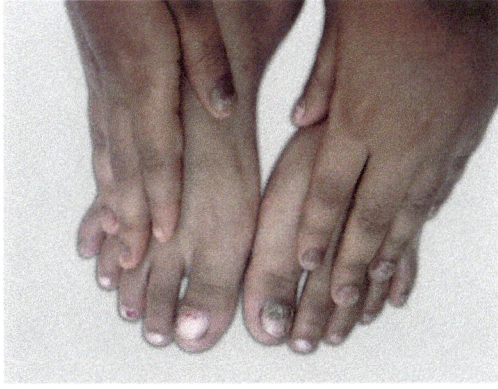

Fig. 4.2L(F): Twenty nail dystrophy in psoriasis

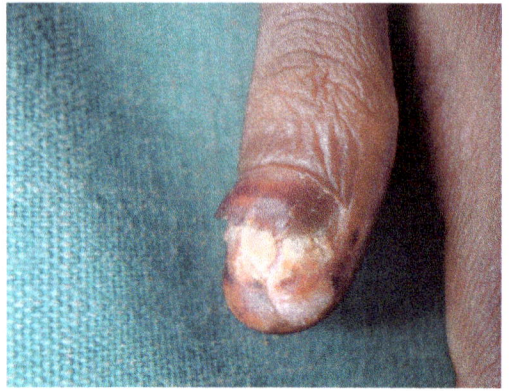

Fig. 4.2L(G): Nail dystrophy in pustular psoriasis

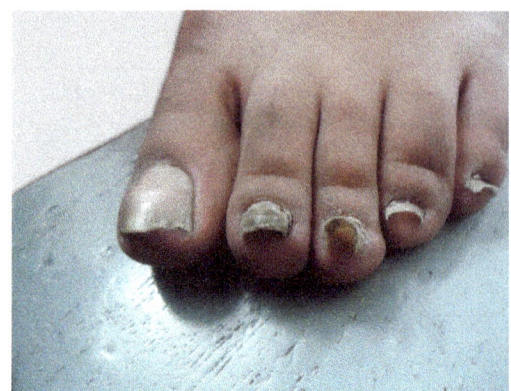

Fig. 4.2L(J): Onycholysis in a case of pustular psoriasis

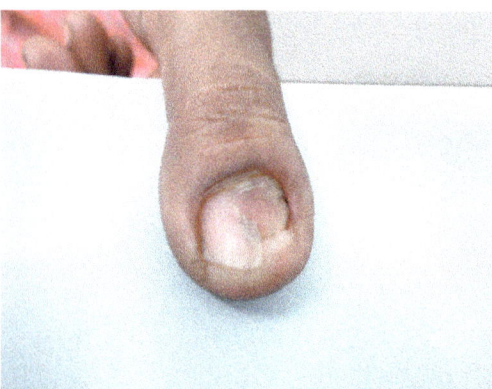

Fig. 4.2L(H): Onycholysis with paronychial changes in a patient with psoriasis

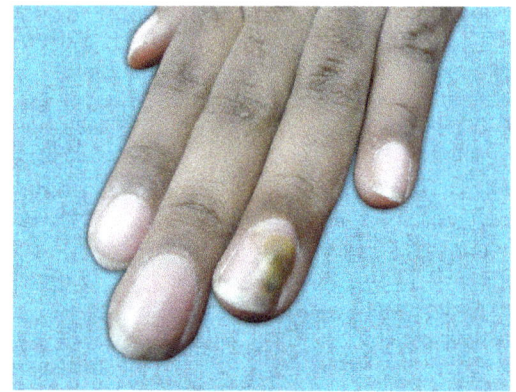

Fig. 4.2L(K): Translucent yellowish discoloration in the nail bed, resembling an oil drop under nail plate

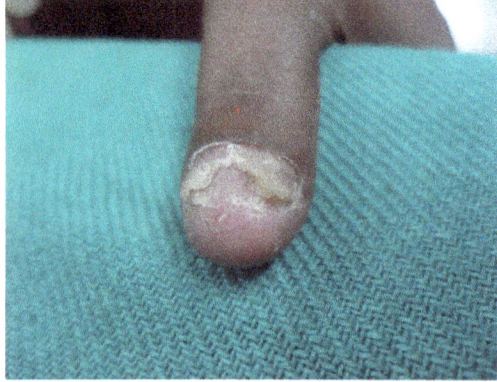

Fig. 4.2L(I): Severe isolated nail psoriasis without skin lesions

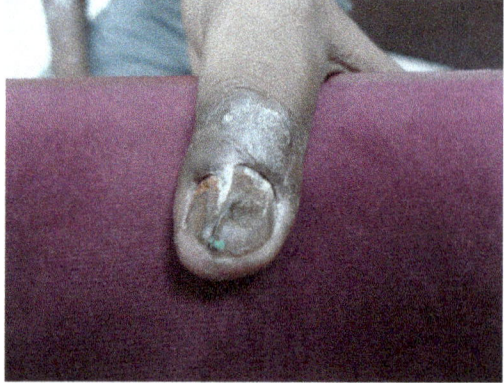

Fig. 4.2L(L): Crumbling and severe dystrophy of the nail mimicking pterigium in psoriasis

Clinical Aspects

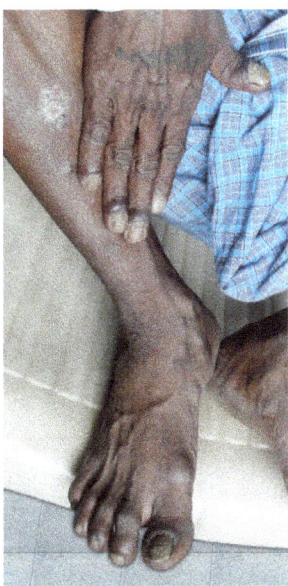

Fig. 4.2L(M): Pitting and paronychia in patient with psoriasis

of patients.[38] Concurrent nail involvement along with skin psoriasis is seen nearly 80% of patients with psoriasis. Nail involvement is seen more frequently in those patients with positive Koebner's phenomenon when compared to those without Koebner's phenomenon. It was also found that nail involvement is more common in males and obese individuals. The association of nail psoriasis with arthropathic psoriasis is highly variable. Nail changes are more frequently seen in type 2 psoriasis.[39] Fingernails are more commonly affected than the toenails due to psoriasis. Nail involvement can cause significant cosmetic handicap, restriction of daily activities, and pain in some. In 2009, Ortonne et al. devised the nail psoriasis quality of life scale-NPQ10-to evaluate the impact of nail psoriasis on quality of life which showed that 86% patients considered nail psoriasis as bothersome, 87% as unsightly, and 59% as painful.[40] Such an impact of nail

> **BOX 4.6: Nail involvement in psoriasis**
> - Corresponding to anatomical site:
>   - Pitting, beau's lines: Proximal nail matrix
>   - Oil drop sign: Nail bed
>   - Leukonychia: Mid matrix
>   - Subungual hyperkeratosis: Hyponychium
>   - Onycholysis: Nail bed and nail hyponychium
>   - Dystrophy, crumbling: Nail plate
>   - Splinter hemorrhage: Papillary capillary
>   - Spotted lunula: Distal matrix
> - Other manifestations of nail psoriasis:
>   - Acropustulosis
>   - Paronychia
>   - Psoriatic onycho-pachydermoperiostitis

psoriasis definitely warrants an insight into its clinical manifestations and treatment options by the treating dermatologist. Nail involvement is much less in children when compared to adults. This may be due to the time lag between the onset of skin lesions and the development of nail changes. Nail involvement in psoriasis is given in Box 4.6.

Corresponding to Anatomical Site

Pitting

Pitting, the most common manifestation of nail psoriasis affects the fingernails more commonly than the toenails. These are superficial depressions in the nail plate that indicate abnormalities in the proximal nail matrix and are a result of the loss of parakeratotic cells from the surface of the nail plate. The length of a pit is suggestive of the length of time the matrix was affected by the psoriatic lesion and a deeper pit is suggestive of involvement of intermediate and ventral matrix along with the dorsal matrix. Pitting may be arranged in transverse or longitudinal rows or it may be disorganized. Elkonyxis refers to punched out hole in the nail plate resulting from large pit. More than twenty pits in finger nails are suggestive of psoriasis.

Beau's Lines

Beau's lines are transverse depressed lines in the nails due to transient arrest in growth resulting from intermittent inflammation. Transverse grooves are formed in the same way as pits when the psoriatic lesion affects a wider area of the nail matrix.

Oil spot or Salmon Patch

Oil spots in the nail result from focal nail bed parakeratosis which leads to focal onycholysis, where serum and cellular debris accumulate and become entrapped. There is usually a yellowish brown margin visible between the white oily spot or salmon patch lesion and the normal pink nail. Extension of an oil spot to the distal free edge may lead to onycholysis.

Leukonychia

Leukonychia or white nail plate is due to foci of parakeratosis within the body of the nail plate. It occurs when psoriasis-induced parakeratosis affects only the intermediate and ventral matrices that form the undersurface of a nail plate, as opposed to the dorsal nail matrix. In these situations, the affected area appears leukonychic (whitish) because of the internal desquamation of parakeratosis cells, as opposed to the materialization of pits externally.

Subungual Hyperkeratosis

Subungual hyperkeratosis affects the nail bed and the hyponychium. Excessive proliferation of the nail bed can lead to onycholysis. Unlike pitting, toenails are more frequently affected than the fingernails. It results from rising of the nail plate off the nail bed as a result of deposition of cells that have not undergone desquamation. This accumulated tissue is friable and is liable to be infected by Candida and Pseudomonas leading to either yellow or green discoloration.

Onycholysis

Onycholysis is functional distal separation of the nail plate from its underlying nail bed. It causes traumatic uplifting of the distal nail plate leading to secondary microbial colonization. There are two likelihoods in the process of onycholysis. One possibility is due to psoriasis affecting the distal nail bed or hyponychium and the other is due to the distal extension of oil spots. The whitish discoloration is due to the entrapped air in the distal end. While, a yellowish hue is a result of accumulation of serum exudates.

Nail Dystrophy Crumbling and Plate Thickening

It suggests an extensive involvement of the entire nail matrix by the psoriatic process. Nail plate crumbling is a result of weakening of the nail plate, due to disease process.

Splinter Hemorrhages

Splinter hemorrhages are longitudinal black lines due to minute foci of capillary hemorrhage between the nail bed and the nail plate. This analogous to the Auspitz sign in the skin. They are considered as nonspecific findings of nail psoriasis by some authors.

Spotted Lunula

Spotted lunula presents as redness of the pale arched area at the bottom of the nail which occurs as a result of congestion of subungual capillaries.

Other Manifestations of Nail Psoriasis

Acropustulosis

Acropustulosis is a manifestation of pustular psoriasis, wherein the nail plate may be lifted off by sterile pustules in the nail bed and matrix resulting in onycholysis and subsequently complete destruction of the nail plate. In the severe form like acrodermatitis continua of Hallopeau, there can be resorptive osteolysis of the digits.

Paronychia

Psoriasis of the periungual skin can manifest as psoriatic paronychia along with nail changes, and at times may indicate associated PsA.

Psoriatic Onycho-pachydermoperiostitis[41]

Psoriatic onycho-pachydermoperiostitis (POPP) is characterized by psoriatic onychodystrophy or onycholysis, soft tissue thickening over distal phalanx, and periosteal reaction with absence of distal interphalangeal joint (DIP) involvement. Together, these lesions result in a typical drumstick-like deformity of the digits. POPP can be extremely painful and frequently causes significant functional impairment. It has been recognized as an uncommon subset of PsA. POPP commonly affects great toe nails, however may involve nails of any digit.[42]

Severity of nail psoriasis can be assessed using nail psoriasis severity index (NAPSI). NAPSI can be used when there is a major functional or cosmetic impact or to assess the therapeutic response before and after treatment is initiated specifically for nail disease. NAPSI is a numeric, reproducible, objective, simple tool for evaluation of nail psoriasis. This scale is used to evaluate the severity of nail bed psoriasis and nail matrix psoriasis by area of involvement in the nail unit. NAPSI is used to assign a score to each nail for nail bed and nail matrix psoriasis where nail plate is divided into quadrants by imaginary longitudinal and horizontal lines. Nail plate is assessed for nail matrix psoriasis by the presence of any feature of nail matrix psoriasis, including nail pitting, leukonychia, red spots in the lunula, and crumbling in each quadrant of the nail. Nail bed psoriasis is assessed by the presence of any features of nail bed psoriasis, including onycholysis, oil drop (salmon patch) dyschromia, splinter hemorrhages, and nail bed hyperkeratosis in each quadrant of the nail score is 0 if the findings are not present, 1, 2, 3, 4 if they are present in 1, 2, 3, all 4 quadrant/s of the nail, respectively. Thus, each nail has a matrix score (0-4) and a nail bed score (0-4), and the total nail score is the sum of those 2 individual scores (0-8) sum of the total score of all involved fingernails is the total NAPSI score for that patient at that time. If a more sensitive scale is needed, the nail can be given a separate score for all 8 features in each quadrant. The resulting is a 0-32 scale for the nail. A modified version (mNAPSI) was developed to enhance the face validity and feasibility of this tool.[43]

Diagnosis of Nail Psoriasis

It is difficult to make a diagnosis of isolated nail psoriasis when diagnostic procedures are used to confirm the clinical suspicion. Simple tests like examination of the nail clipping under potassium hydroxide mount should be performed to differentiate from and exclude tinea unguium which can be further supported by fungal culture. The following investigations will help in the diagnosis of nail psoriasis. Investigations used in nail psoriasis are given in Box 4.7.

Dystrophic nails in psoriasis patients are more predisposed to fungal infections. The mycological examination of all psoriasis patients with nail deformities is considered obligatory because of the great number of psoriasis patients diagnosed with onychomycosis.

Genital Psoriasis[44-47]

Genital psoriasis affects males and females, children and adults. In children, genital

BOX 4.7: Investigations used in nail psoriasis
- Nail biopsy
- Dermoscopy
- Videodermoscopy
- Capillaroscopy
- Ultrasound
- Doppler technique
- Optical coherence tomography
- Confocal laser scanning microscopy
- To exclude infections:
  - Nail clipping and KOH examination, fungal culture
  - Bacterial culture

psoriasis is most common under the age of 2, when it presents as psoriatic napkin eruption.

Scientific evidence shows that involvement of the genital skin occurs in 29–40% of patients with psoriasis.[44] When there is inverse psoriasis, the genital area is usually involved in up to 79% of the patients.[45] The most common type of psoriasis in the genital region is inverse psoriasis. This type of psoriasis first shows up as smooth, dry, red lesions. It usually lacks the scale associated with plaque psoriasis. In most cases, genital psoriasis can accompany plaque psoriasis lesions on other parts of the body, but it has also been reported as being isolated to the genital skin; this form of presentation is rare and occurs in only 2–5% of psoriatic patient.

Patients with genital psoriasis may also experience pruritus and/or a burning sensation in the affected area, which can range from minimal-marked. Due to the Koebner's phenomenon, genital psoriasis may be worsened by irritation from urine and feces, tight fitting clothes, and sexual intercourse.

Clinical Features

Genital psoriasis may be part of a more generalized psoriasis. Psoriasis has multi-factorial genetic and environmental causes. These are not fully understood. In the genital area, specific factors to consider include: colonization by bacteria and yeasts (*Candida albicans*) and injury to the skin, causing new plaques of psoriasis to develop (Koebner's phenomenon).

Psoriasis in the genital area may also be worsened by contact with irritants, such as urine, feces, tight-fitting clothes, and friction associated with sexual intercourse.

There are various regions of the genital area that can be affected by psoriasis [Figs 4.2M(a to k)]:

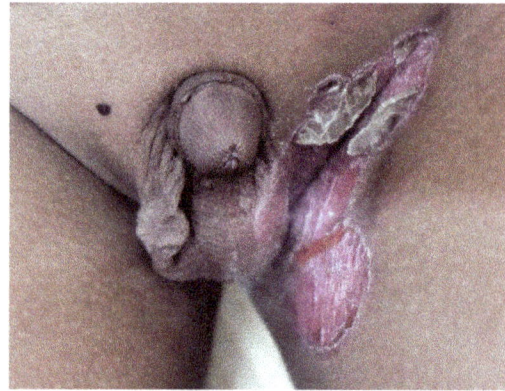

Fig. 4.2M(A): Psoriasis involving the groin in a child

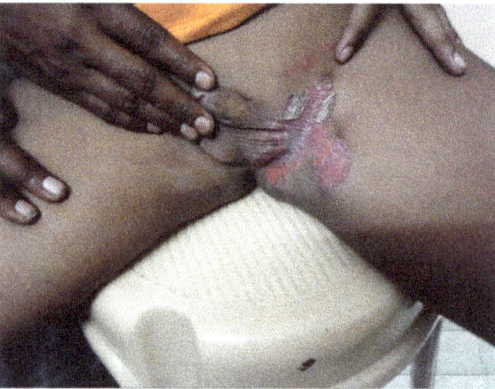

Fig. 4.2M(B): Psoriasis involving the groin. Note the fissure

Clinical Aspects

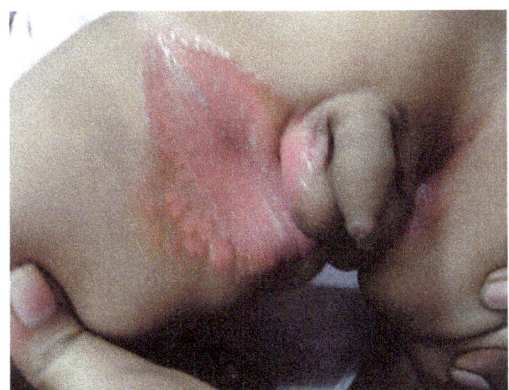

Fig 4.2M(C): Psoriasis involving the groin, thigh, and the scrotal skin

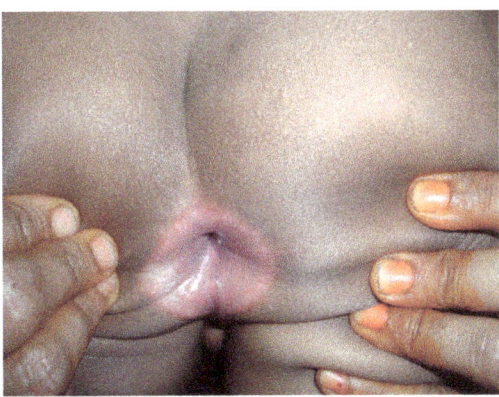

Fig. 4.2M(F): Involvement of perianal area in an infant with genital psoriasis

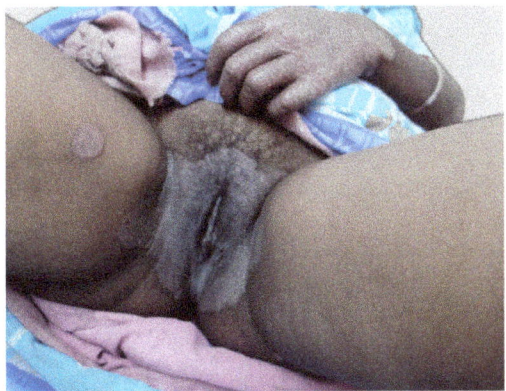

Fig. 4.2M(D): Scaly plaque over the labia. Note the classical psoriatic plaque over the thigh

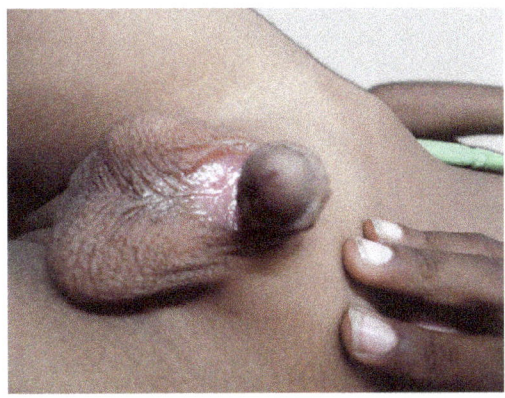

Fig. 4.2M(G): Genital psoriasis with super added candidal infection

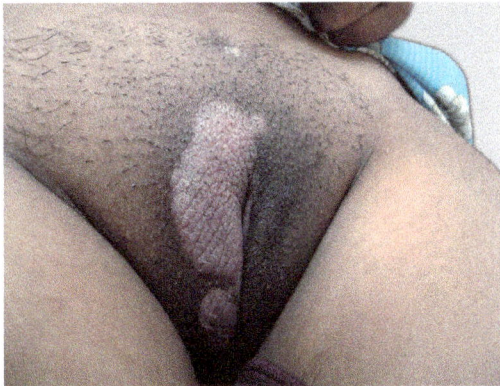

Fig. 4.2M(E): Psoriatic plaque over the labium. Note the pink hue and lichenification secondary to scratching

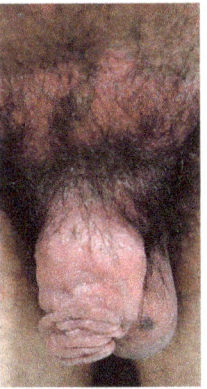

Fig. 4.2M(H): Classical erythematous plaques involving the penile and scrotal skin

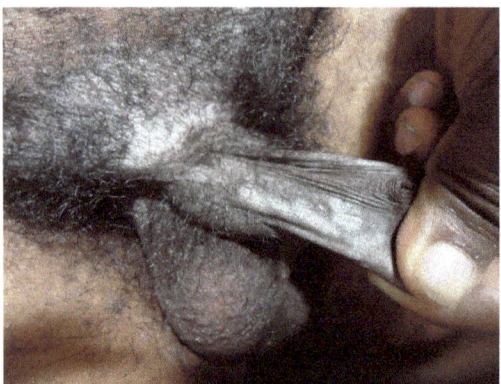

Fig. 4.2M(I): Dry scaly plaque of psoriasis

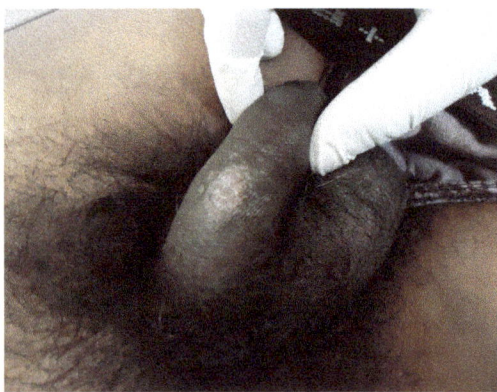

Fig. 4.2M(J): Isolated genital involvement easy to miss. Patient later developed extensive psoriasis vulgaris

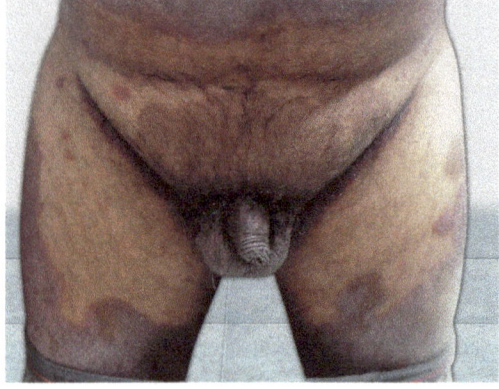

Fig. 4.2M(K): Involvement of genital skin as part of psoriasis vulgaris

Pubis

Psoriasis over the pubic region presents as an erythematous scaly plaque. Sometimes, this can mimic dermatophytes infection due to itching.

Female Genitals

Inverse psoriasis in genital skinfolds usually presents itself as erythematous, irregular, well-demarcated, thin, and often symmetrical plaques in the vulva and vagina, with poor or nondesquamation because of the local conditions and lacks the typical scaling of plaque psoriasis in other skin zones. However, minimal scaling can be seen on the more keratinized regions of the genital skin. The appearance of vulvar psoriasis is often symmetrical smooth, nonscaly redness and can vary from silvery, scaling patches adjacent to the outer parts of the labia majora to moist grayish plaques or glossy red plaques without scaling in the skinfolds.

Scratching this area may cause an infection, create dryness, and result in thickening of the skin, and further itching. Genital psoriasis usually affects the outer skin of the vagina because psoriasis does not normally affect mucous membranes. In general, genital psoriasis does not affect the urethra. Female genital skin can be involved as part of psoriasis vulgaris. Psoriatic plaques can be seen elsewhere in the skin.

Male Genitals

In male patients, both scrotal and penile skin may be affected. The glans penis is the area of male genital skin that is most commonly affected.

Occasionally, the entire penis, scrotum, and inguinal folds are involved. Psoriasis of the penis may appear as many small, red patches on the glans, or shaft. The skin may be scaly or smooth and shiny. Genital psoriasis affects both circumcised and uncircumcised males.

Whereas in uncircumcised males, the well-defined, nonscaling plaques are most common under the prepuce and on the proximal glans, in circumcised male patients the lesions are usually present on the glans and corona. Psoriatic genital lesions of the glans and corona in circumcised males can be scalier than those usually seen in genital skin.

Upper Thighs

Psoriasis on the upper thighs often consists of many small, round patches that are red and scaly. Psoriasis in between the thighs is easily irritated, especially if the thighs rub together and can complicate frictional keratosis, commonly seen in obese individuals. The symptoms worsen on prolonged walking or running.

Creases Between Thigh and Groin

Psoriasis generally appears as nonscaly and reddish-white in the creases between the thigh and groin. The skin may have fissures that can get infected presenting as intertrigo.

Anus and Surrounding Skin

Psoriasis on or near the anus is itchy and presents as red, nonscaly patch. Psoriasis in this area may be confused with perianal dermatitis. Presence of hemorrhoids can complicate and delay diagnosis of psoriasis. Under such circumstances, symptoms of anal psoriasis may include bleeding, pain during bowel movements, and excessive dryness and itching.

Buttocks Crease

Psoriasis in the buttocks crease may be red and nonscaly or red with very heavy scales. The skin in this area is not as fragile as that of the groin.

Based on Disease Manifestation

Based on disease manifestation, psoriasis can be graded in order to select or modify therapy and for assessing the disease outcome. The following working classification of psoriasis into six stages of clinical presentation will help both the clinician and the patient well informed of the disease status which will enable plan investigations and treatment effectively.[15,48] Grading of psoriasis based on disease manifestation is given in Box 4.8.

Under each subset are included certain characteristics of psoriasis which are listed below.

Latent Psoriasis

- In-remission and minimal psoriasis
- Stable remission with no psoriatic lesions
- Signs of borderline psoriasis (e.g., nail pitting, severe dandruff)
- A few isolated lesions negligible to patient.

Mild Psoriasis (Fig. 4.2N)

- Involving less than 10% of body
- Surface area (or PASI <10).
- Good control of lesions with topical therapy.

BOX 4.8: Grading of psoriasis based on disease manifestation

- Latent psoriasis
- Mild psoriasis
- Moderate psoriasis
- Moderate-severe psoriasis
- Severe psoriasis
- Psoriasis with guarded prognosis

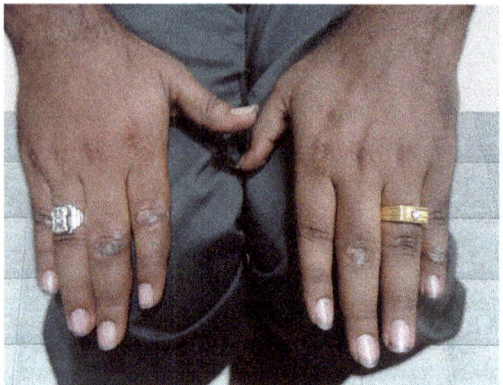

Fig. 4.2N: Mild psoriasis with less than 10% body surface area involvement

Moderate Psoriasis [Figs 4.2O(a and b)]

- Skin involvement more than 10% of BSA
- Topical therapy still possible without having the need for systemic therapy.

Moderate-severe Psoriasis [Figs 4.2P(a to c)]

- Skin involvement more than 10% of BSA and topical therapy fail to control disease
- Skin involvement less than 10%, but lesions in difficult areas (such as involvement of face, hands or feet)
- Having distressing or disabling effects incapacitating daily routine or day-day work.

Severe Psoriasis [Figs 4.2Q(a and b)]

- Skin involvement more than 20% (or PASI >20) with need for systemic treatment.
- Skin involvement 10–20%
- Lesions in difficult areas
- Distressing or disabling effects
- Unstable psoriasis
- PsA.

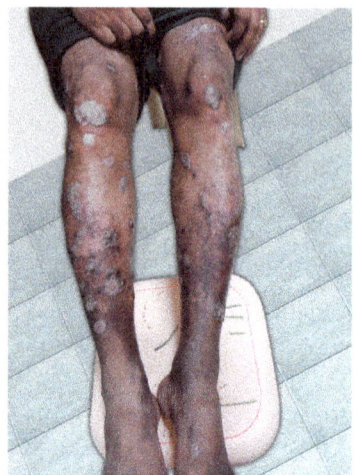

Fig. 4.2O(A): Moderate psoriasis

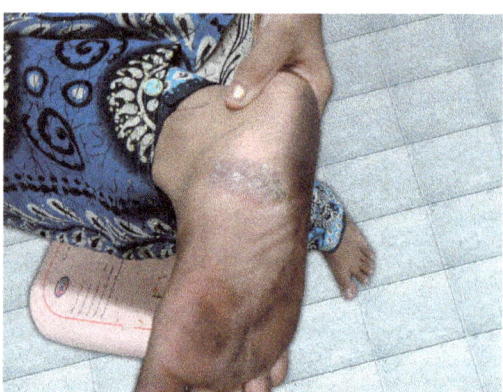

Fig. 4.2O(B): Moderate psoriasis to be considered as severe since the plantar involvement is affecting the routine work of the patient and hence warrants systemic therapy

Psoriasis with Guarded Prognosis (Fig. 4.2R)

- Impending skin failure
- Generalized pustular psoriasis (von Zumbusch type)
- Psoriatic erythroderma.

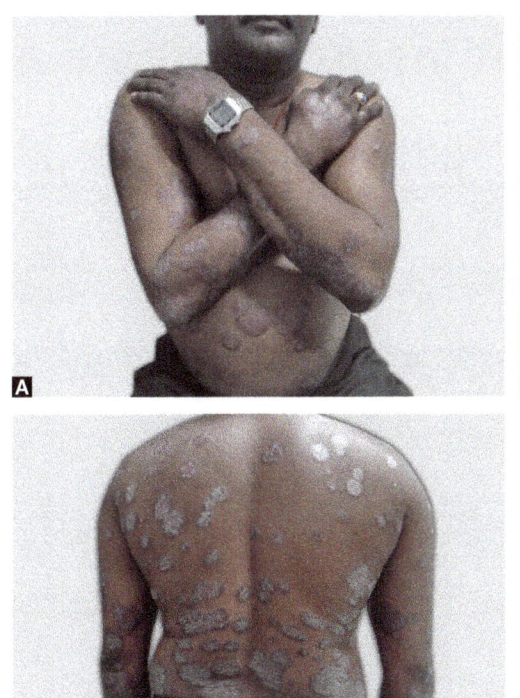
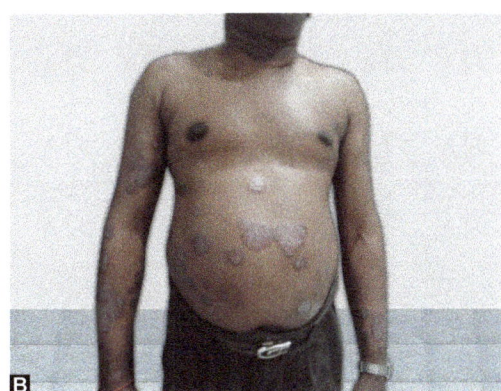

Figs 4.2P(A to C): Moderate-severe psoriasis where early initiation of systemic therapy will help control the disease and prevent other complications

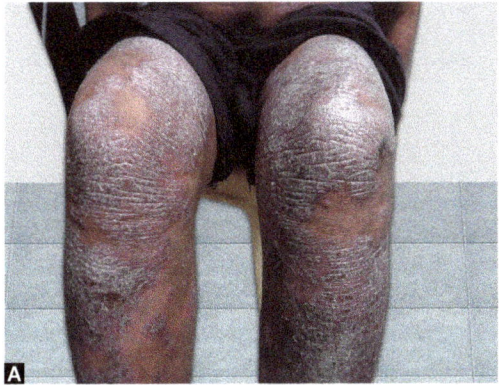
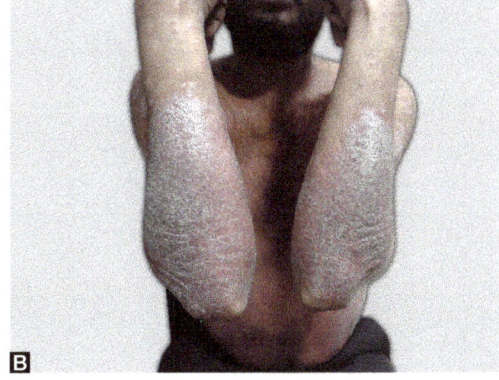

Figs 4.2Q(A and B): Severe psoriasis which needs systemic therapy

The different configurations of psoriasis are:
- Psoriasis gyrate: in which curved linear patterns predominate [Figs 4.2S(a and b)]
- Annular psoriasis: in which ring-like lesions develop secondary to central clearing (Fig. 4.2T)

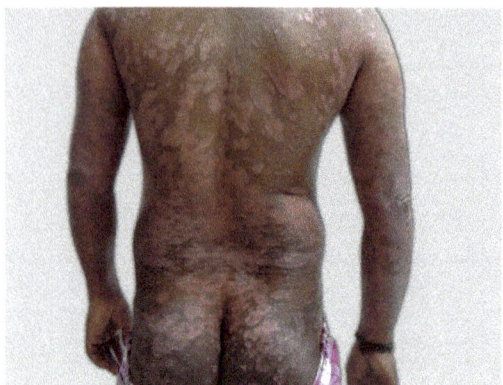

Fig. 4.2R: Severe psoriasis that is unstable whose prognosis is guarded

- Psoriasis follicularis: in which minute scaly papules are present at the openings of pilosebaceous follicles (Fig. 4.2U)
- Rupioid psoriasis are small plaques (2–5 cm in diameter) and highly hyperkeratotic, resembling limpet shells (Fig. 4.2V)
- Ostraceous psoriasis: psoriasis refers to hyperkeratotic plaques with relatively concave centers, similar in shape to oyster shells (Fig. 4.2W)
- Rarely zebra-like manifestations are observed in erythrodermic psoriasis which will need constant and regular follow-up (Fig. 4.2X).

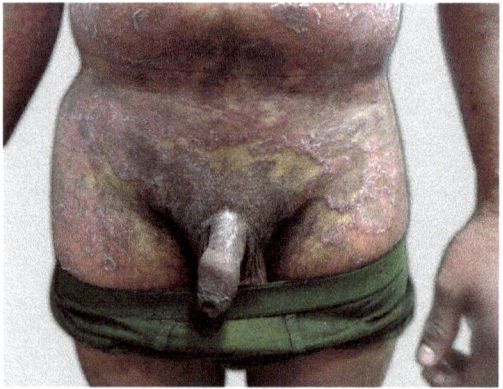

Fig. 4.2S(A): Annular plaques with few gyrate lesions in a severe form of psoriasis

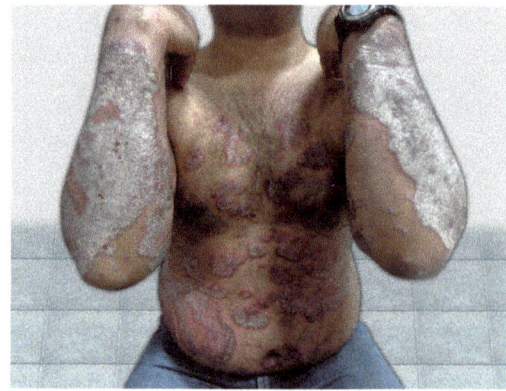

Fig. 4.2T: Annular psoriasis with large plaque type psoriasis

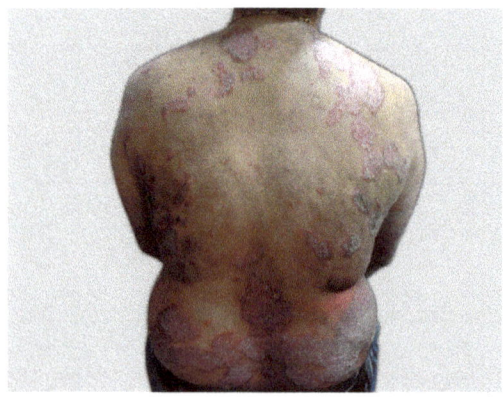

Fig. 4.2S(B): Annular psoriasis showing ring-like lesions

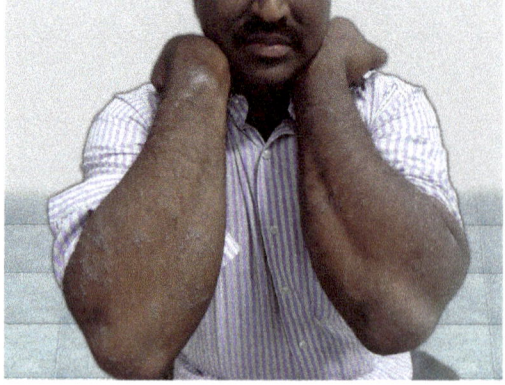

Fig. 4.2U: Follicular psoriasis

Clinical Aspects

DISEASE ASSOCIATION

Studies have reported association between psoriasis and many other diseases that includes both cutaneous and systemic [Figs 4.3(a to e)]. The common etiological factor involved in psoriasis and atopy being the T cell, the association between psoriasis and atopy has been well documented. Lichen planus, vitiligo, bullous pemphigoid are known to be associated with psoriasis. Infections due to bacteria, fungi, especially dermatophytes, virus including HIV are well documented to be occurring in

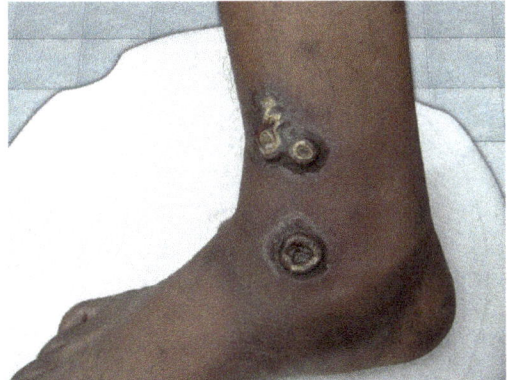

Fig. 4.2V: Rupioid lesions in a patient with Reiter's syndrome

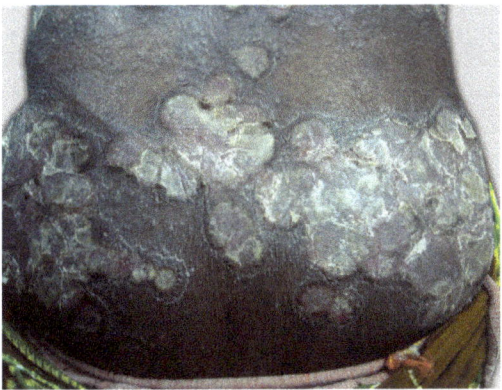

Fig. 4.2W: Note hyperkeratotic plaques with concave center resembling oyster shell

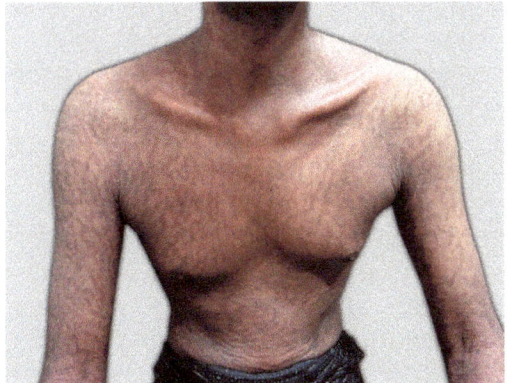

Fig. 4.2X: Unusual presentation of erythrodermic psoriasis

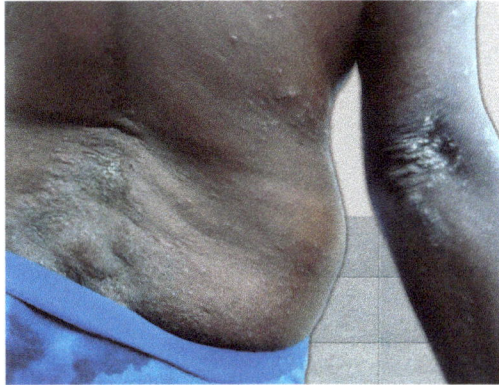

Fig. 4.3A: Psoriasis in association with atopic dermatitis. Note the oozing plaque over the lower back and keratotic scaly plaque over the elbow

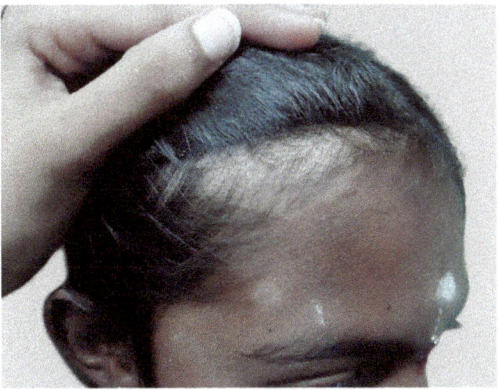

Fig. 4.3B: Psoriasis occurring over a vitiliginous patch

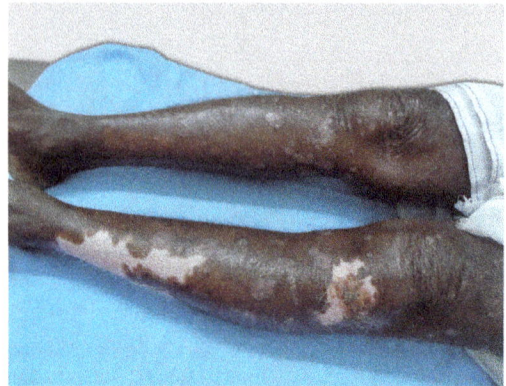

Fig. 4.3C: Psoriasis with vitiligo

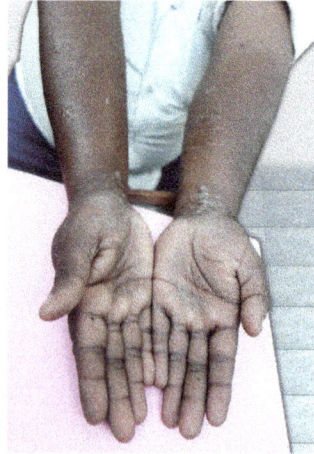

Fig. 4.3D: Lichen planus psoriasis overlap-histology showing features of both

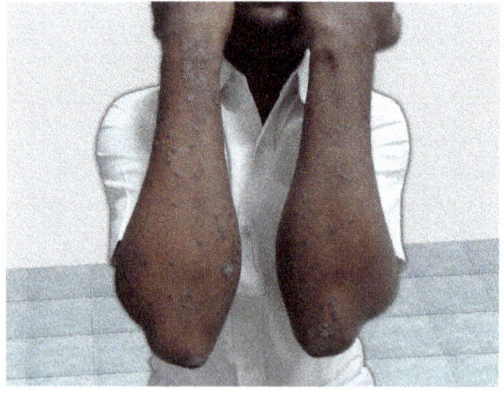

Fig. 4.3E: Psoriasis with lichen planus

increased frequency in psoriasis. Gout and hypocalcemia are documented metabolic associations of psoriasis.

Pustular psoriasis is associated with many diseases like, Crohn's disease, apart from various arthritis or arthropathies including chronic recurrent multifocal osteomyelitis, pustular arthroosteitis, axial and peripheral arthritis. A significant incidence of hyperthyroidism and hypothyroidism, and the presence of thyroid antibodies has been found in association with pustular psoriasis. The association and increased incidence of diabetes other comorbidities and malignancies is dealt with later.

Synovitis, acne, pustulosis palmaris, hyperostosis and osteomyelitis (SAPHO) syndrome is a chronic disorder that involves the skin, bone, and joints, first described by Chamot and co-workers in 1987. The joint involvement is closely linked to psoriatic arthropathy. SAPHO syndrome is characterized by variable bone changes (hyperostosis, arthritis, aseptic osteomyelitis) of the chest wall, sacroiliac joints, and long bones. Dermatologic manifestations include PPP, hidradenitis suppurativa and pustular psoriasis, dissecting cellulitis of the scalp, Sweet syndrome, and Sneddon-Wilkinson disease. Skin and osseous involvement may occur simultaneously or be separated by as long as 20 years.

Though psoriasis is said to be benefitted by phototherapy, in some, the disease is exacerbated with light exposure. In a cross-sectional survey, the prevalence of photosensitive psoriasis was 5.5%. Skin type I, familial history of photosensitivity, advanced age, and psoriasis affecting the hands were all significantly associated with photosensitivity.[49]

Crohn's disease is also reported to be more frequently observed in psoriatic patients. Psoriatic patients, predominantly

Clinical Aspects

> **BOX 4.9: Complications due to psoriasis**
> - Itching
> - Eczematization
> - Infection
> - Arthritis
> - Alcoholism
> - Nephritis and renal failure
> - Hepatic failure
> - Apical pulmonary fibrosis
> - Amyloidosis
> - Complications of erythroderma.

those with severe disease with psoriasis are at an increased risk of developing malignancy particularly nonmelanoma skin cancer, lymphohematopoietic cancers and solid tumors. The risk increases in those treated with phototherapy and systemic agents. The association of metabolic syndrome in patients with psoriasis is dealt with separately.

Complications due to psoriasis by itself are rare, however, the complications due to system involvement and treatment are quite common. Complications due to psoriasis are listed in Box 4.9.

Itching

Intensity of itching can range from complete absence to severe pruritus. It is more common in unstable forms. Itching can be very intense in erythrodermic psoriasis which is sometimes difficult to control. Since degree of itching reflects the emotional state of the patient and, if severe, may be a symptom of anxiety or depression.

Eczematization

Eczematization of the plaque is very common in anatomical sites like the palms and soles. Irritant topical application can lead to eczematization.

Infection

At least 50% of psoriatics are carriers of Staphylococci, especially on the lesions. Psoriasis involving the flexures can be secondarily infected with *Staphylococcus aureus*, especially if there had been fissures. Secondary infection of psoriatic lesions is a problem during topical steroid therapy used under occlusive dressings, which can lead to folliculitis and furunculosis.

It is not uncommon to see flexural psoriasis to be secondarily infected by candida overgrowth, Superadded dermatophytes infections are not uncommon with psoriatic nails.

Arthritis

Psoriatic arthritis is now increasing in incidence. PsA is dealt with separately in the following section.

Alcoholism

Alcoholism is known to exacerbate psoriasis. Interestingly, heavy drinking was found significantly more common in men which could be a symptom of stress caused by severe skin disease.

Nephritis and Renal Failure

Poststreptococcal mesangiocapillary glomerulonephritis and renal failure brought about by acute tubular necrosis are rare complications of psoriasis.

Hepatic Failure

Hepatic failure can be secondary to systemic treatment given in psoriasis. Severe abnormalities of liver function may occur in erythrodermic and or pustular psoriasis. In pustular psoriasis, the raise in liver enzymes is invariably transient and reverts to normal once the disease is effectively controlled.

Apical Pulmonary Fibrosis

Apical pulmonary fibrosis is a rare complication reported in association with a case of psoriatic spondylitis.

Amyloidosis

Secondary amyloidosis is a rare sequel of arthropathic, generalized pustular and severe nonpustular psoriasis. Renal failure may result from amyloidosis.

Complications of erythroderma have been dealt earlier in the chapter.

PSORIATIC ARTHRITIS

Arthropathic psoriasis or PsA is an inflammatory "entheso-arthro-osteopathy" occurring in subjects with psoriasis or with a predisposition to psoriasis. It may involve peripheral and/or axial osteoarticular compartments and may be responsible for extra-articular manifestations. PsA has been defined as an inflammatory arthritis, usually seronegative, associated with psoriasis. PsA can be viewed as a chronic inflammatory condition with significant heterogeneity in clinical manifestations, including skin and nail psoriasis, enthesitis, dactylitis, axial arthritis, and peripheral arthritis warranting early detection and control of inflammation to check mutilation. The disease will be discussed under the following topics:
- Risk factors
- Onset
- Types
- Classification
- Clinical manifestations
- Diagnosis or criteria
- Course of disease in PsA
- Predictors of disease progression in PsA
- Protective factors for disease progression.

Risk Factors

With the increase in the prevalence of psoriasis in the recent days, the prevalence of PsA is also on the raise. There is no documented evidence to precisely blame a single component to be the risk factor in the development of PsA.[50] However, results of many researches point toward a combination of factors and their interplay making an individual develop PsA. The disease develops due to a combination of genetic, immunologic, and environmental factors. Positive family history is noted in as high as 40% of people with PsA. If an identical twin has PsA, the other twin is very likely to have or to develop the condition. Exposure to certain infections may also contribute to the development of PsA. Some experts believe there is a link between streptococcal infection and the development of psoriasis and PsA, although the link has not been proven. PsA also occurs more commonly in people infected with the HIV than in the general population. Comparable to Koebner's phenomenon in the skin, some patients develop PsA in an injured joint.

Onset

Onset typically occurs in patients 30-50 years of age.[51] The peak age of onset of arthritis in one series was 40-60 years. Psoriatic skin lesions precede onset of PsA by an average of 10 years in approximately 70% of patients PsA can precede the development of psoriasis in a small proportion of patients. Simultaneous onset of both PsA and psoriasis occurs in 11-15% of subjects.[52] Onset of PsA in old age has a more severe onset and more a destructive outcome than does PsA that affects younger subjects. The course of PsA is usually characterized by flares and remissions. Skin lesions were found to precede arthritis in nearly two-thirds of patients; arthritis antedated skin lesions in one-fifth, and in nearly 16%, skin and joint involvement occurred almost simultaneously. According to Anandarajan et al., the occurrence of psoriasis followed by PsA, PsA followed by psoriasis, and simultaneous occurrence are 70, 15, and 15, respectively.[53]

The correlation between severity of skin psoriasis and arthropathic involvement has not been consistent. Nor does the severity of the psoriasis relate to the pattern of joint involvement. But, it is consistently reported that pustular psoriasis patients are more prone for joint involvement.

Types

Wright identified five clinical patterns among patients with PsA. The patterns of PsA involvement are as follows:
- Asymmetrical oligoarticular arthritis
- Symmetrical polyarthritis
- Distal interphalangeal arthropathy
- Arthritis mutilans
- Spondylitis with or without sacroiliitis.

The exact frequency of the patterns is not known as there are different definitions that are being used. The disease patterns likely change over time in the same individual such that with longer duration of PsA, patients tend to develop the polyarticular pattern. Arthritis mutilans is the least common but most severe type of psoriatic occurring in about 5% with PsA. This form of the disease results in widespread destruction of the joints. When this affects the hands, it can cause a phenomenon sometimes referred to as "telescoping fingers". Similar changes can occur in the feet. Thus, the varied patterns may not be helpful in the classification of PsA when the disease is already established.

Classification

For a simpler approach, PsA can be classified into three main groups:
- Asymmetrical arthritis usually, but not always, involving a small number of joints with few erosions, infrequent deformity, and good preservation of function
- Two symmetrical polyarthritis, frequently erosive, deforming, and functionally disabling, but distinguished from RA by association with distal interphalangeal joint involvement, spondylitis, and negative rheumatoid factor (titer <1: 80)
- Predominant spondylitis, similar to ankylosing spondylitis, possibly accompanied by peripheral arthritis but behaving independently of it.

Clinical Manifestations

Psoriatic arthritis is a chronic, progressive, inflammatory disorder of the joints and skin belonging to a group of disorders known as spondyloarthritis, the clinical manifestations of which include distal interphalangeal arthritis, dactylitis, enthesitis, axial involvement (sacroiliitis, spondylitis), and synovitis (Figs 4.4A to J). Severity of the disease may range from mild nondestructive disease to a severe mutilating malady which can lead to rapidly destructive arthropathy.

Symptoms of Psoriatic Arthritis Include

- Swelling of over region of the joints or even the entire finger
- Pain and tenderness in the joints
- Difficulty moving or stiffness in the joints and/or in the back. About half of all patients have morning stiffness lasting more than 30 minutes
- Skin lesions either as papules, plaques or pustules with classical findings

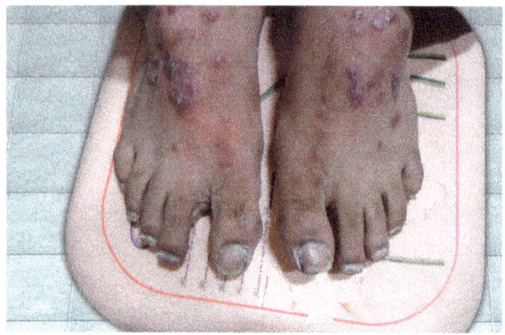

Fig. 4.4.A: Note the nail changes. This patient subsequently developed psoriatic arthropathy

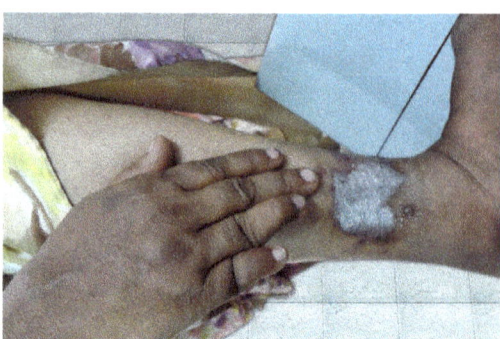

Fig. 4.4D: Symmetrical arthropathy

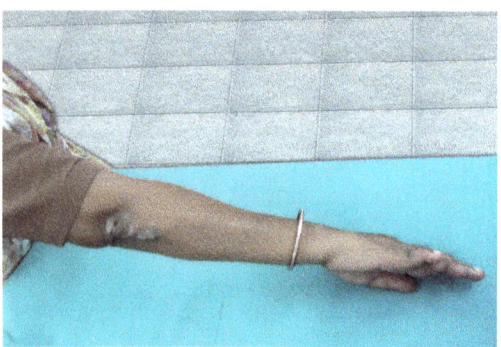

Fig. 4.4.B: Showing oligoarthritis

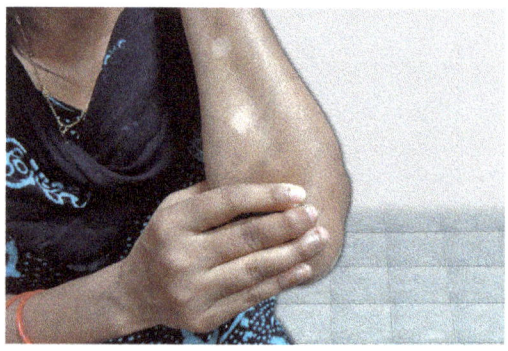

Fig. 4.4E: Patient had sacroiliitis

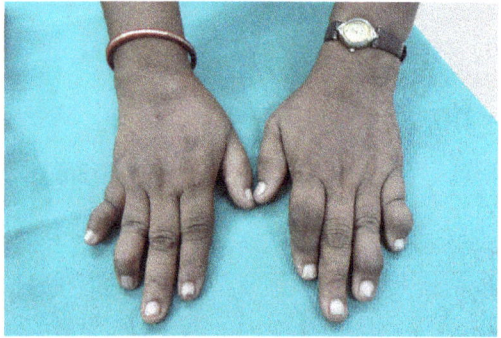

Fig. 4.4C: Symmetrical arthropathy in a patient with no skin lesions of psoriasis

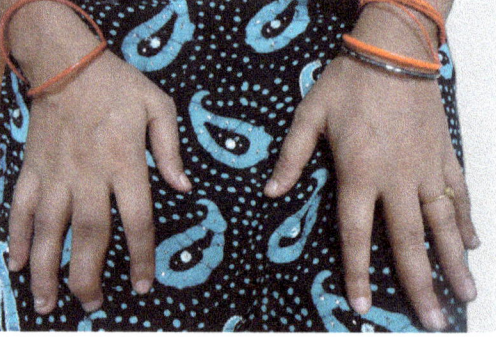

Fig. 4.4F: This patient had sacroiliitis with asymmetrical psoriatic arthritis

- Nail changes, such as pitting, subungual hyperkeratosis, nail plate discoloration, and crumbling
- In some patients with PsA, stiffness and immobility are more troublesome than joint pain

Clinical Aspects

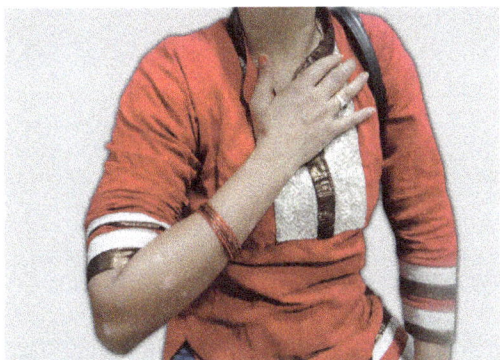

Fig. 4.4G: Note the fusiform swelling. She was seronegative with a positive family history

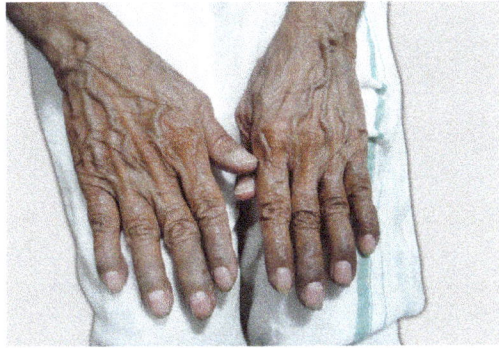

Fig. 4.4H: Had involvement of both peripheral and axial joints

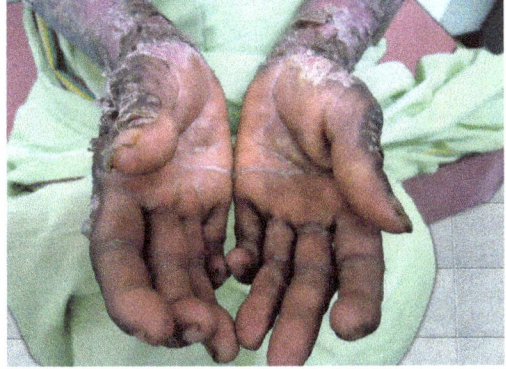

Fig. 4.4I: Pustular psoriasis with arthropathy

- Pain and redness indicating inflammation of the eye structures due to uveitis or iritis
- Symptoms of associated comorbidities, if present.

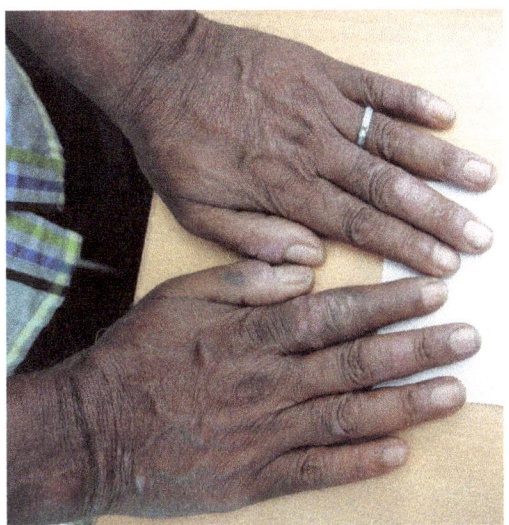

Fig. 4.4J: Note the swollen joints of psoriatic arthritis

Psoriatic arthritis is usually rheumatoid factor negative but the clinical features may mimic and be confused with RA from which it can still be differentiated. PsA is equi-gender while RA has a female preponderance. Apart from the involvement of skin and nail, main features of PsA include dactylitis, enthesopathy, peripheral arthritis and DIP involvement, and spondylitis. Erythema and tenderness over the joints may be the presenting feature of enthesitis.[54] Involvement of distal joints is more common with PsA and the joint distribution tends to occur in a ray pattern involving all the joints of a single digit whereas the same joints on both side are involved in RA. This may explain the tendency to asymmetry that occurs even in the polyarticular disease in PsA. Nail psoriasis and psoriasis of the skin are the extra-articular features of PsA while rheumatoid nodules are seen in RA. Rheumatoid factor, which is detected in more than 80% of patients with RA may be detected in about 13% of patients with PsA. There is severe joint lysis leading to shortening of digits resulting in telescoping.[55-61]

Differentiating points between PsA and RA are given in Table 4.2.

Osteoarthritis, especially in females may mimic PsA and can be confused with the same. Differentiating points given in the following table may help in making a diagnosis of PsA. Differentiating points between PsA and RA are given in Table 4.3.

Psoriatic arthritis can occur without skin lesions. But in majority of cases, PsA is associated with involvement of skin, nail. Main clinical findings of PsA are listed in Box 4.10.

Clinical Findings of Psoriatic Arthritis

Skin

In every patient with PsA, both skin and joints are affected, at some point. Most people have recognized psoriasis, followed by arthritis. In about 15% of PsA, there is no initial skin involvement. Sever involvement of the skin may indicate joint involvement since the more severe the skin symptoms are, the greater the likelihood a person will have PsA.

Nail Psoriasis

Nail lesions are very common and help distinguish between patients who have PsA and those who have RA, and between patients with psoriasis who have arthritis and those who do not have arthritis. Nail lesions occur in about 40–45% of patients with psoriasis uncomplicated by arthritis and about 87% of patients with PsA.[62] Characteristic features of nail psoriasis in these patients include nailplate pitting, crumbling, nail bed hyperkeratosis, oil-drop discoloration, and onycholysis. While psoriasis and RA may coexist with a prevalence of 3:10,000, it appears that the presence of 20 or more pits distinguishes patients with PsA from those with RA and psoriasis.[63]

Enthesitis

Enthesitis is inflammation of the tendon insertions and is a hallmark feature of PsA.

Pathogenesis of enthesitis is not fully elucidated. There are different schools of thought on the pathogenesis. Some believe that it arise at sites of high mechanical stress

TABLE 4.2: Differentiating points between PsA and RA

Features	PsA	RA
Gender	F = M	F > M
Axial involvement	yes	No
DIP involvement	yes	No
Digit involvement	Single digit all joints, shortening leading to telescoping of digits	Same joint on both hands
Symmetry	Asymmetry > Symmetry	Symmetry > Asymmetry
Erythema	More	less
Spinal involvement	Common	Rare
Enthesitis	Yes	No
Dactylitis	Yes	No
Erosion and new bone formation	Yes	No
Tenderness	Less	
Extra-articular manifestation	Psoriasis of nail and skin	Rheumatoid nodule
RA factor	13%	80%

PsA, psoriatic arthritis; RA, rheumatoid arthritis; DIP, distal interphalangeal; F, female; M, male.

Clinical Aspects

TABLE 4.3: Differentiating points between PsA and OA

Features	PsA	OA
Age of onset	Even children	Old age
Gender	F = M	F >M (under 45 years M >F)
Type of arthritis	Inflammatory	Degenerative
Axial involvement	Yes	Rare
DIP involvement	Yes	DIP followed by PIP
Digit involvement	Single digit all joints, shortening leading to telescoping of digits	DIP followed by PIP of multiple digits, osteophyte formation
Symmetry	Rare	Variable
Erythema	More	Less
Spinal involvement	Common	Rare
Enthesitis	Yes	No
Dactylitis	Yes	No
Erosion and new bone formation	Yes	No
Pain	Less	Worsens during activity, gets better during rest.
Extra articular manifestation	Psoriasis of nail and skin, pustular psoriasis	Heberden's nodes: DIP Bouchard's nodes: PIP(rare), Ganglion cysts

PsA, psoriatic arthritis; OA, Osteoarthritis; DIP, distal interphalangeal; PIP, proximal interphalangeal; F, female; M, male.

BOX 4.10: Main clinical findings of psoriatic arthritis

- Psoriasis of skin and nails
- Dactylitis
- Enthesopathy
- Peripheral arthritis
- Distal interphalangeal involvement
- Spondylitis
- Other manifestations
- PsA sine psoriasis

while relate it to systemic over expression of cytokines interleukin-23. It was also observed that isolated peripheral enthesitis may be the only rheumatologic sign of PsA in a subset of patients.

Dactylitis

Dactylitis presents as diffuse swelling of a digit, also referred to as "sausage digit". It is one of the cardinal features of PsA, occurring in up to 40% of patients. It affects feet more than the hands and is associated with increased radiological damage.

Distal Interphalangeal Joint Arthritis

Distal interphalangeal joint arthritis is a hallmark feature of PsA, and may occur in approximately 50% of cases and is frequently associated with dactylitis and nail involvement.

Asymmetric Oligoarthritis

Asymmetric oligoarthritis has a male pre-dominance affecting more than 4 joints with a reported prevalence of 14–70%. Joints of the hands and/or feet are often involved in addition to involvement of the lower limb joints.

Symmetric Polyarticular Arthritis

Symmetric polyarticular arthritis has a prevalence of up to 63%, depending on the PsA population studied. The characteristic features of symmetric polyarticular arthritis include:
- Female predominance
- Involvement of more than or equal to 5 joints involved
- Involves typically the smaller joints of the hands and feet, in addition to larger joints
- Erosions are more frequently found
- May closely mimic RA and is difficult to clinically differentiate from RA
- Usually rheumatoid factor negative.

Spondylitis

Psoriatic arthritis is classified with the spondyloarthropathies because of the presence of spondylitis in up to 40% of patients, the occurrence of extra-articular features common to the spondyloarthropathies (mucous membrane lesions, iritis, urethritis, diarrhea, aortic root dilatation), and association with human leukocyte antigen (HLA)-B27. PsA may be distinguished from the other spondyloarthropathies by the presence of peripheral arthritis, asymmetrical distribution of the spinal involvement (both sacroiliac joints and syndesmophytes), lower level of pain, and limitation of movement.[64]

It has a male predominance with an estimated frequency of up to 5%. Axial involvement is seen in 20–40% of PsA. Since the symptoms can easily be ignored, psoriatic patients with related complaints should be subjected to rigorous clinical and radiographic examination.

Arthritis Mutilans

Arthritis mutilans affects less than 5% of PsA cases having a female predominance. It is characterized by marked deformity and joint destruction leading to shortening of the digits. The important feature includes erosion on two sides of the joint and osteolysis. Patients with arthritis mutilans should be thoroughly investigated as it can be associated with long disease.

Other Manifestations

Cervical spine, temporomandibular joint, sternal joint are other rare joints involved in psoriasis. Extra-articular features like subcutaneous nodule as in RA are not seen in PsA. In contrast, inflammatory eye lesions like Reiter's disease and cardiac involvement similar to that seen in ankylosing spondylitis has been reported.

Poriatic Arthritis Sine Psoriasis

Forms of PsA lacking skin involvement are designated as PsA sine psoriasis.

Diagnostic Criteria

The clinical spectrum of PsA is wide because of the different targets of the disease, which include the axial skeleton, peripheral joints, peripheral entheses, and tenosynovial sheaths (i.e., dactylitis), each of which can be involved in isolation or in combination.

Early diagnosis of PsA should help starting treatment in the early phases of development with the aim of modifying the natural course of the disease. However, it is a challenge to make an early diagnosis of PsA, especially in the absence of skin or nail psoriasis, and the physician must be careful enough to avoid unnecessary examinations and elude risky and unhelpful therapies. It is crucial in a research setting as the results of many researches are highly variable and there in not yet a single protocol that can be accepted worldwide.

In the past, in the field of spondyloarthritis, early diagnosis has not been a priority, especially in the absence of drugs able to modify disease course. The scenario completely changed at the beginning of the new millennium with the introduction of the anti-tumor necrosis factor-α blocking agents. Today, the early diagnosis of both ankylosing spondylitis and PsA has become a challenging task.

The original diagnostic criteria of Moll and Wright are the simplest and the most frequently used in current studies. The criteria are:
- An inflammatory arthritis (peripheral arthritis and/or sacroiliitis or spondylitis)
- The presence of psoriasis
- The (usual) absence of serological tests for rheumatoid factor.

Using these diagnostic criteria Moll and Wright described five subgroups of PsA: DIP joint only, asymmetrical oligoarthritis, polyarthritis, spondylitis, and arthritis mutilans.

The classification criteria for psoriatic arthritis (CASPAR) criteria for PsA consist of inflammatory articular disease (joint, spine or entheseal) with at least 3 points from the below categories which has 98.7% sensitivity and 91.4% specificity.

The CASPAR criteria:
- Evidence of current psoriasis, a personal history of psoriasis, or a family history of psoriasis (2 points)
- Typical psoriatic nail dystrophy including onycholysis, pitting, and hyperkeratosis observed on current physical examination (1 point)
- A negative test result for the presence of rheumatoid factor by any method except latex (1 point)
- Either current dactylitis, defined as swelling of an entire digit, or a history of dactylitis recorded by a rheumatologist (1 point)
- Radiographic evidence of juxta-articular new bone formation appearing as ill-defined ossification near joint margins (but excluding osteophyte formation) on plain radiographs of the hand or foot (1 point)

Screening questionnaires and minimal disease activity criteria are used in order to screen patients with PsA and decide on treatment based on the activity and for also follow-up.

Psoriatic arthritis screening and evaluation (PASE):
- The PASE questionnaire fulfills many properties of an effective screening tool
- PASE is brief and self-administered. It is free of discomfort or risk and performs a convenient musculoskeletal review of systems for dermatologists
- It increases the level of PsA detection, which may help curb high healthcare costs associated with missed PsA cases
- The PASE also helps clinicians decide who among many psoriatic individuals with arthralgias will benefit from prompt treatment
- PASE serves only as a screening tool for PsA and does not substitute for a thorough examination.

Minimal disease activity (MDA) criteria, The Group for Research and Assessment of Psoriasis and Psoriatic Arthritis (GRAPPA). A patient is classified as in MDA when they meet 5 of 7 of the following criteria:
- Tender joint count less than or equal to 1
- Swollen joint count less than or equal to 1
- PASI less than or equal to 1 or BSA less than or equal to 3
- Patient pain visual analog scale (VAS) less than or equal to 15

- Patient global activity VAS less than or equal to 20
- Health assessment questionnaire ≤0.5
- Tender entheseal points less than or equal to 1.

Course of Disease in Psoriatic Arthritis

Psoriatic arthritis may be more common than previously described. In addition, the burden of disease is demonstrated both in terms of progression of clinical and radiological damage, and in terms of quality of life and functional status of these patients. Moreover, patients with PsA are at an increased risk of death, which is related to the severity of their disease.[65,66]

Following are some of the observations made in different studies which explicitly tell the relentless progression of the disease. Sometimes despite treatment, the disease deteriorates.

- Joint damage may occur early, in up to 47% of patients within two years of onset[1]
- Up to 20% develop a severely destructive, disabling form of arthritis[2]
- Joint involvement may become more polyarticular with time[3]
- In a case-control study, PsA patients had radiographic damage comparable with RA patients matched for age, sex, and disease duration[4]
- PsA also associated with a reduced life expectancy with a standardized mortality ratio of 1.62.[2]

The risk for premature death is related to previously active and severe disease, the level of medication, the presence of erosive disease, and a high sedimentation rate at presentation to clinic. Earlier descriptions of PsA suggested that the disease was less severe than that seen in RA. However, over the past three decades, it has become clear that PsA is much more aggressive than previously thought. About 20% of the patients develop a very destructive disabling form of arthritis. A recent study of early-onset PsA showed that within 2 years of onset, 47% of patients demonstrated at least one erosion.[65] It has been reported that there is a group of patients who may achieve remission, defined as no actively inflamed joints for a period of 12 months. These tend to be men with a lower number of actively inflamed joints at presentation. However, after an average of 2.6 years, 52% of these patients had flares, and only 6% sustained a complete prolonged remission on no medications and without evidence of clinical or radiological damage.[67]

Predictors of Disease Progression in Psoriatic Arthritis[68,69]

The following elements can be considered at clinical evaluation that predicts progression:
- More severe disease
  - High number of joints involved (≥5)
  - Longer PsA duration (≥1 year)
  - High extent of disability
  - High joint damage
  - Elevated baseline C-reactive protein (CRP)
- Polyarticular onset
- Presence of dactylitis
- Poor clinical response to treatment
- Higher number of past medications (≥2) including MTX, disease-modifying antirheumatic drugs, and corticosteroids
- HLA-B27 in the presence of HLA-DR7, HLA-B39, and HLA-DQw3 in the absence of HLA-DR7, were predictive of subsequent damage.

Protective Factors for Disease Progression

- Low erythrocyte sedimentation rate
- HLA-B22 was protective.

Psoriatic Arthritis in Children

Psoriatic arthritis in children is clinically heterogeneous. Up to 20% of childhood arthritis cases are diagnosed as PsA. The onset of PsA in children often occurs between the ages of 7 and 13 years and can produce irreversible joint destruction.[70,71]

Juvenile PsA is a relatively rare form of juvenile idiopathic arthritis (JIA) representing less than 10% of all JIA cases. Its prevalence has been estimated between 1 and 10 children per 33,000 with an annual incidence of between 1 and 20 in 1,000,000.[72]

The two forms of PsA encountered in children are:
- That resembles an oligoarticular arthritis with a risk of uveitis is more common in girls with onset at around 6 years of age
- The one that resembles a spondylarthropathy is most common in boys and manifests later.

The diagnostic criteria include:
- Presence of a form of arthritis and psoriasis, or
- Presence of arthritis associated with at least one of the following signs:
  o Dactylitis
  o Ungual pitting or onycholysis
  o Family history of psoriasis in the parents or a first-degree relative.

Exclusion criteria include:
- HLA-B27 positivity in males with onset of arthritis after 6 years of age
- Positive rheumatoid factor IgM in two test samples taken 3 months apart
- Presence of ankylosing spondyloarthritis, enthesitis and arthritis, sacroiliitis with an inflammatory enteropathy or acute anterior uveitis in the patient or a family history or one of these conditions in a parent or first-degree relative
- Presence of systemic arthritis in the patient.

Juvenile PsA is sometimes thought of as part of the spectrum of juvenile chronic arthritis summarized above but others regard it as a separate disease to be distinguished from these, having more in common with reactive arthritis and juvenile ankylosing spondylitis.

The Vancouver criteria for diagnosis of PsA in childhood are a useful guide:

Definite PsA
- Arthritis with three of the four following minor criteria:
  o Dactylitis (pink swollen "sausage" finger or toe)
  o Nail pitting or onycholysis (splitting and breaking up of nail)
  o Psoriasis-like rash
  o Family history of psoriasis in first or second degree relatives.

Probable PsA
- Arthritis with two of the four criteria listed above.

There is a tendency for girls to be more likely to be to be affected than boys. Simultaneous onset of rash and arthritis is rather uncommon. As in the adult variety, the end joints of the fingers are commonly involved. Generally, in juvenile chronic arthritis, this does not happen but tendons are often inflamed. Of the joints involved the knee seems most common in children.

According to Stall et al., in juvenile PsA, the age at onset is biphasic, with peaks occurring at approximately 2 years of age and again in late childhood. Compared with children ages 5 years and older, younger patients are more likely to be female, exhibit dactylitis and small joint involvement, with an increased tendency to progress to polyarticular disease. These children express antinuclear antibodies. Whereas, older children tend to manifest enthesitis, axial joint disease, and persistent oligoarthritis. Uveitis is equally represented in both age groups. Despite a higher utilization of MTX therapy, younger patients required longer duration of treatment to achieve clinical remission.[73]

Following are some of the observations about juvenile PsA (PsA that affects children):[74]

- Juvenile PsA accounts for some cases of arthritis in children
- This often occurs in 9–10 years old girls. It is usually mild, but occasionally it is severe and lasts into adulthood
- In half of affected children, only one joint is affected. The joints at the ends of the fingers or toes are involved in about half of affected people as well
- The tendons are inflamed in a significant percentage of affected children. Nails are involved in a majority of affected children, and little pits can often be seen on the nails
- Bone-growth problems and shortening due to inflammation may occur in almost half of affected children
- Sacroiliitis (inflammation of the sacroiliac joint in the pelvis) or arthritis of the hip occurs in some affected children
- Onset of psoriasis and arthritis at the same time occurs more often in children than adults. Arthritis occurs before psoriasis in half of affected children.

Psoriasis, which is now accepted as a systemic disease affecting mainly the skin and joint with a potential to affect almost all other systems should be meticulously examined and carefully assessed. It is essential that the time of first onset whether early or late, the morphologic aspects of elementary lesions; degree of inflammation whether mainly inflammatory or hyperkeratotic; extent of disease whether involves single site, many sites or generalized, presence or not of joint involvement, velocity of propagation as stable, unstable or eruptive; associated comorbidities, and other conditions like HIV infection will all have to be assessed before completing the diagnosis. PsA is not uncommon in children which have to be kept in mind while dealing with childhood psoriasis.

CONCLUSION

Clinical assessment is as important as treatment in a patient with psoriasis. Clinician must spend sufficient time to elicit proper history and evaluate a patient including the habits and systemic disorder, if any, with a special attention to the psychological status of the patient. Age of onset, symptoms, triggering and exacerbating factors should be asked for and while examining, the signals of psoriasis be looked for. Every patient must be graded with a scoring system (PASI) and systemic associations be recorded. Of the various types, plaque psoriasis seems to be the commonest. Erythrodermic psoriasis should be considered as a medical emergency and patients with unstable forms should be monitored meticulously. In order to plan treatment, the site of involvement and the severity must be considered. Based on the severity psoriasis can be better categorized as latent, mild, moderate, moderate-severe, severe, and those with guarded prognosis. Complications of psoriasis should always be looked for. Eczematization and infection are the most frequent local complications. Sudden withdrawal of potent topical steroids can lead to pustular eruptions. Systemic complications can involve the kidneys and liver leading to organ failure. PsA is a well known complication of long-standing severe psoriasis and therefore, it is mandatory to look for the features of PsA and diagnose them early. Enthesitis is the earliest manifestation of PsA while arthritis mutilans is a severe form of PsA. PsA in children is not uncommon and is now increasingly seen than before.

REFERENCES

1. Seyhan M, Coskun BK, Saglam H, Ozcan H, Karincaoglu Y. Psoriasis in childhood and adolescence: evaluation of demographic and clinical features. Pediatr Int. 2006;48:525-30.
2. Morris A, Rogers M, Fischer G, Williams K. Childhood psoriasis: a clinical review of 1262 cases. Pediatr Dermatol. 2001;18:188-98.
3. Grjibovski AM, Olsen AO, Magnus P, Harris JR. Psoriasis in Norwegian twins: contribution of genetic and environmental effects. J Eur Acad Dermatol Venereol. 2007;21:1337-43.
4. Henseler T, Christophers E. Psoriasis of early and late onset: characterization of two types of psoriasis vulgaris. J Am Acad Dermatol. 1985;13:450-6.
5. al-Fouzan AS, Nanda A. A survey of childhood psoriasis in Kuwait. Pediatric Dermatol. 1994;11:116-9.
6. Altobelli E, Petrocelli R, Marziliano C, Fargnoli MC, Maccarone M, Chimenti S, et al. Family history of psoriasis and age at disease onset in Italian patients with psoriasis. Br J Dermatol. 2007;156:1400-1.
7. Honig PJ. Guttate psoriasis associated with perianal streptococcal disease. J Pediatr. 1988;113:1037-9.
8. Cassandra M, Conte E, Cortez B. Childhood pustular psoriasis elicited by the streptococcal antigen: a case report and review of the literature. Pediatr Dermatol. 2003;20:506-10.
9. Lazar AP, Roenigk HH. Acquired immunodeficiency syndrome (AIDS) can exacerbate psoriasis. J Am Acad Dermatol. 1988;18:144.
10. Tsankov N, Angelova I, Kazandjieva J. Drug-induced psoriasis. Recognition and management. Am J Clin Dermatol. 2000;1:159-65.
11. Wolf R, Ruocco V. Triggered psoriasis. Adv Exp Med Biol. 1999;455:221-5.
12. O'Brien M, Koo J. The mechanism of lithium and beta-blocking agents in inducing and exacerbating psoriasis. J Drugs Dermatol. 2006;5:426-32.
13. Benoit S, Hamm H. Childhood psoriasis. Clinics in Dermatology. 2007;25:555-62.
14. Drusko B, Rucevic. Psoriasis in childhood. Coll Antropol. 2004;1:211-85.
15. Naldi L, Gambini D. The clinical spectrum of psoriasis. Clin Dermatol. 2007;25:510-8.
16. Nanda A, Kaur S, Kaur I, Kumar B. Childhood psoriasis: An epidemiological survey of 112 patients. Pediatr Dermatol. 1990;7:19-21.
17. Stern RS, Wu J. Psoriasis. In: Arndt KA, LeBoit PE, Robinson JK, Wintroub BU (Eds). Cutaneous Medicine and Surgery. Philadelphia: WB Saunders; 1996 pp. 295-321.
18. Gottlieb AB, Chaudhari U, Baker DG, Perate M, Dooley LT. The natural psoriasis foundation score (NPF-PS) system versus the Psoriasis Area Severity Index (PASI) and Physicians Global Assessment. (PGA): a comparison. J Drugs Dermatol. 2003;2:260-6.
19. Langley RBG, Krueger GG, Griffiths CEM. Psoriasis: epidemiology, clinical features, and quality of life. Ann Rheum Dis. 2005;64:ii18-23.
20. Dhar S, Banerjee R, Agrawal N, Chatterjee S, Malakar R. Psoriasis in children: an insight. Indian J Dermatol. 2011;56(3):262-5.
21. Han MH, Jang KA, Sung KJ, Moon KC, Koh JK, Choi JH. A case of guttate psoriasis following Kawasaki disease. B J Dermatol. 2000;142:548-50.
22. Li W, Man XY. Linear psoriasis. CMAJ. 2012;184:789.
23. Chien P, Rosenman K, Cheung W, Wang N, Sanchez M. Linear psoriasis. Dermatol Online J. 2009;15(8):4.
24. Ashurst PJC. Relapsing pustular eruptions of the hands and feet. Br J Dermatol. 1964;76:169-80.
25. Reitamo S, Erkko P, Remitz A. Palmoplantar pustulosis. Eur J Dermatol. 1992;2:311-4.
26. O'Doherty CJ, MacIntyre C. Palmoplantar pustulosis and smoking. Br Med J. 1985;291:861-4.
27. Iria N, Navarini AA, Yawalkar N. Alitretinoin abrogates innate inflammation in palmoplantar pustular psoriasis. Br J Dermatol. 2012;167;1170-4.
28. Pandhi D, Chowdhry S, Grover C, Reddy B S. Parakeratosis pustulosa-a distinct but less familiar disease. Indian J Dermatol Venereol Leprol. 2003;69:48-50.
29. Baker H, Ryan TJ. Generalized pustular psoriasis. Br J Dermatol. 1968;80:771-93.
30. Dawson TAJ. Tongue lesions in generalized pustular psoriasis. Br J Dermatol. 1974;91:419-24.
31. de Oliveira ST, Maragno L, Arnone M, Takahashi F, Romiti R. Generalized Pustular Psoriasis in Childhood. Pediatric Dermatology. 2010;27(4):349-54.
32. Burden AD. Management of psoriasis in childhood. Clin Exp Dermatol. 1999;24:341-5.
33. Liao P, Rubinson R, Howard R, Sanchez G, Frieden IJ. Annular pustular psoriasis—most common form of pustular psoriasis in children: report of three cases and review of the literature. Pediatr Dermatol. 2002;19:19-25.
34. Zelickson BD, Muller SA. Generalized pustular psoriasis in childhood. J Am Acad Dermatol. 1990;24:186-94.

35. Xiao T, Li B, He CD, Chen HD. Juvenile generalized pustular psoriasis. J Dermatol. 2007;34:573-6.
36. Catsarou-Catsari A, Katsambos A, Theodoropoulus P, Stratigos J. Ophthalmological manifestations in patients with psoriasis. Acta Derm Venereol. 1984;64:557-9.
37. Dogra A, Arora AK. Nail psoriasis: The journey so far. Indian J Dermatol. 2014;59:319-33.
38. Jiaravuthisan MM, Sasseville D, Vender RB, Murphy F, Muhn CY. Psoriasis of the nail: Anatomy, pathology, clinical presentation, and a review of the literature on therapy. J Am Acad Dermatol. 2007;57:1-27.
39. Gudjonsson JE, Karason A, Runardsdottir EH, Antonsdottir AA, Hauksson VB, Jonsson HH, et al. Distinct clinical differences between HLA-Cw 0602 positive and negative psoriasis patients: An analysis of 1019 HLA-C- and HLA-B-typed patients. J Invest Dermatol. 2006;126:740-5.
40. Ortonne JP, Baran R, Corvest M, Schmitt C, Voisard JJ, Taieb C. Development and validation of nail psoriasis quality of life scale (NPQ10). J Eur Acad Dermatol Venereol. 2010;24:22-7.
41. Bongartz T, Härle P, Friedrich S, Karrer S, Vogt T, Seitz A, et al. Successful treatment of psoriatic onychopachydermo periostitis (POPP) with adalimumab. Arthritis Rheum. 2005;52(1):280-2.
42. Mahoney JM, Scott R. Psoriatic onychopachydermoperiostitis (POPP): A perplexing case study. J Am Podiatr Med Assoc. 2009;99:140-3.
43. Cassell SE, Bieber JD, Rich P, Tutuncu ZN, Lee SJ, Kalunian KC, et al. The modified nail psoriasis severity index: validation of an instrument to assess psoriatic nail involvement in patients with PsA. J Rheumatol. 2007;34:123-9.
44. Guglielmetti A, Conlledo R, Bedoya J, Ianiszewski F, Correa J. Inverse psoriasis involving genital skin folds: successful therapy with dapsone. Dermatol Ther. 2012;2(1):15.
45. Wang G, Li C, Gao T, Liu Y. Clinical analysis of 48 cases of inverse psoriasis: a hospital-based study. Eur J Dermatol. 2005;15:176-8.
46. Kim AP. Meeuwis KAP, de Hullu JA, Massuger LFAG, et al. Genital psoriasis: A systematic literature review on this hidden skin disease. Acta Derm Venereol. 2011;91:5-11.
47. Buechner SA. Common skin disorders of the penis. BJU Int 2002; 90:498-506.
48. EMEA. Committee for Proprietary Medical Products. Note for guidance on clinical investigation of medical products indicated for the treatment of psoriasis. CPMP/EWP 2454/02.
49. Ros AM, Eklund G, Odont D. Photosensitive psoriasis. An epidemiologic study. J Am Acad Dermatol. 1987;17:752-8.
50. Gladman DD, Ritchlin C. 2015. Patient information: Psoriatic arthritis (beyond the basics). [Online] Available from www.uptodate.com/contents/psoriatic-arthritis-beyond-the-basics. [Accessed June, 2015].
51. About psoriasis: Statistics. National Psoriasis Foundation. [Online] Available from www.psoriasis.org/netcommunity/learn_statistics. [Accessed May, 2013].
52. Mease P, Goffe BS. Diagnosis and treatment of psoriatic arthritis. J Am Acad Dermatol. 2005;52:1-19.
53. Anandarajah AP, Ritchlin CT. The diagnosis and treatment of early psoriatic arthritis. Nat Rev Rheumatol. 2009;5:634-41.
54. Gladman DD. Clinical aspects of the spondyloarthropathies. Am J Med Sci. 1998;3(16):234-8.
55. Bruce IN, Gladman DD. Psoriatic arthritis: recognition and management. Bio Drugs. 1998;9:271-8.
56. Veale D, Rogers S, Fitzgerald O. Classification of clinical subsets in psoriatic arthritis. Br J Rheumatol. 1994;33:133-8.
57. Cassell SE, Bieber JD, Rich P, Tutuncu ZN, Lee SJ, Kalunian KC, et al. The modified Nail Psoriasis Severity Index: validation of an instrument to assess psoriatic nail involvement in patients with psoriatic arthritis. J Rheumatol. 2007;34:123-9.
58. Khan MA. Update on spondyloarthropathies. Ann Intern Med. 2002;136:896-907.
59. McGonagle D. Imaging the joint and enthesis: insights into pathogenesis of psoriatic arthritis. Ann Rheum Dis. 2005;64(Suppl II):ii58-60.
60. Anandarajah AP, Ritchlin CT. Pathogenesis of psoriatic arthritis. Curr Opin Rheumatol. 2004;16:338-43.
61. Sherlock JP, Joyce-Shaikh B, Turner SP, Chao CC, Sathe M, Grein J, et al. IL-23 induces spondyloarthropathy by acting on ROR-γt+ CD3+CD4-CD8- entheseal resident T cells. Nat Med. 2012;18(7):1069-76.
62. Gladman DD, Anhorn KA, Schachter RK, Mervart H. HLA antigens in psoriatic arthritis. J Rheumatol. 1986;13:586-92.
63. Eastmond CJ, Wright V. The nail dystrophy of psoriatic arthritis. Ann Rheum Dis. 1979;38:226-8.
64. Marsal S, Armadans-Gil L, Martinez M, Gallardo D, Ribera A, Lience E. Clinical, radiographic and HLA associations as markers for different patterns of psoriatic arthritis. Rheumatology (Oxford). 1999;38:332-7.
65. Kane D, Stafford L, Bresnihan B, FitzGerald O. A prospective, clinical and radiological study of early psoriatic arthritis: an early synovitis clinic experience Rheumatology (Oxford). 2003;42:1460-8; Gladman DD, Antoni C, Mease P, Clegg DO, Nash P. Psoriatic arthritis: epidemiology, clinical features, course, and outcome. Ann Rheum Dis. 2005;64(Suppl II):14-7.

66. Jones SM, Armas JB, Cohen MG, Lovell CR, Evison G, McHugh NJ, et al. Psoriatic arthritis: outcome of disease subsets and relationship of joint disease to nail and skin disease. Br J Rheumatol. 1994;33(9):834-9; Rahman P, Nguyen E, Cheung C, Schentag CT, Gladman DD, et al. Comparison of radiological severity in psoriatic arthritis and rheumatoid arthritis. J Rheumatol. 2001;28(5):1041-4.
67. Zachariae H, Zachariae R, Blomqvist K, Davidsson S, Molin L, Mork C, et al. Quality of life and prevalence of arthritis reported by 5795 members of the Nordic Psoriasis Associations. Data from the Nordic Quality of Life Study. Acta Derm Venereol. 2002;82:108-13.
68. Gladman DD, Farewell VT. Progression in psoriatic arthritis: role of time varying clinical indicators. J Rheumatol. 1999;26(11):2409-13.
69. Gladman DD, Mease PJ, Choy E HS, et al. Analysis of risk factors for radiographic progression in psoriatic arthritis (PsA): subanalysis of ADEPT. Program and abstracts of the American College of Rheumatology (ACR) 71st Annual Meeting; 2007; Boston, Massachusetts.
70. Brockbank JE, Stein M, Schentag CT, Gladman DD. Dactylitis in psoriatic arthritis: a marker for disease severity? Ann Rheum Dis. 2005;64:188-90.
71. Belazarian L. New insights and therapies for teenage psoriasis. Curr Opin Pediatr. 2008;20:419-24.
72. Beattie PE, Lewis-Jones MS. A comparative study of impairment of qualifies of life in children with skin disease and children with other chronic childhood diseases. Br J Dermatol. 2006;155:145-51.
73. Deslandre CJ. 2007. Juvenile psoriatic arthritis expert reviewer(s). [Online] Available from: http://www.orpha.net/consor4.01/www/cgi-bin/OC_Exp.php?lng=EN&Expert=85436 [Accessed July, 2015].
74. Shiel WC. 2015. Psoriatic arthritis overview. [Online] Available from: http://www.emedicinehealth.com/psoriatic_arthritis/article_em.htm [Accessed July, 2015].

CHAPTER 5

Pediatric Psoriasis

INTRODUCTION

Psoriasis is a T cell-mediated chronic inflammatory disorder of the skin seen in about 3.5% of the population.[1] One-third of psoriasis cases in a dermatology center are seen in pediatric age group.[2] Pediatric psoriasis consists broadly of three age groups of psoriatic patients:
- Infantile psoriasis, a self-limited disease of infancy
- Psoriasis with early onset
- Pediatric psoriasis with psoriatic arthritis (PsA).[3]

Timely diagnosis and appropriate management can not only arrest progression of the disease but also minimize the psychosocial burden imposed by this illness. Thereby, disfiguring states and its evolution into a metabolic syndrome requiring extensive treatment can well be averted. This review will cover almost all aspects of psoriasis including the rare clinical forms like infantile psoriasis and congenital erythrodermic psoriasis (CEP) and present the latest update especially on the etiopathogenesis and treatment options.

Psoriasis may occur at any age and pediatric age is no exemption. Childhood psoriasis has to be regarded as a frequent chronic inflammatory skin disorder, early diagnosis of which will help in better control of the disease. Therapy is demanding with regard to the specific juvenile metabolism, physical development and the number of years of exposure to ultraviolet (UV) light in future. The increased skin penetration of topical drugs and tendency for irritant reactions makes the topical therapy not so easy while dealing with children. These factors have to be considered whenever long-term treatment at an early age is contemplated that has to be critically judged. The impact on the quality of life as well as development of the afflicted children and their parents is evident. Hence, counseling should be given top priority in the management protocol. This section will discuss psoriasis in children under the following topics:
- Epidemiology
- Etiopathogenesis
- Pathology
- Clinical aspects
- Associations and comorbidities

- Treatment
- Psychological aspects and rehabilitation.

EPIDEMIOLOGY

One-third of adults with psoriasis, report onset in childhood. Ethnic variation is not clear, with some studies quoting incidence highest in Caucasians, Blacks, then Asian populations.[4] It is alarming to note that 40,000 children under 10 years of age were afflicted by psoriasis.[5] The distribution of psoriasis in children is almost equal in boys and girls. However, female preponderance has been observed by some authors.[4] The occurrence of psoriatic diaper rash in younger children and its inclusion increases the incidence of psoriasis in children under two.[4] The exact age distribution is not clear though according to some studies nearly 30% of patients with psoriasis develop the disease before the age of 18.[6] It is of interest to note that in the age group less than 20 years, the frequency of psoriasis was 20% higher in girls than in boys, in contrast to adults.[7] Compared with 37% in adult-onset patients, 49% of pediatric-onset patients had first-degree family members affected with psoriasis.[2] Some studies have reported familial incidence in childhood cases of psoriasis as high as 89%.[8] Nearly, two-thirds of children manifest with plaque-type psoriasis vulgaris.[3] Involvement of joints with PsA is less prevalent in younger patients; however, it does occur in childhood disease and should be considered in the differential of pediatric arthritis. Psoriasis of childhood shows an annual prevalence of 0.71% and accordingly, has to be regarded as a frequent chronic inflammatory skin disorder of this age. German studies revealed an annual prevalence of 1.7% in persons less than 18 years of age, a single year prevalence of 0.71% and a cumulative prevalence of 1.37%. Similar population-based data with a prevalence of psoriasis of 1.5% were found in Great Britain.[5]

However, the true prevalence of childhood psoriasis in India is not known as the available literature is insufficient. It is observed that there is a rise in the prevalence of psoriasis in all its aspects, in the recent days than before. This includes overall prevalence, prevalence of childhood psoriasis, arthropathic psoriasis, and metabolic comorbidities associated with psoriasis.

ETIOPATHOGENESIS

Psoriasis is a systemic, immune-mediated disorder, characterized by inflammatory skin and joint manifestations. The exact pathogenesis of psoriasis has not been completely elucidated.

However, it is known to have a genetic basis, as 23.4–71% of children will have a family history of psoriasis[3] and psoriasis is more common in identical than fraternal twins (65–72% vs. 15–30%). Human leukocyte antigen (HLA)-Cw6 has been known to be a susceptibility gene in psoriasis.[9]

Major gene for psoriasis susceptibility is thought mainly to be located on chromosome 6, the site of HLA class I (associated with early onset disease) and II (late onset disease) antigens which are thought to produce differing subtypes of the disease. Individuals with the Cw0602 allele are four times more likely to develop guttate psoriasis.[4] A series of genes have been isolated in which mutations have been associated with psoriatic disease, including interleukin (IL) 12-B9 (1p31.3), IL-13 (5q31.1), IL-23R (1p31.3), HLA-BW6, psoriasis susceptibility locus 6 (PSORS6), signal transducer and activator of transcription (STAT)2/IL-23A (12q13.2), tumor necrosis factor-α-induced protein 3 (TNF-α-IP3) (6q23.3), and TNF-α-IP3 interacting protein 1 (TNIP1) TNIP1 (5q33.1).

These genes play a role in T helper (Th) 2 cell and Th17 cell activity which have been noted in psoriatic lesions.[10,11]

Several attempts have been made to detect psoriasis susceptibility loci by linkage studies. Up to now, at least 12 loci are known PSORS1-12.[12] Interestingly, a strong association exists in early-onset psoriasis for the HLA-Cw6 allele.[13]

Precipitating factors are more important in pediatric than in adult-onset psoriasis.[2] They largely include trauma, infections, drugs, and stress. Streptococcal pharyngitis or perianal streptococcal dermatitis typically provokes guttate psoriasis. Infection with human immunodeficiency virus (HIV) can induce or exacerbate psoriasis.[14]

Children with obesity and overweight get more adipose tissue deposited. This adipose tissue, especially in those with central obesity, is a vigorous endocrine organ capable of secreting multiple pro-inflammatory adipocytokines, such as IL-6, IL-1, TNF-α11, and adiponectin[7] which play an important role in the pathogenesis of psoriasis. Serum and skin levels of TNF-α and IL-6 are increased in psoriasis and are positively correlated with disease severity. Obesity is a risk factor for psoriasis and can increase the severity of psoriasis.[15,16] There is a strong correlation between psoriasis and autoimmune diseases and atopy. Coexistence of psoriasis with any of the above been reported.

Expression of the disease clinically depends on the capacity of the child's epidermis to express the same. This is a complex process, linked to interaction of cells of the epidermis, dermis, immune system, and humoral elements. The inherent phenotype has a capacity of the keratinocyte for hyperproliferation and altered differentiation, both of which are genetically controlled. A genetic aberration can, therefore, trigger the cascade of inflammatory events in the evolution of the disease.

PATHOLOGY

From a histological point of view, psoriasis is a dynamic dermatosis that changes during the evolution of an individual lesion. Lesions are usually diagnostic only in early stages or near the margin of advancing plaques. Hyperkeratosis, parakeratosis, Munro's microabscesses, spongiform pustule of Kogoj, diminished or absent granular layer, regular acanthosis, papillomatosis, tortuosity and dilatation of papillary capillaries, and chronic inflammation in the upper dermis are the common features seen in psoriasis. However, Munro's microabscesses and Kogoj's micropustules are diagnostic clues of psoriasis, but they are not always present in all cases at all stages. All other features can be found in various types of eczemas and other dermatoses.[17] Depending on type, site, and stage of the disease, histological features tend to differ. Leclerc-Mercier et al., have studied various histological patterns in infantile erythroderma, and classified them into psoriasiform, spongiform, and ichthyosiform.[18] The psoriasiform pattern included:

- Psoriasiform epidermal hyperplasia
- Parakeratosis
- None or mild spongiosis

Psoriasiform epidermal hyperplasia comprised confluent parakeratosis, hyperkeratosis, hypogranulosis, and suprapapillary thinning of the epidermis, regular acanthosis often with clubbed rete ridges. According to Walsh et al., the mean accuracy of the histopathological diagnoses was less than 55%, even in adult erythroderma.[19] In the case of psoriatic erythroderma, particularly in infants, Netherton Syndrome (NS) was the closest histological mimicker. Prior to the availability of lymphoepithelial Kazal-type inhibitor (LEKTI) antibody nearly one fifth of the cases of NS being misdiagnosed as psoriasis most often.[20] Determination of the underlying cause is usually a challenge for clinicians, considering the poor specificity of clinical signs. Consequently, the diagnosis is often delayed by 11 months.[21]

The most consistent feature of CEP, according to the authors, was acanthosis and dilatation of papillary capillaries with neutrophilic squirting in to the epidermis.

Psoriasis and atopic dermatitis (AD) were once believed to be mutually exclusive. In a prospective study undertaken by Beer et al., 16.7% of AD patients had psoriasis and 9.5% of psoriasis patients had AD. In consecutive occurrences, psoriasis generally followed AD. The ratio of concurrent to consecutive incidences was 3:1. The two diseases are shown not to be mutually exclusive and may coexist in the same individual.[22] Distinct populations of T cells are defined by their unique patterns of cytokine production.[23] Keratinocytes of patients with AD and psoriasis show an intrinsically abnormal and different chemokine production profile and favor the recruitment of distinct leukocyte subsets into the skin.[24] However, in spite of their differences, both AD and psoriasis share epidermal hyperplasia, aberrant immunity, and skin barrier anomalies.

Genetic studies of both psoriasis and AD suggest that defects affecting cells of the skin need to be as seriously considered as defects in adaptive immunity. The epidermal differentiation complex has been implicated in both AD and psoriasis.[25] It transcribes within terminally differentiating keratinocytes and contains many genes that may modify immune processes in the epithelium. The colocalization of AD to psoriasis loci indicates that AD is influenced by genes that modulate dermal responses, independently from atopic mechanisms. The histological findings of both diseases occurring simultaneously as early as in infancy definitely adds further evidence to the association between psoriasis and AD.[26]

Histological confirmation of psoriasis is not always mandatory as most of the cases are clinically diagnosed even in children. However, early skin biopsy is helpful in the diagnosis of neonatal and infantile erythroderma where the etiology of erythroderma can be many and timely diagnosis will help to manage the child better.

CLINICAL ASPECTS

Psoriasis in children is not uncommon. A positive family history, precipitating trigger factors, and age of onset can all, to some extent, predict the prognosis of the disease in children. A positive family history has been reported in 23.4–71% of children with psoriasis.[27,28] Identical twins have more chances of manifesting psoriasis than fraternal twins.[30]

Age of Onset

With reference to the age of onset, psoriasis can be divided into "pediatric-onset psoriasis" (POP) and to "adult onset psoriasis" (AOP).[9] Variations exist between studies regarding the age of onset of childhood psoriasis. According to Stefanaki et al. majority of the children were 9-10 years as they represented 40% of their study population.[30] According to Stefanaki, the peak age of onset is between 8 and 12 years which they compared and stated to be the same with studies from China, Denmark, and India, in which most of the children had an onset of disease at 8–12 years of age, contrary to the reports from

Middle East and Australia where the onset was before 5 years of age.[31] Such differences may be attributable to the referral pattern, and also due to inadequate documentation and statistics as children are being treated by neonatologists, pediatricians, and family and adolescent physicians apart from dermatologists, in various set ups. A positive family history was obtained in only 16% of study conducted by Stefanaki et al. Family history of psoriasis predicts early disease onset.[32] While the mean age at manifestation lies between the 8th and 12th year of life, manifestation at all ages is possible which is evident by the fact that rare forms like congenital psoriasis and psoriasis in infancy are reported in literature. Childhood psoriasis can be associated with a seronegative arthritis, with two subtypes of juvenile PsA with differences in age of manifestation, sex distribution, the pattern of joint involvement, and therapeutic response.[5]

Triggering and Exacerbating Factors

Precipitating factors are more important in pediatric, than in adult-onset psoriasis.[2] They largely include trauma, infections, drugs, and stress. Positive family history, preceding infections, particularly with streptococci, or a psychosocial stress situation are found more frequently in children with psoriasis.[5] The appearance of psoriatic lesions in uninvolved skin at sites of former trauma is known as isomorphic response or Koebner's phenomenon. Any form of trauma including physical, chemical, thermal, surgical, or inflammatory trauma can result in exacerbation of psoriasis. Streptococcal pharyngitis or perianal streptococcal dermatitis typically provokes guttate psoriasis and childhood pustular psoriasis can be elicited by the streptococcal antigen.[33,34] Infection with HIV can induce or exacerbate psoriasis.[35] Whereas the use of β-blocking agents and lithium is a well-known trigger of psoriasis in adult patients, antimalarials and withdrawal of oral or topical corticosteroids (TCS) play a more important role in rebound or induction of childhood psoriasis.[36-38] In addition, several studies emphasize the influence of psychological and psychosomatic factors like stress or lack of social support in modifying the course of psoriasis.[15] Inflammatory focus was the most frequent trigger factor observed by Barisic-Drusko and Rucevic.[39]

Type I psoriasis has an early onset and therefore, it may be appropriate to group all children under type I psoriasis and consider those children with a positive family history and who are positive for HLAs-Cw6, B57, DR7 to have severe presentation and course.[13] According to Morris et al., no gender difference has been observed in childhood psoriasis, whereas Stefanaki et al., have observed a female-to-male ratio of 1.4:1 in a study of 125 children.[30] Many authors have observed girls to be affected more than boys.[6,15,40] The clinical types of psoriasis are more or less the same as in adults with some variation in the incidence of different types. Plaque type psoriasis, scalp psoriasis, guttate psoriasis, nail psoriasis, flexural psoriasis, napkin psoriasis, unstable psoriasis, pustular psoriasis are the types of psoriasis commonly encountered in children. Congenital psoriasis, congenital psoriatic erythroderma and infantile psoriasis are rare forms of psoriasis seen in the first year of life. Erythrodermic psoriasis and PsA are less frequent when compared to adulthood psoriasis. Mucosal involvement has been rare in Indian children.[41] Psoriasis can, hence, be considered as a disease manifesting from "womb to tomb".

The disease in children is more pruritic, and the lesions are relatively thinner, softer,

and less scaly.[15] The classical erythematous scaly papule or plaque will mostly give a clue to diagnosis. The following features are pertinent and helpful in the clinical diagnosis of psoriasis:[42]
- The isomorphic response or Koebner's phenomenon, which is occurrence of lesions in areas of trauma
- The Auspitz sign—pinpoint bleeding at the base of scale that has been removed
- Presence of nail pitting, which can aid in diagnosis of the disease
- Altered pigmentation with lesional clearance.

The first two findings are useful to assess the disease activity.

Grading

Severity grading for psoriasis is usually based on surface area and severity.

Psoriasis area and severity index (PASI) is the most widely used tool for the measurement of severity of psoriasis. PASI combines the assessment of the severity of lesions and the area affected into a single score in the range 0 (no disease) to 72 (maximal disease).

Within each area, the severity is estimated by three clinical signs: erythema (redness), induration (thickness), and desquamation (scaling). Severity parameters are measured on a scale of 0–4, from none to maximum.

The sum of all three severity parameters is then calculated for each section of skin, multiplied by the area score for that area and multiplied by weight of respective section (0.1 for head, 0.2 for arms, 0.3 for body, and 0.4 for legs).

A simpler way to assess the severity would be mild, moderate, and severe which are represented as less than 3%, 3–10%, and more than 10% body surface area (BSA), respectively.[43]

Clinical Subtypes

Clinical subtypes of juvenile psoriasis can be broadly grouped into three categories, namely psoriasis vulgaris and its variants, psoriasis pustulosa, and special forms of psoriasis.

The subtypes include the following:
- Psoriasis vulgaris or plaque-type psoriasis
  o Guttate psoriasis
  o Napkin psoriasis
  o Psoriasis capitis
  o Psoriasis faciei
  o Psoriasis inversa
- Psoriasis pustulosa
  o Pustulosis palmoplantaris
  o Generalized pustular psoriasis (GPP)
- Special forms
  o Psoriatic erythroderma
  o PsA
  o Psoriatic nail disease
  o SAPHO (synovitis, acne, pustulosis, hyperostosis, and osteitis)

Plaque Psoriasis

Plaque-type psoriasis is by far the most common clinical type of psoriasis in children accounting from 30% to 60% of the total pediatric cases studied 56.8% (Figs 5.1A to J).[30]

Classical plaque is characterized by erythema and silvery white scales. However, in dark skinned children, both erythema and scaling are not so obvious. The common sites involved include scalp, postauricular area, elbows, knees, umbilical region, and buttocks. Scalp was the most common initial site affected (50.3%).[40] In an Indian study, leg was the most frequently affected site than the scalp involvement.[44] Facial involvement in children is a frequent observation in majority of the reports, which varies from 18% to 46%.[28,45]

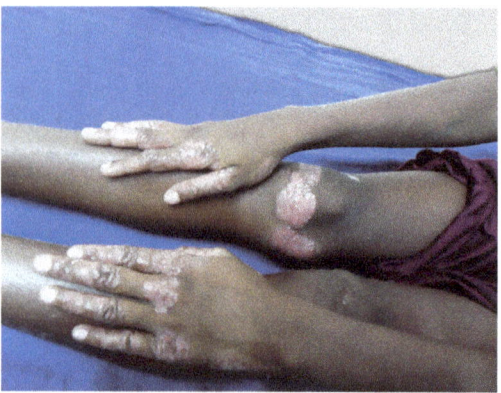

Fig. 5.1A: Classical erythematous plaque with silvery white scales over the extensor aspect of the knees and hands in a boy having psoriasis vulgaris

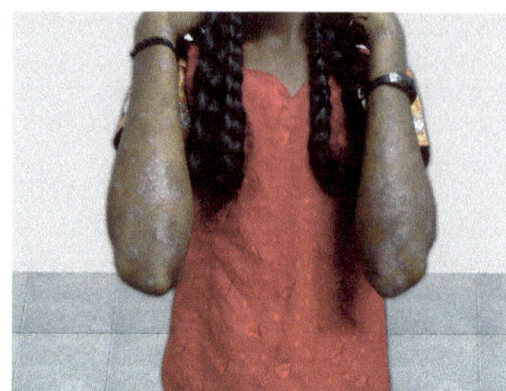

Fig. 5.1D: Girl with plaque psoriasis involving more than 20% body surface area

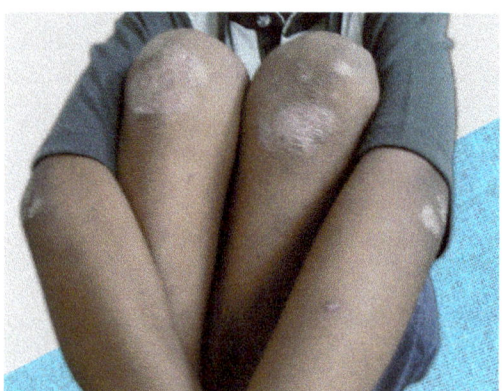

Fig. 5.1B: Knees and elbows showing silvery white psoriatic plaques

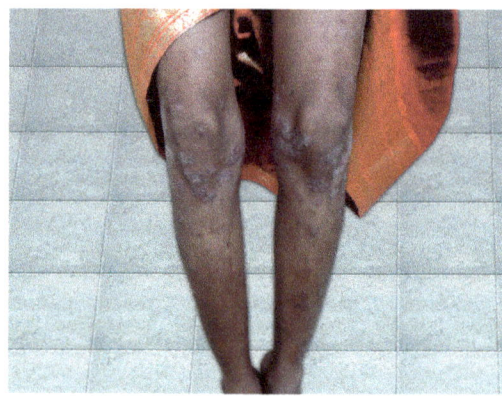

Fig. 5.1E: Same girl as in Fig. 5.1D. This child will require systemic therapy. Avoid psoralen and ultraviolet A

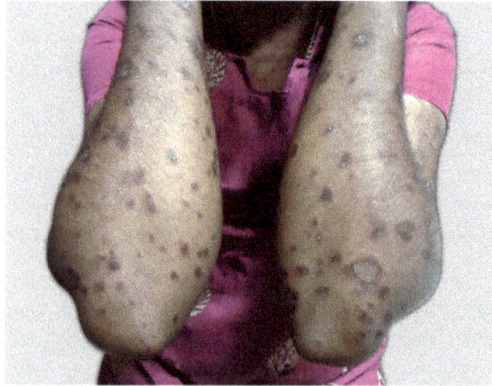

Fig. 5.1C: Multiple erythematous plaque with silvery scales

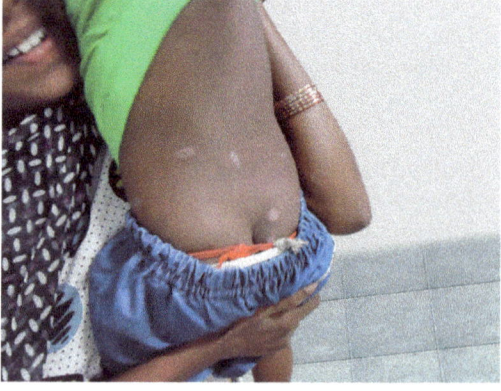

Fig. 5.1F: Infant with plaque lesions

Pediatric Psoriasis

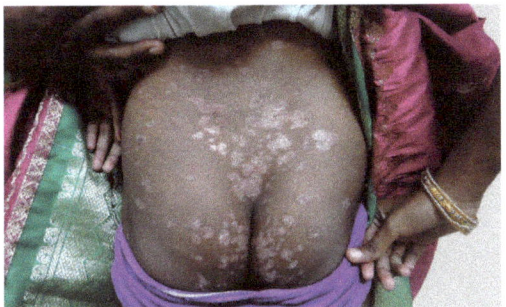

Fig. 5.1G: The lower back is another oft-affected area in psoriasis as seen in this picture

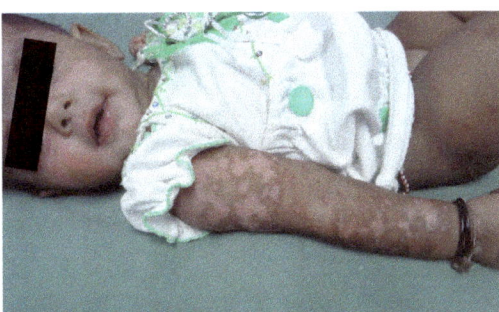

Fig. 5.1J: Classical plaque type psoriasis in an infant who should be watched for evolution to erythrodermic psoriasis

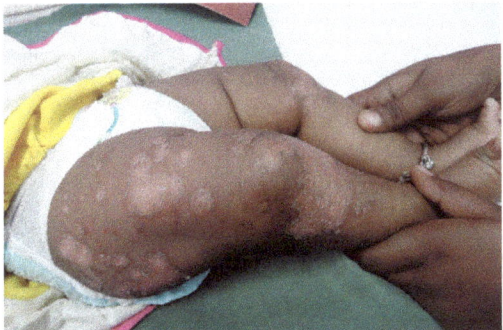

Fig. 5.1H: Severe type of plaque psoriasis in an infant

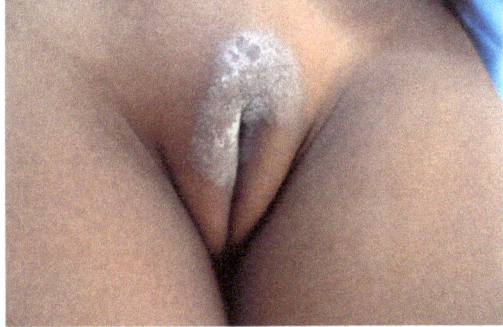

Fig. 5.1I: Odd site of plaque psoriasis where potent topical steroid should be avoided

- More generalized thickening and scaling of the palms and soles (keratoderma).

Plantar psoriasis, the one with highest discomfort, was observed in about 12.8% of children with psoriasis in an Indian study conducted in 419 children by Kumar et al., (Figs 5.2A to D).[5]

Guttate Psoriasis

Guttate psoriasis is characterized by eruption of small scaly papules in a widespread fashion involving the trunk, abdomen, and back (Figs 5.3A to D). History of recent pharyngitis is invariably present in the majority of the children and in up to 85% of children, associated streptococcal infection could be proved.[28,31] Guttate psoriasis can evolve into plaque type psoriasis in some children. Very early papules of guttate psoriasis, when the scaling is not evident, can be mistaken for early papules of acute lichen planus (Fig. 5.3E).

Scalp Psoriasis

Scalp is the most common site involved in majority of children affected by psoriasis (Figs 5.4A to I).[28,31] Scalp can be involved either as an isolated site of affection or as part of plaque type psoriasis, pustular psoriasis, and erythrodermic psoriasis. The scaling and erythema typically transgress

Plantar Psoriasis

Nonpustular variants of psoriasis predominantly affecting the palms and soles take two forms:
- Erythematous scaly plaques typical of psoriasis elsewhere in the body

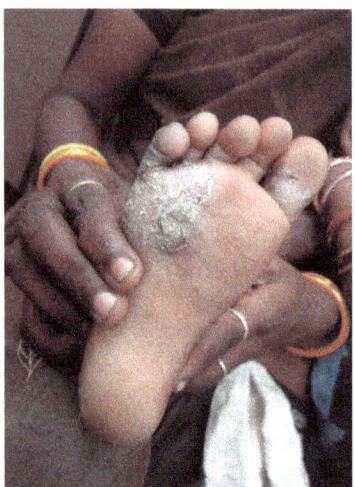

Fig. 5.2A: Single plaque of plantar psoriasis in a child

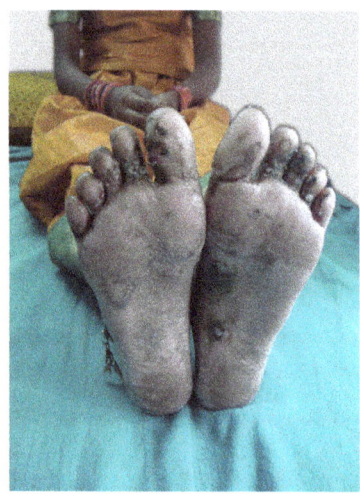

Fig. 5.2C: Plantar psoriasis in a girl with no other lesion

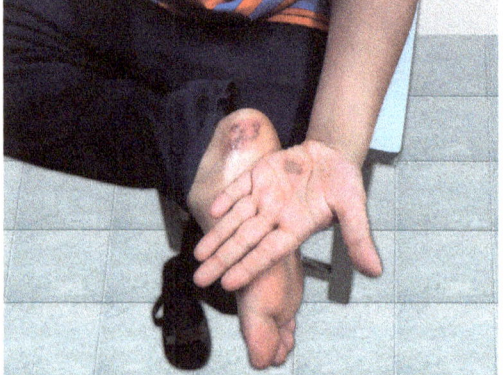

Fig. 5.2B: Early lesions of palmoplantar psoriasis in a 12-year-old

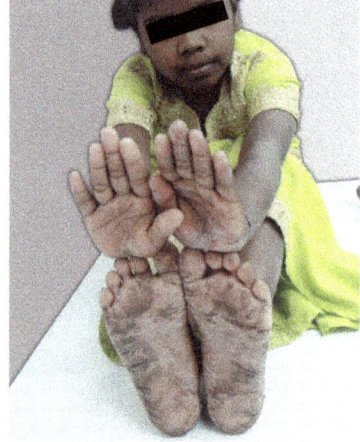

Fig. 5.2D: Classical palmoplantar psoriasis in a child

the frontal hair line, feature that helps in differentiating from seborroheic dermatitis. Circumscribed scaly plaques are sometimes the only presentation of scalp psoriasis. Plaque of pityriasis amiantacea over the scalp is characterized by the presence of asbestos-like scales. Localized hair loss can be seen in children with pityriasis amiantacea (Fig. 5.4J).[13] There can be diffuse hair loss in those with erythrodermic psoriasis. Scalp is the most common site involved in childhood psoriasis as in adults. Itching and hair loss are common symptoms though not a feature seen in all. Hair loss in psoriasis is reversible once the disease is under control.

Flexural or Inverse or Napkin Psoriasis

Flexural psoriasis was observed in up to one-tenth of children with psoriasis. Localization of erythematous, sometimes macerated, thick plaques to the folds of the skin, including axillae and groin can be associated with

Pediatric Psoriasis

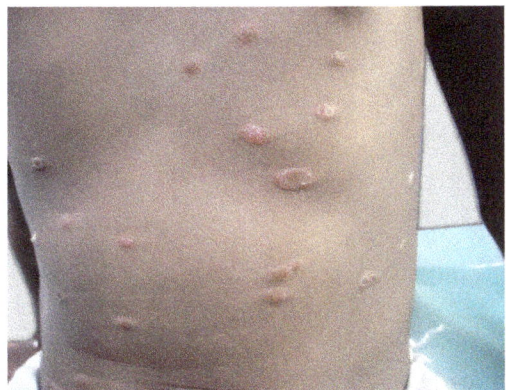

Fig. 5.3A: Drop-like guttate psoriasis on the trunk

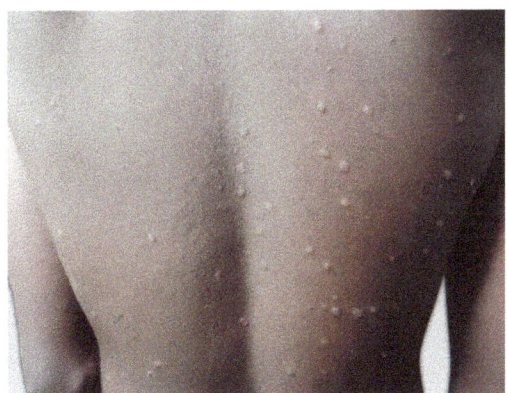

Fig. 5.3D: Older child with classical papules of guttate psoriasis

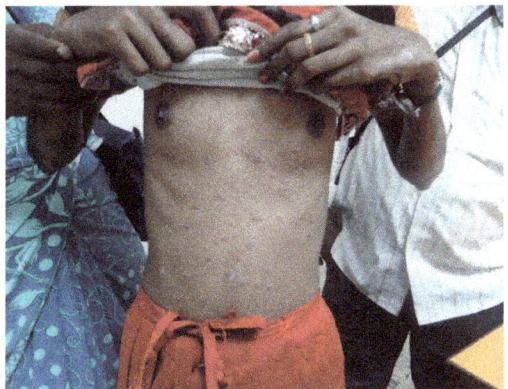

Fig. 5.3B: Child with guttate psoriasis

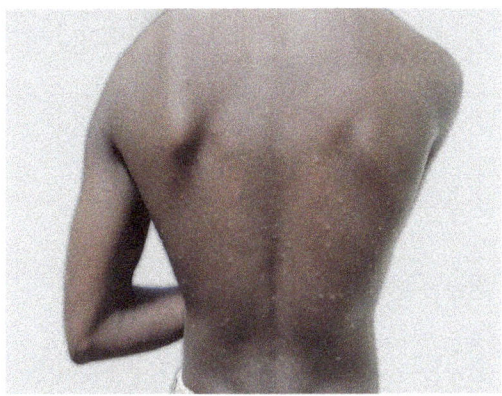

Fig. 5.3E: Early papules of guttate psoriasis easily missed for those of acute lichen planus

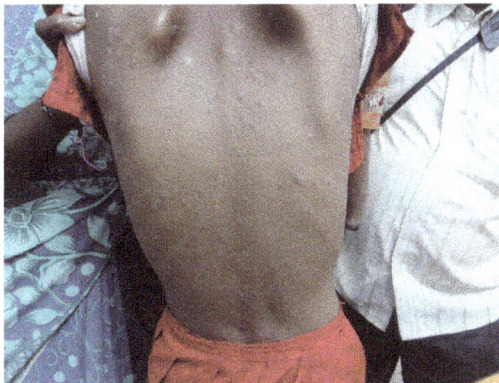

Fig. 5.3C: Same child as in Fig 5.3B who later developed psoriasis vulgaris

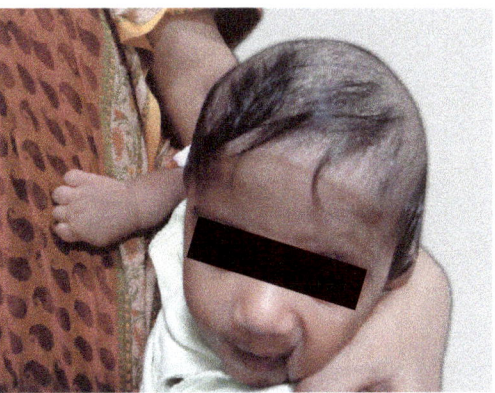

Fig. 5.4A: Scalp psoriasis in an infant

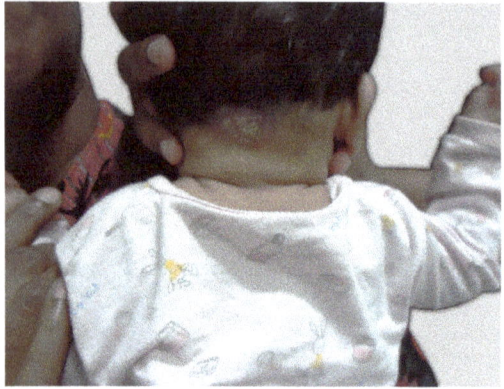

Fig. 5.4B: Scalp scales that extend below the hair line is almost always suggestive of psoriasis

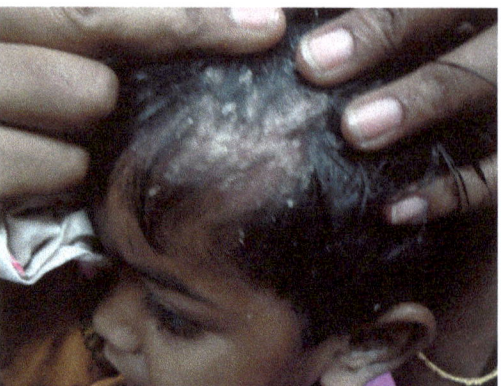

Fig. 5.4E: Thick loose silvery scales as against greasy scales of seborrheic dermatitis

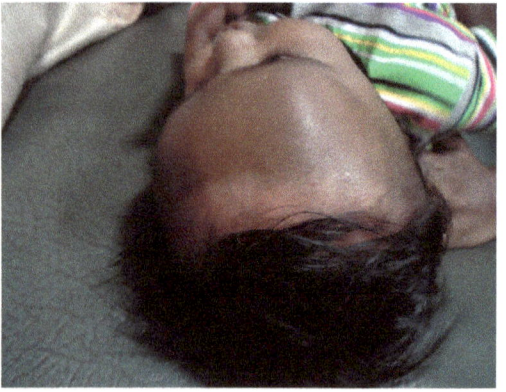

Fig. 5.4C: Note extension of scales beyond the hair line

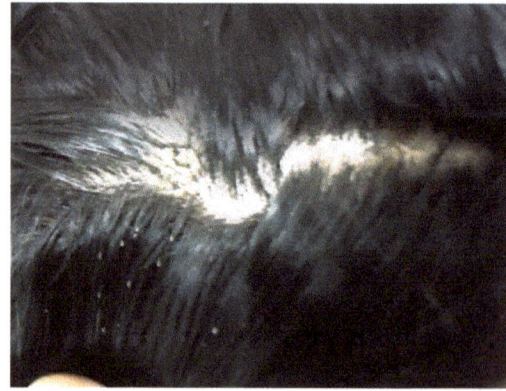

Fig. 5.4F: Large obvious silvery scales of psoriasis on the scalp

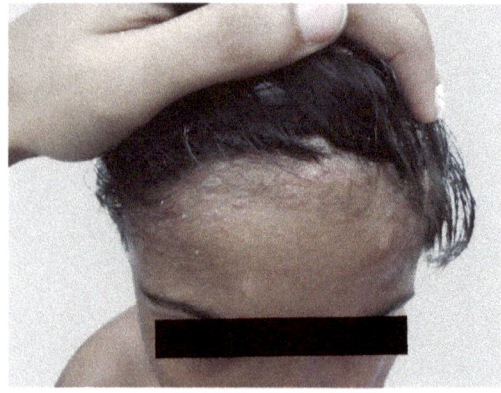

Fig. 5.4D: Scalp psoriasis showing the "psoriatic corona"

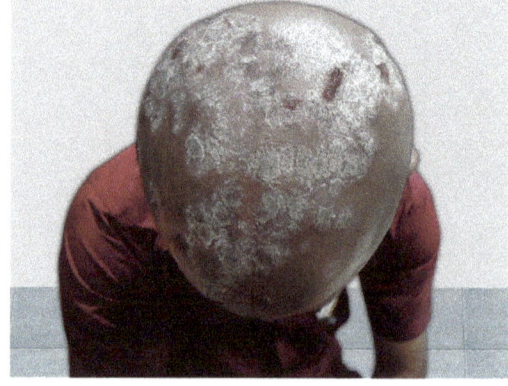

Fig. 5.4G: Severe involvement of scalp in a grown up boy

plaque type psoriasis in other sites. Although clinical diagnosis is often possible, similarity to other diseases may require biopsy for differentiation. Secondary infection with Candida and/or Streptococcus may require cutaneous culture to confirm diagnosis.

In contrast to irritant diaper dermatitis, it is sharply demarcated, brightly red, and involves the inguinal folds. Typically, symptoms respond poorly to conventional treatment of diaper dermatitis. Dissemination with widespread eruption of erythematosquamous lesions on the whole body may follow. A special clinical variant in young children is psoriatic diaper rash, which usually occurs until the age of 2 years. In the series of Morris et al., 13% of the children presented with diaper rash with dissemination and 4% with localized psoriatic diaper rash. Macerated shiny erythema of the groin region including the folds and the genital skin with sharply demarcated, brightly red, erythema involving the inguinal folds will differentiate it from diaper dermatitis where the convexities are more affected sparing the folds (Figs 5.5A to G).[28]

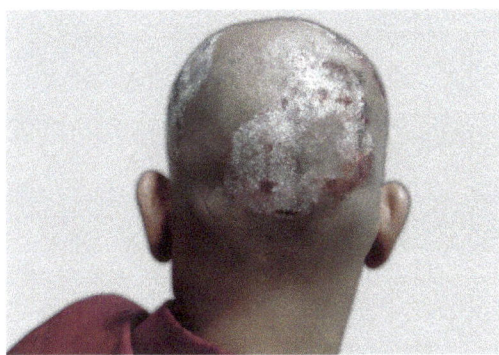

Fig. 5.4H: Same boy as in Fig 5.4G

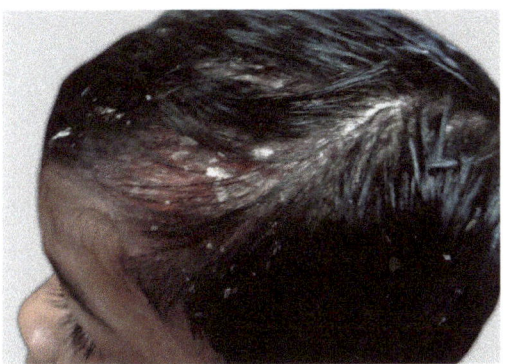

Fig. 5.4I: Thick asbestos-like scales with hairloss in a child with tinea amiantacea

Linear Psoriasis

Erythematous scaly papules or plaques following the lines of Blaschko are typically present since birth (Figs 5.6A to E). Unlike

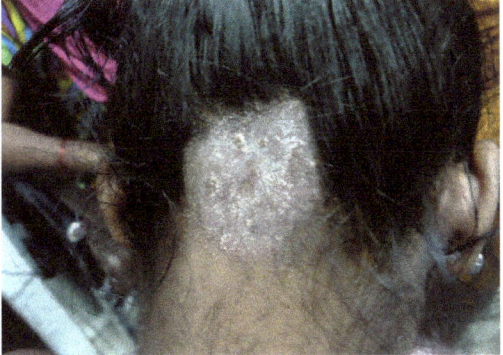

Fig. 5.4J: Localized hair loss in a child with pityriasis amiantacea

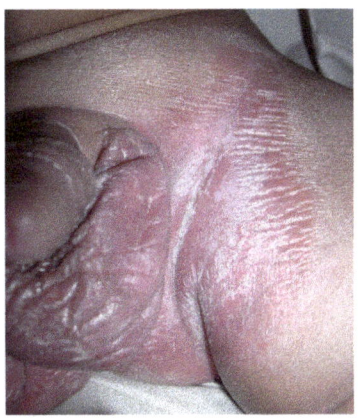

Fig. 5.5A: Classical flexural psoriasis in the napkin area

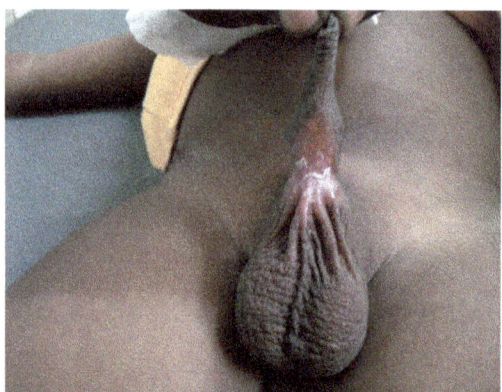

Fig. 5.5B: Flexural psoriasis with no other suggestive lesions over the flexures

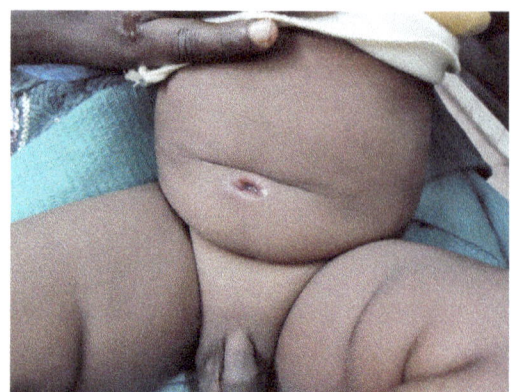

Fig. 5.5E: Erythematous scaly plaque around umbilicus with loose scales signaling psoriasis infant

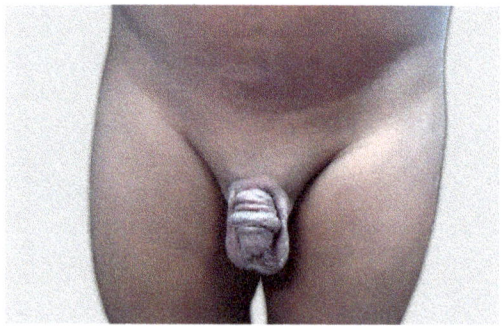

Fig. 5.5C: Well-defined erythematous scaly plaque of psoriasis

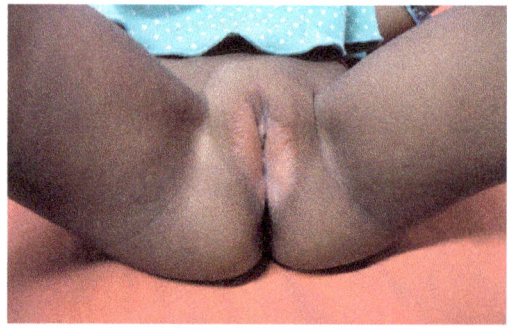

Fig. 5.5F: Psoriasis of the napkin area in a girl child

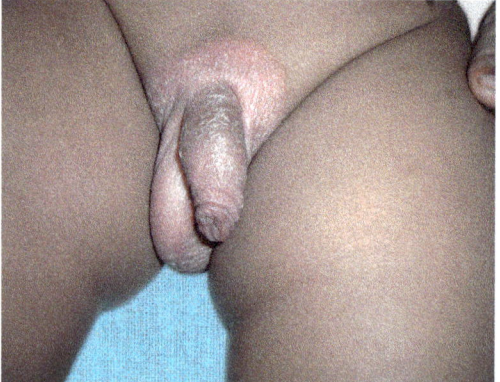

Fig. 5.5D: Psoriasis affecting the genitals

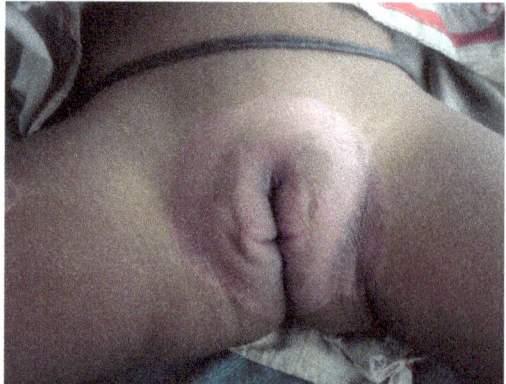

Fig. 5.5G: Infant with napkin psoriasis

inflammatory linear verrucous epidermal nevus, there is no or only mild pruritus. Presence of Koebner's phenomenon and demonstration of Auspitz sign will help in the clinical diagnosis which can be further confirmed with biopsy, the histology of

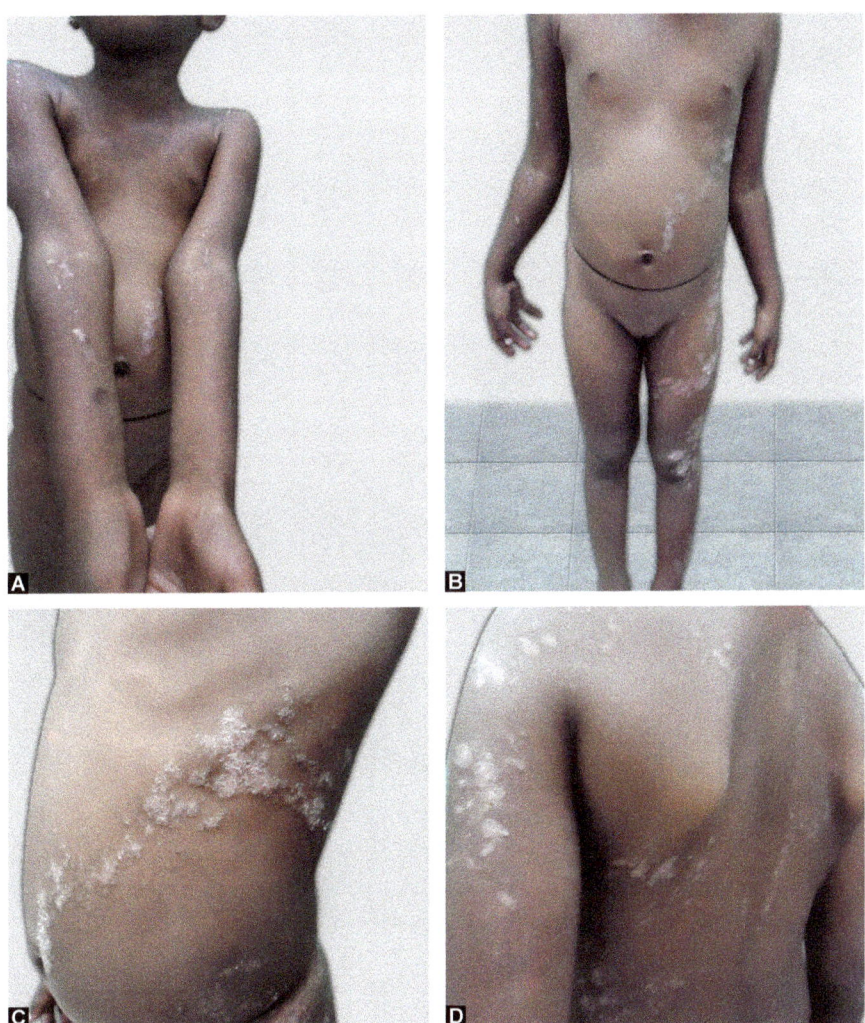

Figs 5.6A to D: Psoriasis along Blaschko's lines

which will show psoriasiform features. Family history for psoriasis is often positive.[5]

Special Forms

Nail Psoriasis

Stefanaki et al., have reported 10.4% of children to present with nail involvement (Figs 5.7A and B).[4] Nail changes in psoriasis may be seen in up to 40%.[5,31,41] Nail pitting is the most common manifestation. Oil drop sign, onycholysis, subungual hyperkeratosis, onychodystrophy, and splinter hemorrhages can also be observed. Nail involvement can precede, coincide with, or succeed psoriasis and may even rarely appear isolated (Figs 5.7C and D). Nail abnormalities are more frequent in PsA and in digital skin involvement.[15]

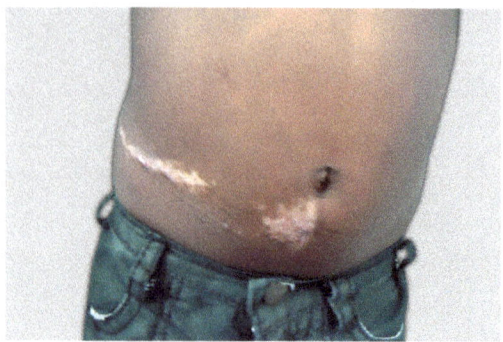

Fig. 5.6E: Linear psoriasis in a child

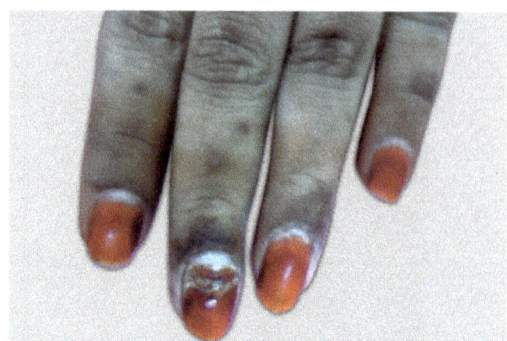

Fig. 5.7C: Nail involvement in a child that precede skin involvement of psoriasis vulgaris

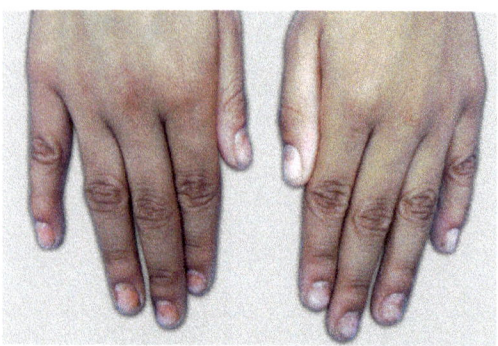

Fig. 5.7A: Nail pitting in a boy with psoriasis

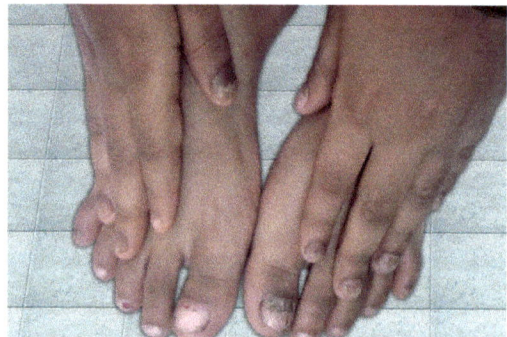

Fig. 5.7D: Asymmetric multiple nail involvement in a child with psoriasis

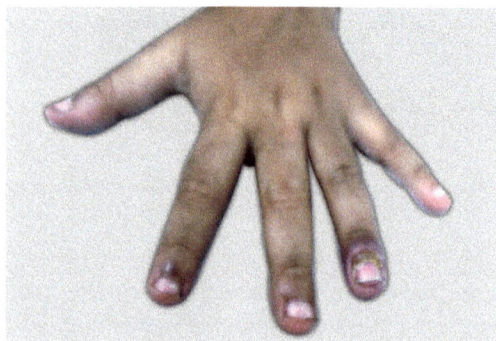

Fig. 5.7B: Nail involvement in a child with psoriasis vulgaris

Mucosal Psoriasis

Involvement of mucosa is seen in up to 7% of children in a study conducted by Alfonza and Nanda.[31] Annular plaques on the tongue may be noted in patients with psoriasis (Fig. 5.8). Geographic tongue is a common presentation of pustular psoriasis.

Erythrodermic Psoriasis

Psoriasis constituted about 18% of erythroderma in children in a study conducted by Sarkar and Garg.[46] Erythrodermic psoriasis is a rare clinical presentation in childhood psoriasis. It may arise from any type, commonly from the plaque type. It may arise from any type of psoriasis. Drugs, environmental, psychological, and metabolic factors can trigger the onset of erythrodermic form of the disease.[47,48] This spectrum of psoriasis is characterized by generalized

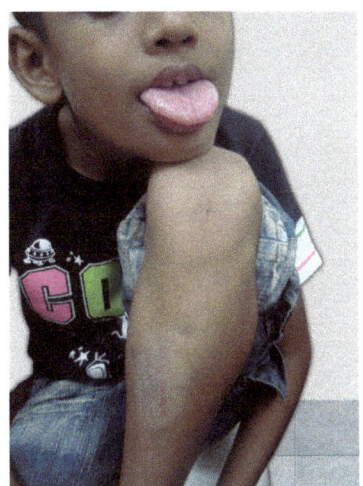

Fig. 5.8: Oral mucosal involvement in a boy with psoriasis

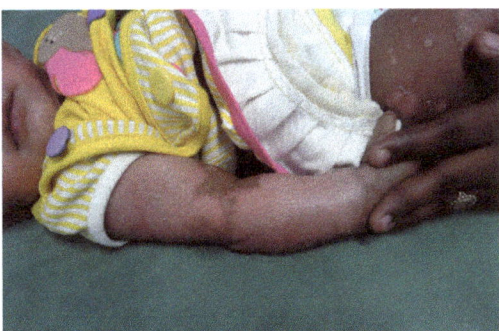

Fig. 5.9A: Plaque psoriasis as in 5.1H evolving to erythrodermic psoriasis

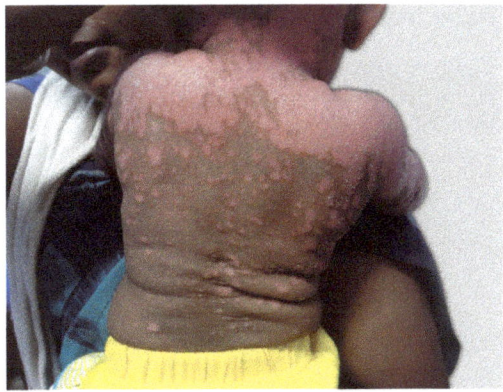

Fig. 5.9B: Same child as in 5.9A with impending erythroderma

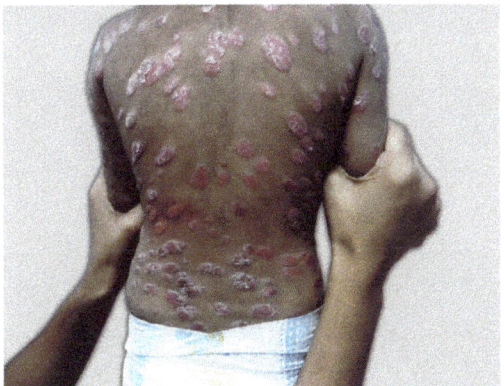

Fig. 5.9C: Unstable psoriasis as seen by the fiery red plaques with irregular margins

erythema, edema, desquamation, and systemic compromise. The child will present with fever, dehydration, malaise, and malnutrition.[49] The overall presentation can range from mild to severe form. The erythrodermic form occurs in about 1.4% of psoriasis cases in children and adolescents.[3,6] Over all, less than 3% of childhood psoriasis manifests with erythroderma (Figs 5.9A to H).[50]

Congenital Psoriasis

Congenital psoriasis, meaning psoriasis present at birth or appearing during the neonatal period, is exceptional (Figs 5.10A to E). Congenital occurrence of psoriasis, defined as the development of any of its clinical variants at birth or during very first days of life is considered very rare.[51] The erythrodermic variant is exceptional. CEP is one of the most rare and severe forms of psoriasis. It was first described in 1966 by Frost and Van Scott who distinguished this entity from nonbullous ichthyosis form congenital erythroderma, with which it might be confused.[52] The neonates with erythroderma are at increased risk of hypernatremic dehydration, severe systemic infections,

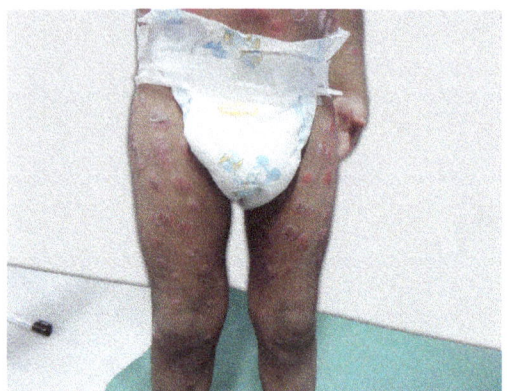

Fig. 5.9D: Same child as in Fig 5.9C with bright-red plaques and irregular margins

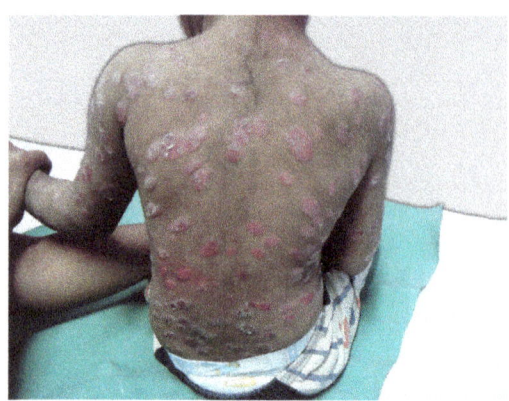

Fig. 5.9G: Same boy as in Fig. 5.9F

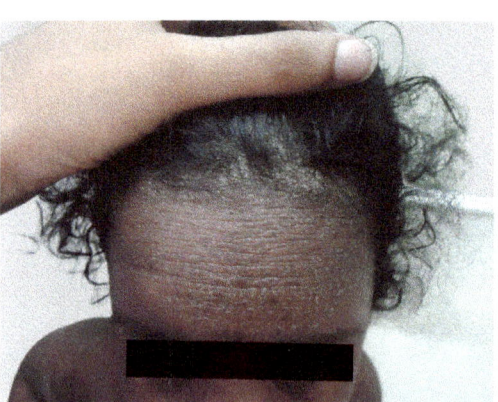

Fig. 5.9E: Involvement of scalp in erythrodermic psoriasis

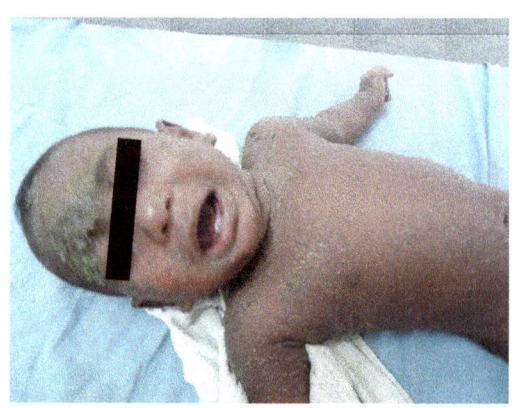

Fig. 5.9H: Child with psoriasis evolved to erythroderma following irritation by local application

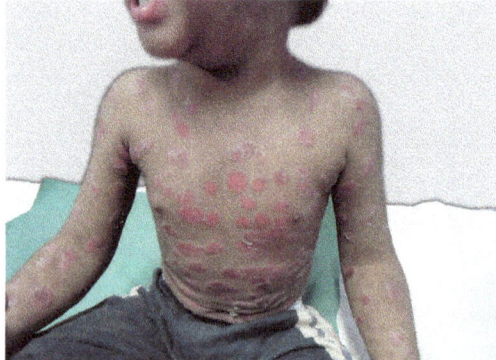

Fig. 5.9F: Rapidly evolving severe plaque type psoriasis in an infant must think of unstable psoriasis

hypoalbuminemia, and hyperpyrexia or hypothermia as a result of consequences of erythroderma. CEP is reported in as young as 5-day-old infant.[53]

Infantile psoriasis

As high as 16% of childhood psoriasis were reported to have started during the first year of life (Figs 5.11A to D).[28] Psoriatic diaper rash, otherwise known as the napkin psoriasis and erythrodermic psoriasis are the two common manifestations during the first year of life. Scalp psoriasis is easily missed as cradle cap or seborroheic dermatitis.[54] The

Pediatric Psoriasis

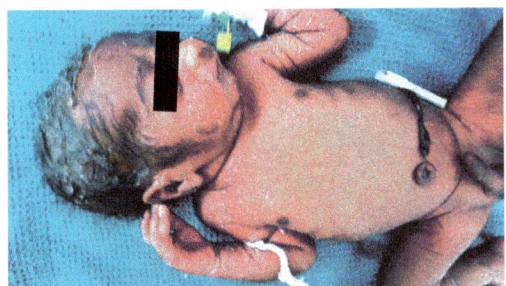

Fig. 5.10A: Congenital erythrodermic psoriasis in a 5-day-old neonate

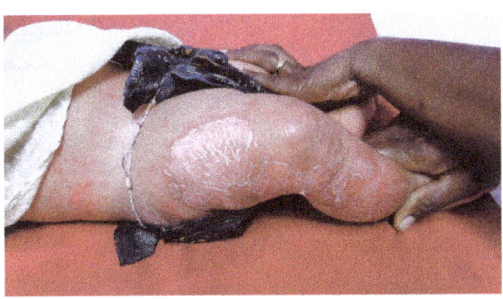

Fig. 5.10D: Same infant as in Fig 5.10C

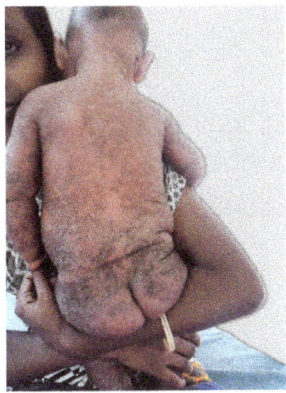

Fig. 5.10B: Congenital erythrodermic psoriasis in an older infant

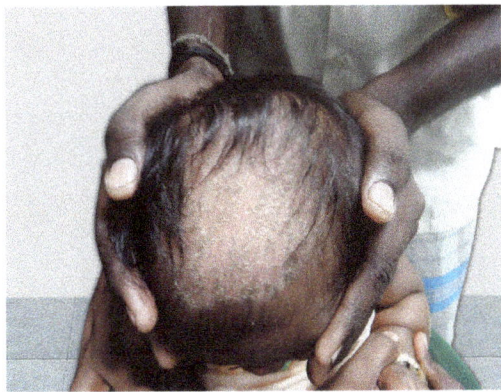

Fig. 5.10E: Classical erythematous plaque over scalp with silvery scale in congenital erythrodermic psoriasis

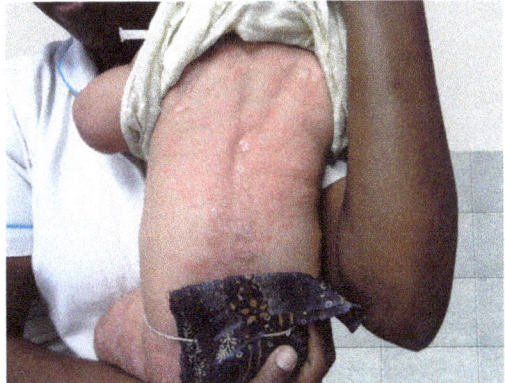

Fig. 5.10C: Classical erythematous plaque over the back with silvery scale in congenital erythrodermic psoriasis in an infant

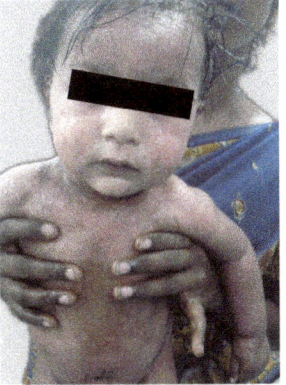

Fig. 5.11A: Infant with erythroderma as presenting feature without history of plaque psoriasis

associated atopic dermatitis can sometimes pose a diagnostic dilemma in erythrodermic form in infants.[55]

Pustular Psoriasis

Pustular psoriasis appears at 2–10 years of age constituting less than 1% of childhood psoriasis (Figs 5.12A to D).[15,56] A review of 1,262 cases of childhood psoriasis found a 0.6% rate of pustular variants.[28] Four clinical patterns of pustular psoriasis have been described in children, namely:
- GPP or von Zumbusch
- Annular pustular psoriasis
- Exanthematicpustular psoriasis
- Localized pustular psoriasis.

Annular form seems to be the commonest presentation of pustular psoriasis. They are

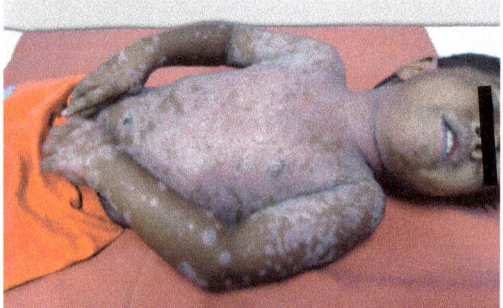

Fig. 5.11B: Plaque psoriasis evolving into erythroderma in infant

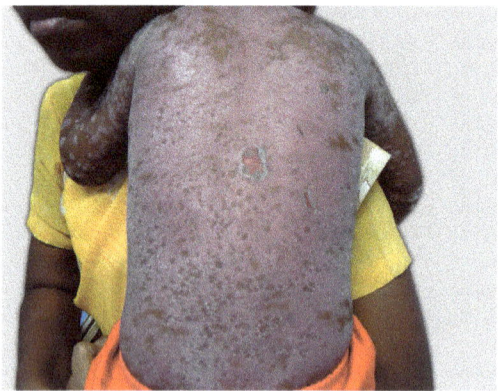

Fig. 5.11C: Same infant as in 5.11B

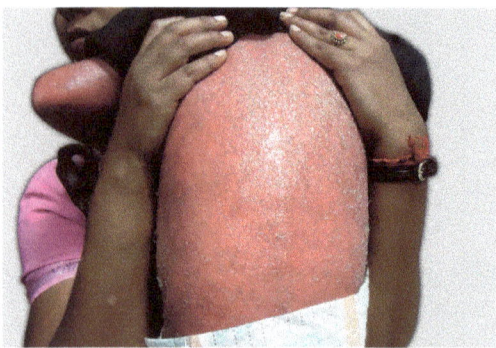

Fig. 5.11D: Erythrodermic psoriasis in an infant

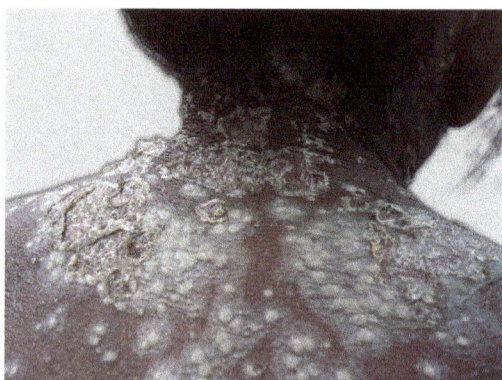

Fig. 5.12A: Superficial pustules coalescing to form lake of pus in a known case of psoriasis after sudden withdrawal of systemic steroids

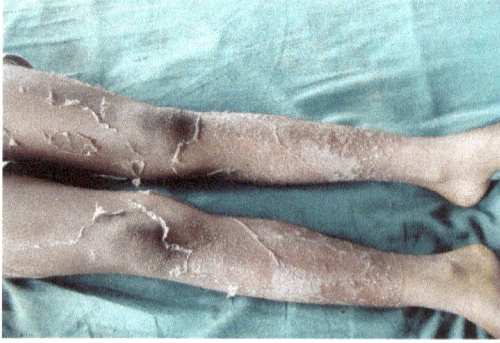

Fig. 5.12B: Same child as in Fig 5.12A showing resolution

Pediatric Psoriasis

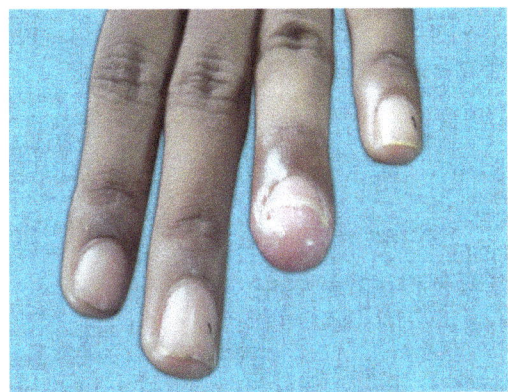

Fig. 5.12C: Fingertip pustular lesion with nail change is an indicator of pustular psoriasis

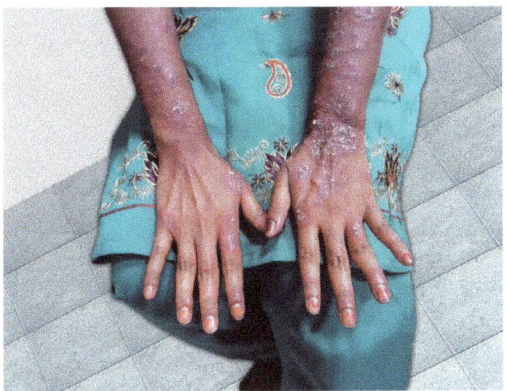

Fig. 5.12D: Pustular psoriasis in an older girl

not necessarily mutually exclusive and mixed variants are also possible.[57]

The clinical pattern of GPP (an acute, episodic, and potentially life-threatening form of psoriasis) classically presents as widespread sheets of sterile pustules on bright erythematous skin that resolves within 3-4 days, with recurrent waves of inflammation. The acute pustulation is typically associated with fever and toxic changes.[34,58,59] Considering the condition of the patients, GPP in children could be further classified as either the severe type or the mild type. Compared with the adult forms, the first manifestation of GPP in children is usually high fever accompanied by generalized pustules. Few of these cases converted to be psoriasis vulgaris.[60] The younger the age of onset, the more severe the patient's condition can be.[58]

Arthropathic Psoriasis

Psoriatic arthritis is relatively uncommon in children; it may occur with either plaque or guttate psoriasis and may precede skin involvement (Fig. 5.13). The estimated prevalence of PsA in all patients with psoriasis differs from 5%-30%.[61,62] 8%-20% of cases of childhood arthritis are diagnosed as PsA.[63] The age of onset of findings in childhood ranges from 9-12 years of age.[64] An incidence of less than 2% was noted in studies conducted by Stefanaki, Fouzan, and Kumar.[5,30,31]

ASSOCIATIONS AND COMORBIDITIES

Psoriasis is commonly found to be associated with conditions like allergic contact dermatitis, eczema, vitiligo, and alopecia areata.[42] It can also be easily mistaken for

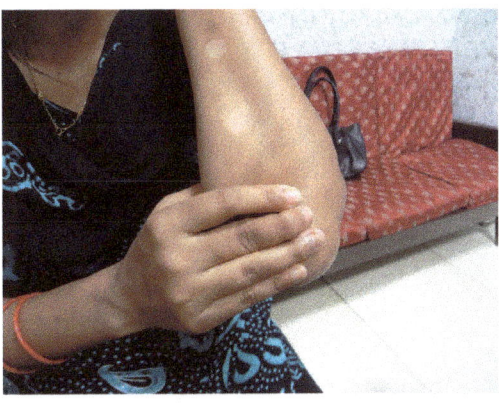

Fig. 5.13: Arthropathy of distal interphalangeal joints with lesion on the extensors in an adolescent girl with psoriasis

seborrheic dermatitis, avitaminosis with which it can coexist (Figs 5.14A to D). The association with atopic dermatitis commonly seen in adults is also seen in children with psoriasis.[55] Psoriatic children have a higher prevalence of obesity. It was also observed that overweight had different effects on childhood patients. Psoriasis in these children was more severe compared with psoriatic children of normal weight.[65] There is a strong association between psoriasis and obesity in children, especially boys.[66] Increased incidence of hyperlipidemia, hypertension, and diabetes, has also been reported to be associated with psoriasis in children and adolescents. It may be considered that in an obese child, disease severity can be a marker of cardiovascular risk. Prevalence of comorbidities in persons in the age range 0–20 years with psoriasis was found to be more than those without psoriasis. The following comorbidities were observed by Augustin et al.: Crohn's disease, hyperlipidemia, diabetes mellitus, arterial hypertension, rheumatoid arthritis, obesity, ischemic heart disease, and ulcerative colitis.[6]

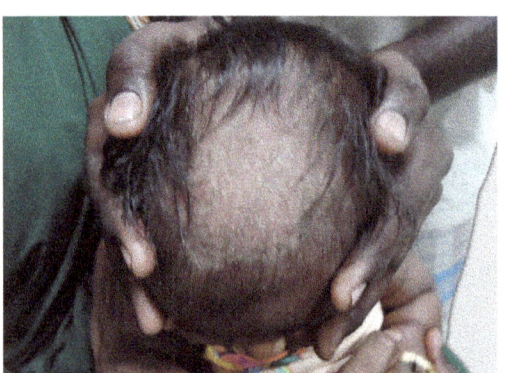

Fig. 5.14A: Severe seborrheic dermatitis in an infant lasting longer than usual may be an indicator of psoriasis as is severe dandruff in an adult

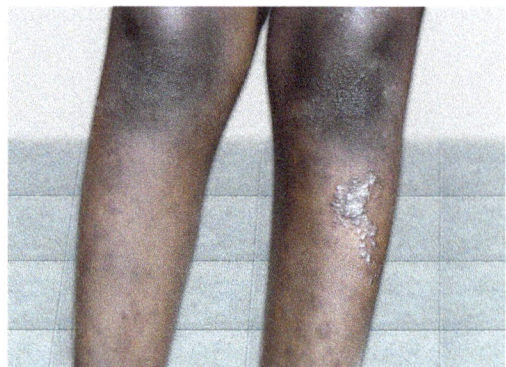

Fig. 5.14C: Follicular psoriasis with phrynoderma

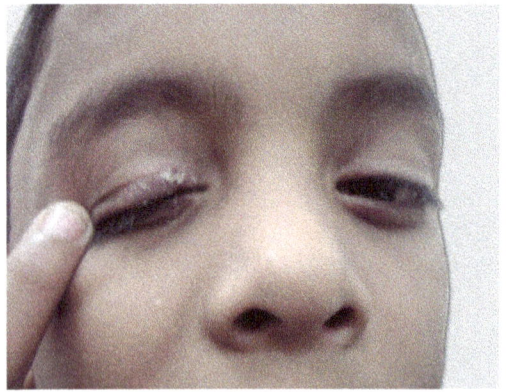

Fig. 5.14B: Psoriasis in a boy mimicking seborrheic dermatitis

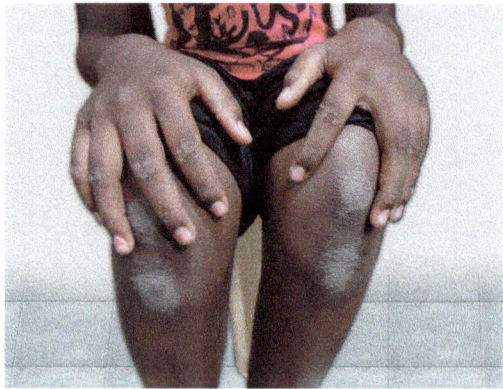

Fig. 5.14D: Psoriasis in a boy with avitaminosis

Recent Research with Respect to Young People and Comorbidities

Increased rates of diabetes, arthritis, Crohn's disease, obesity, hypertension, and high cholesterol were associated with juvenile psoriasis as indicated by recent research with respect to young people and comorbidities. In psoriasis patients under 20 years of age, the overall rate of comorbid conditions is nearly double when compared to their peers who do not have psoriasis.[6] 32% of children and 41% of adolescents with moderate-to-severe psoriasis were overweight which is significantly higher than the general population. Obesity in early adulthood may increase the risk for developing PsA later in life.[67]

TREATMENT

Therapy of childhood psoriasis is demanding with regard to the specific juvenile metabolism, physical development, and skin penetration of topical drugs. Long-term treatment at an early age with any form: topical steroids, methotrexate, other immune suppressive agents, and phototherapy has to be critically judged taking into consideration the chronicity of the disease.

Childhood psoriasis is a cause for concern to the child, parent, and the doctor alike. An effective therapy starts with counseling the patient and parent, explaining to them the nature of the disease, treatment options available, their pros and cons.

This segment will review the treatment of childhood psoriasis under two headings:
- The treatment options available
- Treatment of different types of psoriasis.

Treating a child with psoriasis is a challenge. Success of the treatment partially lies on the compliance of the patient which means that the safety and accessibility of treatment should be considered important.

Treatment options available can be symptomatic and specific. Antihistamines are given to alleviate itching. It would, therefore, be preferable to give sedative antihistamines.

The available treatment options are broadly divided as
- Topical therapy
- Phototherapy
- Systemic therapy
- Other modalities.

Topical Therapy

The limitations of systemic therapy in childhood lead to a distinctly higher role of topical treatment even for moderate-to-severe forms of psoriasis. Despite advancement of modern systemic therapeutic agents including advent of the biologicals, topical therapy seems sensible for vast majority of children with psoriasis. These topical agents can be used exclusively or in combination with systemic therapy depending on the individual requirement. Since psoriasis is a chronic inflammatory disease with remissions and exacerbations, often requiring prolonged therapy, the choice of topical therapy should be made taking into consideration the long-term side effect of therapy with particular reference to steroids and topical immune suppressives. Further attention should be paid to the higher penetration capacity of children's skin as well as to ratio of BSA to body weight and thus, increased resorption of topical therapeutic agents. In childhood psoriasis, complete clearance should not always be the primary goal.

Only topical products containing corticosteroids and anthralin are licensed for children with psoriasis. In case of contemplating on other drugs lacking approval, patient and parents must be comprehensively informed before the initiation of therapy.

Topical therapy is the mainstay for mild or localized disease with a PASI less than 10 or involvement of BSA of less than 20%.

Emollients, moisturizers, keratolytics, tar, anthralin, topical steroids, vitamin D analogs, calcineurin inhibitors, and retinoid are various topical preparations available.

The choice will depend upon the age of the child, type of psoriasis, PASI score, site of involvement, other comorbidities and associations, tolerance, and affordability.

In addition to anti-inflammatory therapy, dermatological basic therapy with keratolytic or keratoplastic and antipruritic topical agents plays an important role. Regular skin care is necessary even during phases of remission. Urea in different concentrations in lipophilic cream base can be useful as emollient, antipruritic and or keratolytics in selected patients.

Emollients

Emollients are the most commonly used in management of childhood psoriasis. White soft paraffin reduces transepidermal water loss, soothe and soften the skin and reduce scaling. They improve the barrier function and stratum corneum hydration, making the epidermis less amenable to trauma and stress, which is one of the trigger factors for the disease exacerbation. It is wise to start treatment with these agents and allow the disease to evolve before embarking to any stronger medications with side effects.

Keratolytics

Keratolytics, such as salicylic acid and urea, reduce scaling and enhance absorption of other drugs. Topical products containing salicylic acid commonly employed for therapy in adults should be used with great care in children as systemic resorption can be very high. Even with small amounts of salicylic acid, central nervous system (CNS) side effects, renal damage as well as fatalities has been reported. Therefore, before school age it should be used only on small areas and in a maximum concentration of 0.5%. Salicylic acid can be used in lesions over the scalp, palms, and soles in children older than 6 years. It is to be avoided in younger children because of the risk of percutaneous salicylate absorption leading to salicylism.[68] Salicylic acid preparations should be avoided before phototherapy as topical salicylic acid reduces the efficacy of ultraviolet B (UVB) phototherapy because of its filtering effect.

Tar

Coal tar, which has antipruritic and anti-inflammatory effects, also suppresses deoxyribonucleic acid (DNA) synthesis and acts as antiproliferative agent.[69,70] It can be used alone or in combination with other agents, such as corticosteroids, salicylic acid, and UV therapy. However, it is not to be used on face and flexures and in children below 12 years of age. Tar causes irritation, when combined with UV light in the Goeckerman regimen. Tar is also known to induce chromosomal aberrations in peripheral lymphocytes and bring on release of heat shock proteins.[71]

Dithranol

Dithranol, also known as anthralin, has anti-inflammatory and antiproliferative effects which are attributable to its ability to regulate keratinocyte differentiation and prevent T lymphocyte activation. The drug accumulates in keratinocyte mitochondria, dissipates mitochondrial membrane potential, and induces apoptosis through a pathway dependent on respiratory competent mitochondria.[72] "Short contact therapy" is the preferred method these days in which increasing concentrations of anthralin are applied for a short period (10–30 minutes) till a slight irritation develops, after which the dose and time are held constant till lesions clear.[73]

A significant remission in 81% of children was observed with 1% concentration.[74] It can be combined with UVB phototherapy, as in Ingram regimen, to improve the response. Anthralin 1% or dithranol are rarely used for localized areas and can cause localized irritation.[76] The usage of dithranol has been reducing with advent of new more cosmetically acceptable topical preparations.

Topical Corticosteroids

The remarkable efficacy of TCS in the treatment of inflammatory dermatoses was noted soon after the introduction of hydrocortisone in 1952. TCS are the most frequently employed antipsoriatic topical agents especially in itchy lesions. Topical steroids are suitable for the treatment of childhood psoriasis among all age groups. They have anti-inflammatory, antiproliferative, immunosuppressive, and vasoconstrictive effects. Hydrocortisone and betamethasone are examples of low-potency and high-potency TCS. TCS have been ranked in terms of potency into four groups consisting of seven classes. Class I TCS are the most potent and Class VII are the least potent. Steroids low-potency to mid-potency corticosteroids, class 5–7, are chosen for facial and intertriginous lesions, while mid-potency class 2–4, are chosen for extremities and the scalp,[81] respectively. Only short-term effects and the rapid recurrence of signs and symptoms after discontinuation of therapy are the few disadvantages even with well-tailored therapy. TCS treatment should not be discontinued abruptly for the above reasons and for fear of developing pustular lesions on abrupt withdrawal. Highly potent corticosteroids should not be used over the face, genitals, and in intertriginous regions. While using high potent TCS over other sites in older children, they should not be applied for more than 2 weeks. Topical clobetasol has been approved for use in children aging 12 years and over in some formulations and can be quite effective for use in psoriatic lesions in adolescents.[77] Their inadvertent and long-term use can lead to local infections, skin atrophy, telangiectasia, striae distensae, acneiform eruption, and purpura. Contact dermatitis to the molecule or the vehicle is not uncommon. Rebound and tachyphylaxis are to be remembered while using topical steroids for a prolonged period. It is always advisable to follow the fingertip unit and adhere to the schedule. Side effects of TCS are given in Table 5.1.

Side Effects of Topical Corticosteroids

Systemic side effects are more common in children than adults because of a higher skin surface or body mass ratio. Ointments are to be avoided in flexural, facial, and genital skin. Lotions are preferred for hairy scalp. They can also be combined with other topical agents, such as calcipotriol and tazarotene, to enhance efficacy and reduce irritation. One should remember that the absorption is variable in different anatomical sites as seen

TABLE 5.1: Age and choice of potency of topical corticosteroids to be used

Age	Potency
0–3 months	No topical corticosteroids
3 months–1 year	Class VI, VII
1–2 years	Class IV, V, VI, VII
2–12 years	Class II, III, IV, V, VI, VII
Above 12 years	Class I, II, III, IV, V, VI, VII

below. Skin over the eyelids absorbs the most while that of the sole absorbs the least.
- Eyelids and genitals absorb 30%
- Face absorbs 7%
- Armpit absorbs 4%
- Forearm absorbs 1%
- Palm absorbs 0.1%
- Sole absorbs 0.05%.

Potency of Topical Corticosteroids

The United States (US) system utilizes 7 classes, which are classified by their ability to constrict capillaries. Class I is the strongest, or super potent. Class VII is the weakest and mildest with poor lipid permeability, and cannot penetrate mucous membranes well.

United Kingdom (UK) System of classifying TCS has four classes. Class IV being the strongest, about 600 times potent than the weakest class I TCS, hydrocortisone. US and UK systems of classification of TCS are given in Boxes 5.1 and 5.2. Summary of usage of correct formula of TCS in children are given in Box 5.3. The agewise choice of potency, side effects, and requirement of TCS in fingertip units are given in Table 5.1 to 5.3, respectively.

Topical Vitamin D Analogs

Topical vitamin D analogs have anti-inflammatory and antiproliferative actions. They also induce downregulation and correction of keratinocyte differentiation. Calcipotriol, calcitriol, maxacalcitol and tacalcitol are the various vitamin D analogs useful in the treatment of psoriasis. When combined with betamethasone, the effect is better than either agent used alone. UVB phototherapy increases the efficacy of calcipotriol.[57,78] The most common adverse events are burning and stinging sensation, the drug is safe when the total dose does not exceed the recommended dose of not more than 75 g/week for children above 12 years and 50 g/week for children between 6 and

BOX 5.1: The United States system of classification of topical corticosteroids

- Group I: Very potent; up to 600 times stronger than hydrocortisone
  - Clobetasol propionate 0.05%
  - Betamethasone dipropionate 0.25%
  - Halobetasol propionate 0.05%
  - Diflorasone diacetate 0.05%
- Group II
  - Fluocinonide 0.05%
  - Halcinonide 0.05%
  - Amcinonide 0.05%
  - Desoximetasone 0.25%
- Group III
  - Triamcinolone acetonide 0.5%
  - Mometasonef uroate 0.1%
  - Fluticasone propionate 0.005%
  - Betamethasone dipropionate 0.05%
  - Halometasone 0.05%
- Group IV
  - Fluocinolone acetonide 0.01–0.2%
  - Hydrocortisone valerate 0.2%
  - Hydrocortisone butyrate 0.1%
  - Flurandrenolide 0.05%
  - Triamcinolone acetonide 0.1%
  - Mometasone furoate 0.1%
- Group V
  - Fluticasone propionate 0.05%
  - Desonide 0.05%
  - Fluocinolone acetonide 0.025%
  - Hydrocortisone valerate 0.2%
- Group VI
  - Alclometasone dipropionate 0.05%
  - Triamcinolone acetonide 0.025%
  - Fluocinolone acetonide 0.01%
  - Desonide 0.05%
- Group VII–(least potent)
  - Hydrocortisone 2.5%
  - Hydrocortisone 1%

BOX 5.2: The United Kingdom system of classification of topical corticosteroids

- Class IV: Very potent (up to 600 times as potent as hydrocortisone)
  - Clobetasol propionate
  - Betamethasone dipropionate
- Class III: Potent (50–100 times as potent as hydrocortisone)
  - Betamethasone valerate
  - Betamethasone dipropionate
  - Diflucortolone valerate
  - Hydrocortisone 17-butyrate
  - Mometasone furoate
  - Methylprednisolone aceponate
  - Halometasone 0.05%
- Class II: Moderate (2–25 times as potent as hydrocortisone)
  - Clobetasone butyrate
  - Triamcinolone acetonide
- Class I: Mild
  - Hydrocortisone 0.5%–2.5%

BOX 5.3: Choosing the correct formula for the correct site

- Gel: Hairy areas
- Lotion: Hairy areas, wider surface
- Cream: Face, tender skin
- Ointment: Occlusive effect
- Emulsion: Hairy areas, wider surface

TABLE 5.2: Fingertip units required for effective topical corticosteroids usage

Anatomic area	3–6 months	1–2 years	3–5 years	6–10 years
Face and neck	1	1.5	1.5	2
Arm and hand	1	1.5	2	2.5
Leg and foot	1.5	2	3	4.5
Anterior trunk	1	2	3	3.5
Posterior trunk	1.5	3	3.5	5

12 years. Over use can lead to hypocalcemia. Calcipotriene or calcitriol can be used for pediatric psoriasis, the latter being well tolerated for sensitive skin.[79,80] Clinical response, with vitamin D are evident after 2 weeks of treatment and maximum effects observed after 6-8 weeks (Figs 5.15A and B). Initial mild skin irritation is a common untoward effect which usually fades away during the further course of therapy.

Calcineurin Inhibitors

Topical calcineurin inhibitors act as nonsteroidal immune modulatory drugs. They inhibit IL2 production and subsequent T-cell activation and proliferation by blocking the enzyme calcineurin. Tacrolimus (0.03%, 0.1%) ointment and pimecrolimus (1%) cream are two drugs belonging to this

TABLE 5.3: Side effects of topical corticosteroids

Local side effects	Systemic side effects
• Skin thinning, easy bruising, striae • Hypopigmentation • Purpura, telangiectasia • Susceptibility to skin infections • Perioral dermatitis • Gluteal granulomas • Hypertrichosis • Acneiform eruptions • Contact allergy • Tachyphylaxis	• HPA axis suppression • Cushing's syndrome • Linear growth retardation • Delayed weight gain • Intracranial hypertension • Disbalance of electrolytes • Steroid diabetes • Increased catabolism of proteins • Addisonian crisis

HPA, hypothalamic-pituitary-adrenal.

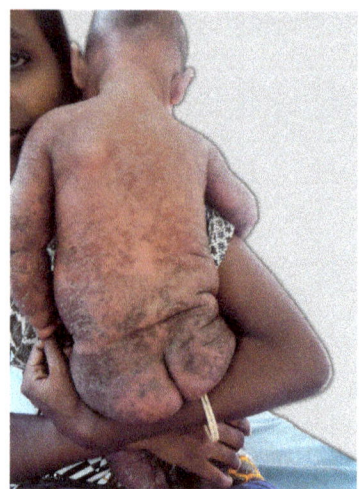

Fig. 5.15A: Infant with psoriasis before treatment with calcipotriol

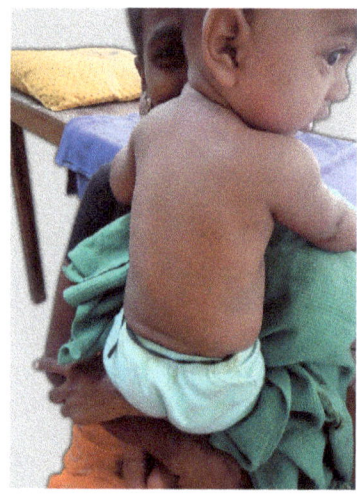

Fig. 5.15B: Same as in Fig. 5.15A after treatment with calcipotriol

class, which, although not food and drug administration (FDA) approved, have proven efficacy. This has recently been documented for treatment of childhood psoriasis.[81,82] They can be used as steroid sparing agents and are also useful for sequential and rotational regimens, so as to avoid long-term adverse effects of topical steroids. They are useful for sites, such as face, flexures, and anogenital region where topical steroids cannot be used safely.[83] Use in children under the age of 2 years is not recommended by the FDA.

Retinoids

Tazarotene is a third-generation retinoid that acts on keratinocyte differentiation, diminishing hyperproliferation, and decreases expression of inflammatory markers. Skin irritation is the most common side effect and its use is thus usually restricted to thicker plaques in the nonintertriginous sites. Tazarotene 0.05% gel has been successfully used to treat nail psoriasis in a child.[84]

Combinations of Topical Agents

It was found that combination of topical agents work better than when they are used alone. Effective combinations in the management of psoriasis help in various ways. They aid to:
- Achieve rapid cure
- Reduce need for prolonged treatment with TCS, thereby reduce its side effect of TCS
- Reduce duration and cost of therapy.

These combinations include:
- Topical corticosteroids with vitamin D3
- Topical corticosteroids with salicylic acid
- Topical corticosteroids with tar
- TCS with UVB
- Dithranol with UVB
- Tar with salicylic acid
- Tar with UVB.

It is worthwhile remembering that calcipotriol should be applied only after irradiation due to its photolytic degradation, as well as its properties as a light filter.

Pretreatment with salicylic acid inactivates calcipotriol and hence, it is advisable not to combine both.

Phototherapy

Ultraviolet radiation in the spectrum of UVA and UVB act by inhibiting DNA synthesis and epidermal keratinocyte proliferation, inducing T cell apoptosis. They also exhibit immunosuppressive and anti-inflammatory property. Broadband UVB (BB-UVB, 290–320 nm), narrowband UVB (NB-UVB, 311 ±2 nm), and UVA (320–400 nm) are the three spectra used in the treatment of psoriasis. Phototherapy is appropriate for carefully selected patients with refractory disease, diffuse (>15–20% BSA) involvement, or focal debilitating palmoplantar psoriasis. Guttate and thin plaque type lesions respond best to phototherapy. NB-UVB is the safest of the three and is used in children above 6 years of age. UVA or psoralens and UVA (PUVA) therapy is not advised in children below 12 years of age. In children, NB-UVB is more convenient and may be less carcinogenic, and given the independence of psoralens-related precautions and adverse effects, NB-UVB is now considered first-line phototherapy in pediatric age group for psoriasis. PUVA bath treatment should be preferred to oral PUVA in older children (>12 years) and adolescents in situations like recalcitrant hand and foot psoriasis because of the advantage of avoidance of gastrointestinal side effects, lack of eye protection required, and shorter photosensitization time.[85] To limit the cumulative UVB dose and thereby, the carcinogenic risk, combination with systemic therapy like acitretin or topical therapy like calcipotriol, tazarotene, and anthralin has been found useful.[86] UV treatment to children must be administered in an appropriate environment with constant supervision by parents and trained professional staff. One has to remember that any form of light therapy has to be commenced in children with enough considerations and thoughtfulness of the child being exposed to UV light-containing sunlight for many more years to come in their life time.

Systemic Therapies

Specific systemic therapy is rarely used in childhood psoriasis (Figs 5.16A to G). Systemic therapy including retinoid, methotrexate, and cyclosporine, biologic is only used in severe forms of the disease, such as erythrodermic, pustular, and arthritic psoriasis. All these therapeutic options can be used as monotherapy or in various combinations.[87]

The indication for systemic therapy is one or more of the following:
- Involvement of BSA more than 20%
- PASI more than 10
- Erythrodermic psoriasis, with or without metabolic complication
- GPP
- Psoriatic arthropathy
- Localized disease not responding to topical therapy alone or with significant psychological morbidity.

Retinoids

Etretinate and acitretin, belonging to second generation retinoid, are the most commonly used systemic retinoid in children. The

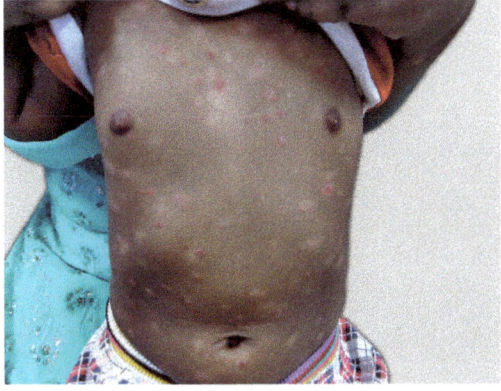

Fig. 5.16A: Child one month after cyclosporine

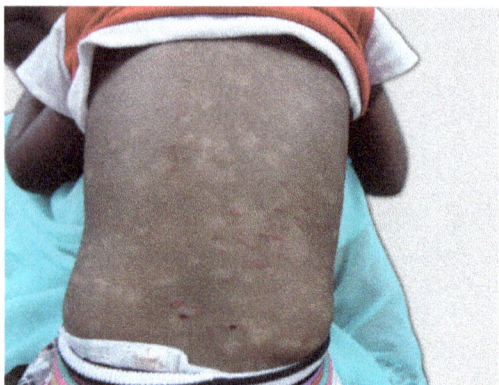

Fig. 5.16B: Same child as in Fig 5.16A

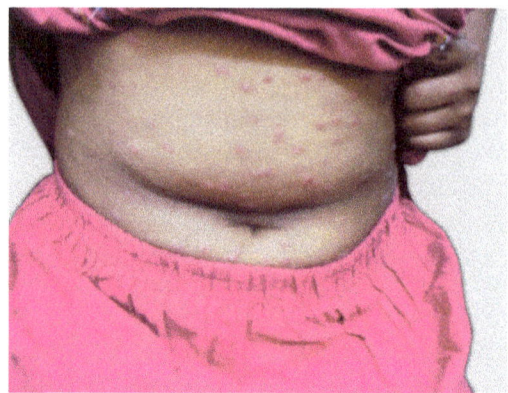

Fig. 5.16E: Older child 1 month after methotrexate

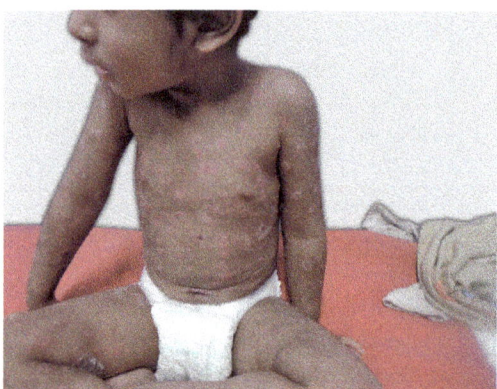

Fig. 5.16C: Same child as in Fig 5.16A, 2 months after cyclosporine

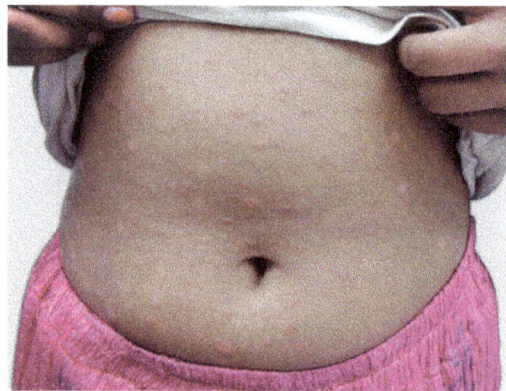

Fig. 5.16F: Same child as in Fig. 5.16E after 2 months

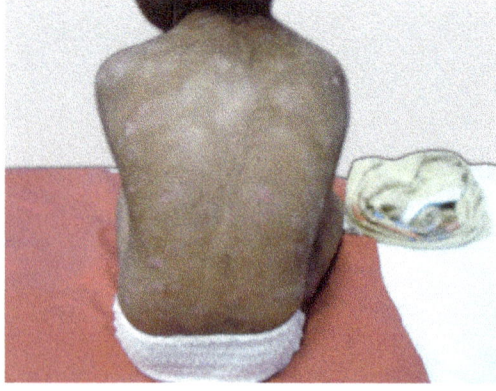

Fig. 5.16D: Same child as in Fig 5.16B, 2 months after cyclosporine

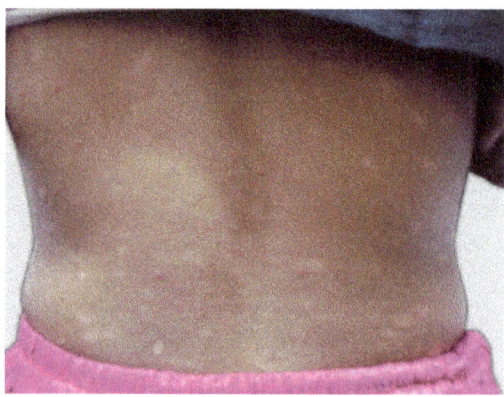

Fig. 5.16G: Same child as in Fig. 5.16F showing the back

modes of action include modulation of the epidermal proliferation and differentiation, and anti-inflammatory activity. To begin with, a low dose is started which can be increased up to 1 mg/kg/day and on improvement, tapered to 0.2 mg/kg body weight. The treatment continued for around 2-3 months postremission. Absorption is increased by milk or fatty foods and when dissolved in edible oils will enhance absorption.[88] The most common adverse effects are xerosis, cheilitis, epistaxis, and reversible alteration in liver enzymes and serum lipids. Premature closure of epiphysis limits its use in children. Retinoids are best avoided while treating girls.

Methotrexate

It is an antimetabolite agent and one of the most commonly used systemic agent for the treatment of psoriasis, because of its efficacy, affordability, and convenient dosing. It is usually given in a dosage of 0.2-4 mg/kg/week.[89] There are various studies documenting the successful use of methotrexate in various forms of juvenile psoriasis. Methotrexate is well tolerated by children. It is effective as a single weekly oral dose of 3.75-25 mg. Most of the children tolerate the drug well; nausea, vomiting are the common side effects.[90] Serious adversities are a rare occurrence. When carefully monitored, methotrexate can be a safe and efficacious treatment option for severe forms of psoriasis in children. Obesity may be a relative contraindication, as associated nonalcoholic fatty liver disease is likely to increase the hepatotoxicity of the drug.[91,92]

Relative Contraindications for Methotrexate Use

- Renal dysfunction (dosage adjustments needed)
- Significantly abnormal results on liver function tests
- Hepatitis
- Cirrhosis
- Significant pulmonary disease
- Blood dyscrasias (severe anemia, leukopenia, thrombocytopenia)
- Excessive alcohol consumption
- Active infectious disease (tuberculosis, pyelonephritis)

Cyclosporine

It's an immunosuppressive drug that primarily acts by inhibiting T cell function and IL-2. Cyclosporine is an effective drug in the management of childhood psoriasis and is generally well tolerated.[93] It is used in a dose range of 3-5 mg/kg and is variably effective. In some patients, it is a true crisis buster. Nephrotoxicity, hypertension, immunosuppression are the major side effects and hence, the drug is reserved only for severe cases.[94,95]

Biologics

The introduction of biologics in the armamentarium of antipsoriatic drugs is indeed a giant leap in the management of refractory pediatric psoriasis where other drugs like retinoids, methotrexate, and cyclosporine cannot be used. Etanercept, an anti-TNF fusion protein, has been the one studied most extensively.[96-98] It has been found to be effective and well tolerated in children and adolescents with moderate-to-severe plaque psoriasis. There are 4 case reports of the use infliximab in childhood psoriasis with good results.[99-101] When providing a child with biologics parents should be cautioned as to the side effects and potential life-threatening complications which can be associated. Being an immunosuppressive drug, the dosing of biologic agent is crucial ensuring that the child's immune system is not suppressed and allows for contacting infectious disease.

Administration of any of the above systemic drugs in a child should always be a team effort of dermatologist and pediatrician along with other specialist like gastroenterologist as whenever necessary.

There is a paucity of data regarding its efficacy and safety in children and adolescents, with only one published case reporting the successful administration of ustekinumab in a 14-year-old male patient with plaque psoriasis who failed to respond to conventional systemic agents as well as etanercept.[102] Ustekinumab's rapid onset of action as well as its convenient dosing schedule make it a promising treatment option, although it is very early to recommend its universal adoption for the treatment of adolescent psoriasis.

Other Modalities

LASER

A pilot study has reported 308 nm excimer lasers to be a safe and effective treatment for localized psoriasis in children as in adults.[103]

Oral antibiotics can be useful in treating psoriasis vulgaris, particularly in the setting of positive oral pharyngeal cultures, presence of perianal bacterial dermatitis, pustular psoriasis.[3,104]

Dietary Supplement

Fish oil, rich in omega-3 fatty acids is the best-known dietary supplement. Oral and intravenous supplementation of omega-3 and, less effectively, omega-6 fatty acids have been found effective in psoriatic adults, possibly through alterations in production and alterations in arachidonic acid (20:4 omega 6) and docosapentanenoic acid.[105]

Indigo naturalis, a traditional Chinese medicine, can be formulated into topical ointment with anecdotal reports of good results in childhood psoriasis, when used for 8 weeks.[106]

Treatment According to Type of Psoriasis

Plaque Type Psoriasis

Treatments must be tailored to the age of the patient, quality of life issues, and surface area affected. Anthralin is an effective treatment of plaque psoriasis either with or without topical steroids. With the advent of newer drugs, the frequency of its use has come down. Topical steroids, calcipotriol, tazarotene are useful and safe if used properly. Salicylic acid can be used along with steroids in thick plaques. Systemic agents like methotrexate and phototherapy may be needed in moderate-to-severe recalcitrant disease.

Scalp Psoriasis

Topical steroid with or without salicylic acid as lotion applied at night followed by steroid or ketoconazole-based shampooing in the morning is helpful. For resistant plaques, tar-based shampoos will help. A combination with NB-UVB and targeted phototherapy will give better results.

Guttate Psoriasis

Oral antibiotics are found to be useful in the treatment of guttate psoriasis. Systemic agents and phototherapy may be needed in moderate-to-severe disease. It should be remembered that guttate psoriasis can evolve into psoriasis vulgaris and hence, the child should be followed up regularly.

Inverse Psoriasis

Nonsteroidal agents like calcineurin inhibitor, low-potency TCS are used with caution. Ointments should be avoided over the folds as they have an occlusive effect which will increase absorption and result in side effects much earlier.

Nail Psoriasis

Psoriatic nail will frequently have super-added fungal infection. It is advisable that fungal infection is treated first. After elimination of the infection, by appropriate treatment, TCS, tazarotene or calcipotriene can be applied to the paronychial skin. Calcipotriol or tazarotene under occlusion covering the nail folds, plate, and under the nail plate are useful. Intralesional triamcinolone can also be used in the same region to reduce the subungual inflammation.

Napkin Psoriasis

Mild TCS with or without topical anticandidal agents can be helpful. Secondary infection, if any should be attended to. Barrier therapy with zinc oxide pastes reduces secondary irritant reactions.

Pustular Psoriasis

Generalized pustular psoriasis responds well to methotrexate in children.[107]

Maintenance of nutrition, fluid electrolyte balance prevention of organ failure should be stressed. Acitretin or isotretinoin (not for adolescent girls), and dapsone can be tried depending on the biochemical parameters. Oral steroids are used only to tide over the acute crisis.

If the disease is localized, topical agents-like steroids will suffice.

Mucosal Psoriasis

Involvement of mucosa is rare except in pustular psoriasis. No therapy is usually needed; however topical medicaments like steroids in an oral base can be used when needed. However, care has to be taken as inadvertent or prolonged use of topical steroid can lead to oral candidosis.

Congenital Erythrodermic Psoriasis

Regardless of underlying disease, the management of neonatal erythroderma includes fluid and electrolyte balance, correction of caloric and protein intake, and prevention and treatment of infections. Specific therapy is started once the diagnosis of underlying disease is established. The infant should be followed up. Topical calcipotriol is effective when emollients are not sufficient enough to clear the lesions.[108]

Arthropathic Psoriasis

The main aims of treating juvenile PsA are to reduce joint inflammation, maintain mobility, and prevent deformity. Physiotherapy is as important as drug treatment. Daily exercises, hydrotherapy (supervised exercise in a warm pool), and day and night splints are all important for long-term joint mobility. The aim of treatment is for the child to have as normal and active childhood as possible. In children with psoriatic arthropathy, methotrexate is the drug of choice.

Bullet Point Summary of Therapy of Juvenile Psoriasis

- Urea is standard in the basic therapy of juvenile psoriasis
- Corticosteroids and vitamin D3 analogs alone or in combination are standard therapeutic agents for topical therapy

- Dithranol is particularly advisable for partly or fully inpatient therapy
- The indication for phototherapy in childhood must be made very strictly
- Acitretin can especially be employed for pustular psoriasis forms in childhood
- Case reports exist for fumaric acid esters in children and adolescents
- Considering experience for other indications, cyclosporine can be used for short-term and methotrexate for middle term therapy of severe juvenile psoriasis
- Among TNF antagonists, etanercept should be favored for juvenile psoriasis based on the status of data and licensing.

PSYCHOLOGICAL ASPECTS AND REHABILITATION

Psoriasis by itself is a disease that causes a lot of psychological stress and vice versa.

Psoriasis was recently shown to have a great impact on quality of life in affected children (Figs 17A to C). Like atopic dermatitis, urticaria, and acne, psoriasis in the pediatric age group can lead to a severe emotional burden to the extent of impairing the health-related quality of life. A study on children and adolescents aged between 5 and 16 years found that in children with psoriasis, the values were as high as in children with atopic dermatitis and higher than in children with urticaria or acne.[109]

The Psychosocial Impact of Psoriasis and Psoriatic Arthritis on Children

The psychological impact of this currently incurable disease can be particularly traumatic for children and adolescents. In children, especially with severe disease, social development that contributes to many

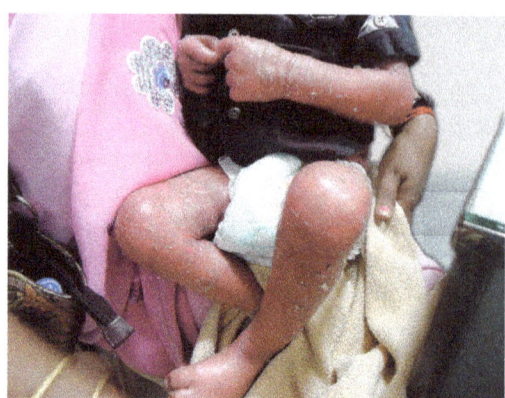

Fig. 5.17A: Boy with erythrodermic psoriasis with severe psychological disturbance

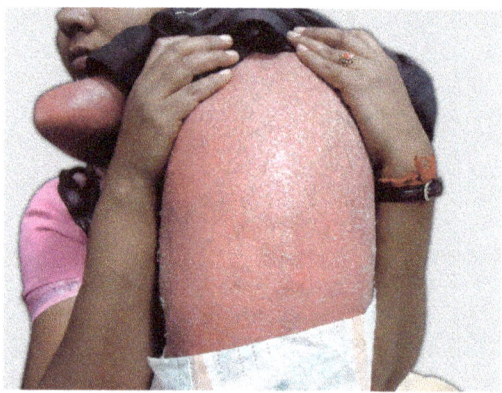

Fig. 5.17B: Same boy as in Fig. 5.17A

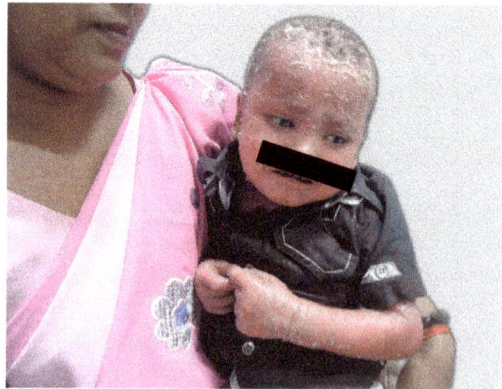

Fig. 5.17C: Same boy as in Figs 5.17A and B. Note the facial expression

developmental milestones is particularly impaired. Children with skin diseases are alienated, called names, teased, and bullied. Children with psoriatic disease also frequently experience discrimination at school or in public facilities, such as swimming pool. Studies suggest that these negative experiences in adolescence may have long-term negative effects on self-esteem and anxiety levels in adulthood.

In children with at least one of 12 different skin diseases, those with psoriasis reported the greatest impairment to quality of life. Additionally, studies found that psoriasis impacts health-related quality of life more than other chronic childhood conditions including epilepsy, diabetes, and alopecia.[109] Studies also reveal that nearly half of children with psoriasis reported being bullied. Children experience teasing, being excluded by peers, name calling, intimidation and in some cases, physical violence. The emotional impacts reported include anxiety, crying, trouble in school, and difficulty sleeping. 61% of surveyed children under the age of 10 years find psoriasis to be a significant problem in everyday life.[110] Children with psoriasis face significant emotional and physical challenges and probably have an increased risk of depression, anxiety, and suicidal tendency comparable with that of adults.[111]

The afflicted children must learn to cope with life and to adapt to their individual health situation. They must be counseled to choose a profession suitable to them in future. Rehabilitation of psoriatic children and adolescents can also supplement therapy and prevent the disease.

Therapy goals of rehabilitation will include:
- Regular treatment of the skin under proper supervision clubbed with climate therapy, nutritional therapy, and psychological interventions
- Help in coping with the disease with respect to the psychosocial consequences of psoriasis
- Help in finding an occupation.

CONCLUSION

Childhood psoriasis signifies a special challenge. The varied etiopathological theories make the disease more diverse. The early onset of the disease and the congenital forms indicate a much stronger genetic background. Awareness of the characteristics of childhood psoriasis will aid clinicians in early diagnosis and management. Further, work into the genetics and more research on pathology and controlled studies on therapy will throw more light on effective management protocol. It is essential to understand the impact of adiposity on childhood psoriasis which can predispose to metabolic comorbidity. Besides proper treatment, counseling and supportive care is an important segment of effective management of childhood psoriasis. Although spontaneous remission is more frequent in pediatric-onset disease than in adult-onset patients, clearance is often followed by recurrence. Hence, the parents, teachers, and all the associates of the affected child should be adequately advised.

Early detection, appropriate management will avoid comorbidities that are likely to develop in adulthood due to chronic inflammation. Aggressive therapy should be considered in children with severe psoriasis in whom intermittent therapy has failed to control the disease.

Psoriasis in children is an underrecognized and undertreated disease that can limit physical activity, impair social interaction, and add a significant psychological burden that has life-long adverse impacts on self-esteem and mental health. The negative physical and psychological impact of psoriasis on the pediatric population is further exacerbated by the fact that there are not enough drugs approved by the FDA to treat psoriasis in children. In addition to facing significant challenges in their youth, children with psoriasis also may expect additional problems when they reach adulthood. Children deserve a normal childhood irrespective of their ailment and children with psoriasis or PsA should not be an exempt.

Given the significant and growing link between psoriasis and the threat of developing comorbidities as they grow into adulthood, the fear of disability, life-threatening complications warranting costly treatment options, a collaborative interdisciplinary approach will go a long way in effectively treating the disease in childhood, which to a great extent control the untoward sequel in adulthood.

REFERENCES

1. Kurd SK, Gelfand JM. The prevalence of previously diagnosed and undiagnosed psoriasis in US adults: results from NHANES 2003–2004. J Am Acad Dermatol. 2009;60:218-24.
2. Raychaudhuri SP, Gross J. A comparative study of pediatric onset psoriasis with adult onset psoriasis. Pediatr Dermatol. 2000;17:174-8.
3. Silverberg NB. Pediatric psoriasis: an update. Therapeutics and Clinical Risk Management. 2009;5:849-56.
4. Sharma V, Orchard D. Paediatric psoriasis. Paediatrics and Child Health. 2011;21(3):126-31.
5. Sticherling M, Augustin M, Boehncke W, Christophers E, Domm S, Gollnick H, et al. Therapy of psoriasis in childhood and adolescence –a German expert consensus. J Dtsch Dermatol Ges. 2011;9(10):815-23.
6. Augustin M, Glaeske G, Radtke MA, Christophers E, Reich K, Schäfer I. Epidemiology and comorbidity of psoriasis in children. Br J Dermatol. 2010;162:633-6.
7. Swanbeck G, Inerot A, Martinsson T, Wahlström J, Enerbäck C, Enlund F, et al. Age at onset and different types of psoriasis. Br J Dermatol. 1995;133:768-73.
8. Farber EM, Mullen RH, Jacobs AH, Nall L. Infantile psoriasis: a follow up study. Pediatr Dermatol.1986;3:237-43.
9. Li Y, Begovich AB. Unraveling the genetics of complex diseases: Susceptibility genes for rheumatoid arthritis and psoriasis. Semin Immunol. 2009;1-10:318-27.
10. Lowes MA, Kikuchi T, Fuentes-Duculan J, Cardinale I, Zaba LC, Haider AS, et al. Psoriasis vulgaris lesions contain discrete populations of Th1 and Th17 T cells. J Invest Dermatol. 2008;128:1207-11.
11. Hüffmeier U, Lascorz J, Becker T, Schürmeier-Horst F,Magener A, Ekici AB, et al. Characterization of psoriasis susceptibility locus 6 (PSORS6) in patients with early onset psoriasis and evidence for interaction with PSORI. J Med Genet. 2009;46(11):736-44.
12. Wagner EF, Schonthaler HB, Guinea-Viniegra J, Tschachler E. Psoriasis: what we have learned from mouse models. Nat Rev Rheumatol. 2010;6:704-14.
13. Henseler T. The genetics of psoriasis. J Am Acad Dermatol. 1997;37:S1-11.
14. Benoit S, Hamm H. Childhood psoriasis. Clinics in Dermatology. 2007;25:555-62.
15. Takahashi H, Tsuji H, Takahashi I, Hashimoto Y, Ishida-Yamamoto A, Iizuka H. Plasma adiponectin and leptin levels in Japanese patients with psoriasis. Br J Dermatol. 2008;159:1207-8.
16. Takahashi H, Tsuji H, Takahashi I, Hashimoto Y, Ishida-Yamamoto A, Iizuka H, et al. Prevalence of obesity/adiposity in Japanese psoriasis patients: adiposity is correlated with the severity of psoriasis. J Dermatol Sci. 2009;54:61-3.
17. Mobini N, Toussaint S, Kamino H. Papulosquamous disorders. In: Elder DE, Elenitsas R, Johnson BL, Murphy GF, Xu X (Eds). Lever's histopathology of skin, 10th edition. New York: Lippincott Williams & Wilkins Co; 2008. pp. 169-203.
18. Leclerc-Mercier S, Bodemer C, Bourdon-Lanoy E, Larousserie F, Hovnanian A, Brousse N, et al. Early skin biopsy is helpful for the diagnosis and management of neonatal and infantile erythrodermas. J Cutan Pathol. 2010;37:249-55.
19. Walsh NM, Prokopetz R, Tron VA, Sawyer DM, Watters AK, Murray S, et al. Histopathology in erythroderma: review of a series of cases by multiple observers. J Cutan Pathol. 1994;21:419-23.
20. Bitoun E, Micheloni A, Lamant L, Bonnart C, Tartaglia-Polcini A, Cobbold C, et al. LEKTI proteolytic processing in human primary keratinocytes, tissue distribution, and defective expression in Netherton syndrome. Hum Mol Genet. 2003;12:2417-30.
21. Pruszkowski A, Bodemer C, Fraitag S, Teillac-Hamel D, Amoric JC, de Prost Y. Neonatal and infantile erythrodermas: a retrospective study of 51 patients. Arch Dermatol. 2000;136:875.
22. Beer WE, Smith AE, Kassab JY, Smith PH, Rowland Payne CM. Concomitance of psoriasis and atopic dermatitis. Dermatology. 1992;184:265-70.

23. Guttman-Yassky E, Nograles KE, Krueger JG. Contrasting pathogenesis of atopic dermatitis and psoriasis- Part II: Immune cell subsets and therapeutic concepts. J Allergy Clin Immunol. 2011;127:1420-32.
24. Giustizieri ML, Mascia F, Frezzolini A, De Pita O, Chinni LM, Giannetti A, et al. Keratinocytes from patients with atopic dermatitis and psoriasis show a distinct chemokine production profile in response to T cell-derived cytokines. J Allergy ClinImmunol. 2001;107:871-7.
25. Cookson WO, Ubhi B, Lawrence R, Abecasis GR, Walley AJ, Cox HE, et al. Genetic linkage of childhood atopic dermatitis to psoriasis susceptibility loci. Nature Genetics. 2001;27:372-3.
26. Parimalam K, Thomas J. Congenital erythrodermic psoriasis with atopic dermatitis: An example of immunogenetic spinoff. Indian J Pathol Microbiol. 2013;56:72-3.
27. Seyhan M, Coskun BK, Saglam H, Ozcan H, Karincaoglu Y. Psoriasis in childhood and adolescence: evaluation of demographic and clinical features. Pediatr Int. 2006;48:525-30.
28. Morris A, Rogers M, Fischer G, Williams K. Childhood psoriasis: a clinical review of 1262 cases. Pediatr Dermatol. 2001;18:188-98.
29. Grjibovski AM, Olsen AO, Magnus P, Harris JR. Psoriasis in Norwegian twins: contribution of genetic and environmental effects. J Eur Acad Dermatol Venereol. 2007;21:1337-43.
30. Stefanaki C, Lagogianni E, Kontochristopoulos G, Verra P, Barkas G, Katsambas A, et al. Psoriasis in children: a retrospective analysis. JEADV. 2011;25:417-21.
31. Al-fouzan AS, Nanda A. A Survey of Childhood Psoriasis in Kuwait. Pediatric Dermatol. 1994;11:116-9.
32. Altobelli E, Petrocelli R, Marziliano C, Fargnoli MC, Maccarone M, Chimenti S, et al. Family history of psoriasis and age at disease onset in Italian patients with psoriasis. Br J Dermatol. 2007;156:1400-1.
33. Honig PJ. Guttate psoriasis associated with perianal streptococcal disease. J Pediatr. 1988;113:1037-9.
34. Cassandra M, Conte E, Cortez B. Childhood pustular psoriasis elicited by the streptococcal antigen: a case report and review of the literature. Pediatr Dermatol. 2003;20:506-10.
35. Lazar AP, Roenigk HH. Acquired immunodeficiency syndrome (AIDS) can exacerbate psoriasis. J Am Acad Dermatol. 1988;18:144.
36. Tsankov N, Angelova I, Kazandjieva J. Drug-induced psoriasis. Recognition and management. Am J Clin Dermatol. 2000;1:159-65.
37. Wolf R, Ruocco V. Triggered psoriasis. Adv Exp Med Biol. 1999;455:221-5.
38. O'Brien M, Koo J. The mechanism of lithium and beta-blocking agents in inducing and exacerbating psoriasis. J Drugs Dermatol. 2006;5:426-32.
39. Barisic- Drusko V, Rucevic I. Psoriasis in childhood. Coll Antropol. 2004;1:211-85.
40. Wu Y, Lin Y, Liu HJ, Huang CZ, Feng AP, Li JW. Childhood psoriasis: A study of 137 cases from central China. World J Pediatr. 2010;6:260-4.
41. Nanda A, Kaur S, Kaur I, Kumar B. Childhood psoriasis: An epidemiological survey of 112 patients. Pediatr Dermatol. 1990;7:19-21.
42. Stern RS, Wu J. Psoriasis. In: Arndt KA, LeBoit PE, Robinson JK, Wintroub BU, (Eds). Cutaneous Medicine and Surgery. Philadelphia: WB Saunders; 1996.
43. Gottlieb AB, Chaudhari U, Baker DG, Perate M, Dooley LT. The natural psoriasis foundation score (NPF-PS) system versus the Psoriasis Area Severity Index (PASI) and Physicians Global Assessment. (PGA): a comparison. J Drugs Dermatol. 2003;2:260-6.
44. Dhar S, Banerjee R, Agrawal N, Chatterjee S, Malakar R. Psoriasis in children: an insight. Indian J Dermatol. 2011;56(3):262-5.
45. Atherton DJ, Kahana M, Russell-Jones R. Naevoid psoriasis. Br J Dermatol. 1989;120:837-41.
46. Sarkar R, Garg VK. Erythroderma in children. Indian J Dermatol Venereol Leprol. 2010;76:341-7.
47. Dika E, Bardazzi F, Balestri R, Maibach HI. Environmental factors and psoriasis. Curr Probl Dermatol. 2007;35:118-35.
48. Fry L, Baker BS. Triggering psoriasis: the role of infections and medications. Clin Dermatol 2007;25(6):606-15.
49. Naldi L, Gambini D. The clinical spectrum of psoriasis. Clin Dermatol. 2007;25(6):510-8.
50. Sarkar R. Neonatal and infantile erythroderma:The Red Baby. Indian J Dermatol. 2006;51:178-82.
51. Salleras M, Sanchez-Regaña M, Umbert P. Congenital erythrodermic psoriasis: case report and literature review. Pediatr Dermatol. 1995;12(3):231-4.
52. Frost P, Van Scott EJ. Ichthyosiform dermatoses. Classification based on anatomic and biometric observation. Arch Dermatol. 1966;94:113.
53. Parimalam K, Thomas J. Congenital Erythrodermic psoriasis—A case report. The Indian J Bio research. 2012;82:1-5.
54. Thomas J, Kumar P. Childhood Psoriasis– a challenge to all. Ind J Pract Ped. 2011;13(1):98-100.
55. Kumar P, Thomas J, Dineshkumar D. Histology of infantile erythrodermic psoriasis – a study of eight cases. Indian J Dermatol. 2015;60(2):213.
56. de Oliveira ST, Maragno L, Arnone M, Takahashi F, Romiti R. Generalized pustular psoriasis in childhood. Pediatric Dermatology. 2010;27(4):349-54.
57. Liao P, Rubinson R, Howard R, Sanchez G, Frieden IJ. Annular pustular psoriasis – most common form of pustular psoriasis in children: report of three cases and review of the literature. Pediatr Dermatol. 2002;19:19-25.
58. Zelickson BD, Muller SA. Generalized pustular psoriasis in childhood. J Am Acad Dermatol. 1990;24:186-94.

59. Xiao T, Li B, He CD, Chen HD. Juvenile generalized pustular psoriasis. J Dermatol. 2007;34:573-76.
60. Judge MR, McdonaldA, Black MM. Pustular psoriasis in childhood. Clin Exp Dermatol.1993;18:97-9.
61. Espinoza LR, Cuellar ML, Silveira LH. Psoriatic arthritis. Curr Opin Rheumatol. 1992;4:470-8.
62. Zachariae H. Prevalence of joint disease in patients with psoriasis: implications for therapy. Am J Clin Dermatol. 2003;4:441-7.
63. Southwood TR, Petty RE, Malleson PN, et al. Psoriatic arthritis in children. Arthritis Rheum. 1989;32:1007-13.
64. Shore A, Ansell BM. Juvenile psoriatic arthritis—an analysis of 60 cases. J Pediatr. 1982;100:529-35.
65. Zhu KJ, He SM, Zhang C, Yang S, Zhang XJ. Relationship of the body mass index and childhood psoriasis in a Chinese Han population: A hospital-based study. J Dermatol. 2011;39(2):181-3.
66. Boccardi D, Menni S, La Vecchia C, Nobile M, Decarli A, Volpi G, et al. Overweight and childhood psoriasis. Br J Dermatol. 2009;161:484-6.
67. Soltani-Arabshahi R, Wong B, Feng BJ, Goldgar, DE, Duffin KC, Krueger GG. Obesity in Early Adulthood as a Risk Factor for Psoriatic Arthritis. Archives of Dermatology. 2010;146:721-6.
68. Fluhr JW, Cavallotti C, Berardesca E. Emollients, moisturizers and keratolytic agents in psoriasis. Clin Dermatol. 2008;26:380-6.
69. Smith CH, Jackson K, Chinn S, Angus K, Barker JNWN. A double blind, randomized, controlled clinical trial to assess the efficacy of a new coal tar preparation (Exorex®) in the treatment of chronic, plaque type psoriasis. Clin Exp Dermatol. 2000;25:580-3.
70. Thami GP, Sarkar R. Coal tar: Past, present and future. Clin Exp Dermatol. 2002;27:99-103.
71. Borska L, Andrys C, Krejsek J, Hamakova K, Kremlacek J, Ettler K, et al. Genotoxic hazard and cellular stress in pediatric patients treated for psoriasis with the Goeckermann regimen. Pediatr Dermatol. 2009;26: 23-7.
72. McGill A, Frank A, Emmett N, Turnbull DM, BirchMachin MA, Reynolds NJ. The antipsoriatic drug anthralin accumulates in keratinocyte mitochondria, dissipates mitochondrial membrane potential, and induces apoptosis through a pathway dependent on respiratory competent mitochondria. FASEB J. 2005;19:1012-4.
73. Lebwohl M, Ali S. Treatment of psoriasis. Part 1. Topical therapy and phototherapy. J Am Acad Dermatol. 2001;45:487-98.
74. Zvulunov A, Anisfeld A, Metzker A. Efficacy of shortcontact therapy with dithranol in childhood psoriasis. Int J Dermatol. 1994;33:808-10.
75. Farber EM, Nall L. Childhood psoriasis. Cutis. 1999; 64:309-14.
76. Kiken DA, Silverberg NB. Atopic dermatitis in children, part 2: treatment options. Cutis. 2006;78:401-6.
77. Kimball AB, Gold MH, Zib B, Davis MW. Clobetasol Propionate Emulsion Formulation Foam Phase III Clinical Study Group. Clobetasol propionate emulsion formulation foam 0.05%: review of phase II open-label and phase III randomized controlled trials in steroid-responsive dermatoses in adults and adolescents. J Am Acad Dermatol. 2008;59:448-54.
78. Rim JH, Choe YB, Youn JI. Positive effect of using calcipotriol ointment with narrowband Ultraviolet B phototherapy in psoriatic patients. Photodermatol Photoimmunol Photomed. 2002;18:131-4.
79. Oranje AP, Marcoux D, Svensson A, Prendiville J, Krafchik B, Toole J, et al. Topical calcipotriol in childhood psoriasis. J Am Acad Dermatol. 1997;36:203-8.
80. Liao YH, Chiu HC, Tseng YS, Tsai TF. Comparison of cutaneous tolerance and efficacy of calcitriol 3 µg g^{-1} ointment and tacrolimus 0·3 mg g^{-1} ointment in chronic plaque psoriasis involving facial or genitofemoral areas: a double-blind, randomized controlled trial. Br J Dermatol. 2007;157:1005-12.
81. Brune A, Miller DW, Lin P, CotrimRussi D, Paller AS. Tacrolimus ointment is effective for psoriasis on the face and intertriginous areas in pediatric patients. Pediatr Dermatol. 2007;24:76-80
82. Mansouri P, Farshi S. Pimecrolimus 1 percent cream in the treatment of psoriasis in a child. Dermatol Online J. 2006;12:7.
83. Jain VK, Aggarwal K, Jain K, Bansal A. Narrow-band UV-B phototherapy in childhood psoriasis. Int J Dermatol. 2007;46:320-2.
84. Diluvio L, Campione E, Paternò EJ, Mordenti C, El Hachem M, Chimenti S. Childhood nail psoriasis: A useful treatment with tazarotene 0.05%. Pediatr Dermatol. 2007;24:332-3.
85. Holme SA, Anstey AV. Phototherapy and PUVA photo-chemotherapy in children. Photodermatol Photoimmunol Photomed. 2004;20:69-75.
86. Pasić A, Ceović R, Lipozencić J, Husar K, Susić SM, Skerlev M, et al. Phototherapy in pediatric patients. Pediatr Dermatol. 2003;20:71-7.
87. Ceović R, Pasić A, Lipozencić J, Murat-Susić S, Skerlev M, Husar K, et al. Treatment of childhood psoriasis. Acta Dermatol Venereol Croat. 2006;14(4):261-4.
88. Pang ML, Murase JE, Koo J. An updated review of acitretina systemic retinoid for the treatment of psoriasis. Expert Opin Drug Metab Toxicol. 2008;4:953-64.
89. Cordoro KM. Topical therapy for the management of childhood psoriasis: Part I. Skin Therapy Letter. 2008;13:1-3.
90. Kumar B, Dhar S, Handa S, Kaur I. Methotrexate in childhood psoriasis. Pediatr Dermatol. 1994;11(3):271-3.

91. Collin B, Vani A, Ogboli M, Moss C. Methotrexate treatment in 13 children with severe plaque psoriasis. Clin Exp Dermatol. 2009;34(3):295-8.
92. Kalb RE, Strober B, Weinstein G, Lebwohl M. Methotrexate and psoriasis: 2009 National Psoriasis Foundation Consensus Conference. J Am Acad Dermatol. 2009;60:824-37.
93. Perrett CM, Ilchyshyn A, Berth-Jones J. Cyclosporin in childhood psoriasis. J Dermatol Treat. 2003;14(2):113-8.
94. Alli N, Gónger E, Karakayali G, Lenk N, Artóz F. The use of cyclosporin in a child with generalized pustular psoriasis. Br J Dermatol. 1998;139:754-5.
95. Pereira TM, Vieira AP, Fernandes JC, SousaBasto AJ. Cyclosporin A treatment, in severe childhood psoriasis. J Eur Acad Dermatol Venereol. 2006;20:651-6.
96. Paller AS, Siegfried EC, Langley RG, Gottlieb AB, Pariser D, Landellsl. Etanercept treatment, for children and adolescents with plaque psoriasis. N Engl J Med. 2008;358:241-51.
97. Trueb RM. Therapies for childhood psoriasis. Curr Probl Dermatol. 2009;38:137-59.
98. Kress DW. Etanercept therapy improves symptoms and allows tapering of other medications in children and adolescents with moderate to severe psoriasis. J Am Acad Dermatol. 2006;54:S126-8.
99. Pereira TM, Vieira AP, Fernandes JC, Antunes H, Basto AS. AntiTNFalpha therapy in childhood pustular psoriasis. Dermatol. 2006;213:350-2.
100. Farnsworth NN, George SJ, Hsu S. Successful use of infliximab following a failed course of etanercept in a pediatric patient. Dermatol Online J. 2005;11:11.
101. Menter MA, Cush JM. Successful treatment of pediatric psoriasis with infliximab. Pediatr Dermatol. 2004;21:87-8.
102. Fotiadou C, Lazaridou E, Giannopoulou C, Ioannides D. Ustekinumab for the treatment of an adolescent patient with recalcitrant plaque psoriasis. Eur J Dermatol. 2011;21:117-8.
103. Pahlajani N, Katz BJ, Lozano AM, Murphy F, Gottlieb A. Comparison of the efficacy and safety of the 308 nm excimer laser for the treatment of localized psoriasis in adults and in children: A pilot study. Pediatr Dermatol. 2005;22:161-5.
104. Pacifico L. Acute guttate psoriasis after streptococcal scarlet fever. Pediatr Dermatol. 1993;10:388-9.
105. Grattan C, Burton JL, Manku M, Stewart C, Horrobin DF. Essential fatty- acid metabolites in plasma phospholipids in patients with ichthyosis vulgaris, acne vulgaris and psoriasis. Clin Exp Dermatol. 1990;15:174-6.
106. Lin YK, Yen HR, Wong WR, Yang SH, Pang JH. Successful treatment of pediatric psoriasis with Indigo naturalis composite ointment. Pediatr Dermatol. 2006;23:507-10.
107. Kumar P, Nithya P, Saratha K P, Mythili P C, Manoharan K. Effect of methotrexate in juvenile generalized pustular psoriasis. J of Applied Medicine and Surgery. 2012;1(3):28-31.
108. Parimalam K, Thomas J. Infantile erythrodermic psoriasis: successful treatment with topical Calcipotriol. e-Journal of the Indian Society of Teledermatology. 2011;5(2)9-14.
109. Beattie PE, Lewis-Jones MS. A comparative study of impairment of quality of life in children with skin disease and children with other chronic childhood diseases. Br J Dermatol. 2006;155:145-51.
110. National Psoriasis Foundation Psoriasis and Children Issue Brief January 2012. [online] Available from http://www.psoriasis.org/document.doc?id=348. [Accessed October, 2015].
111. Kurd SK, Troxel AB, Christop P, Gelfand JM. The risk of depression, anxiety and suicidality in patient with psoriasis: a population-based cohort study. Archives of Dermatology. 2010;146(8):891-5.

CHAPTER 6

Psoriasis and Pregnancy

INTRODUCTION

It is well established that psoriasis fluctuates during pregnancy, likely due to the hormonal changes in estrogen and progesterone resulting in a state of altered immune surveillance (Fig. 6.1). The majority of women usually experience an improvement in their cutaneous disease during pregnancy. According to a study by Murase et al., 55% of the patients reported improvement during pregnancy, 21% no change, and 23% reported worsening.[1] However, only 9% of patients reported improvement, 26% no change, and 65% reported worsening postpartum. In patients with 10% or greater body surface area involvement who reported improvement, lesions decreased by 83.8% during pregnancy. Similar data were obtained by Raychaudhuri et al.[2] Of the 91 pregnant women involved in the study, 51 (56%) improved, 24 (26.4%) worsened, and 16 (17.6%) had no change during pregnancy. Relapse during the early postpartum period was common. The mechanism by which psoriasis tends to improve during pregnancy is not well understood. However, there is now data to suggest that the upregulation of T helper (Th) 2 cytokines during pregnancy counteracts the effects of proinflammatory Th1 cytokines which are key players in the pathogenesis of psoriasis.

Women with psoriasis generally progress through conception, pregnancy, and birth just like anyone else.

Rates of pregnancy and spontaneous abortion were found to be similar in both, in pregnant women with inflammatory skin

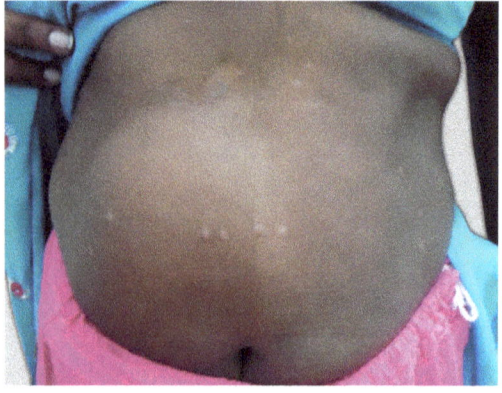

Fig. 6.1: Mild psoriasis in pregnancy, therapy will suffice

diseases and women without inflammatory skin diseases. However, studies have shown that women with severe psoriasis (defined as those who had received photochemotherapy or systemic therapy within 2 years before delivery) had a higher risk for the delivery of low birth weight infants compared with mothers without psoriasis.

But, it was noted that receiving systemic therapy during pregnancy did not appear to contribute to the increased risk of low birth weight; rates of low birth infants were similar among mothers who received systemic medications during pregnancy and those who did not, indicating that psoriasis by itself due to the chronic inflammatory process increases the risk of low birth weight babies, which was also proved in a retrospective cohort study which identified psoriasis as an independent risk factor for spontaneous abortions, induced abortions, premature rupture of membranes, and infant macrosomia.[3]

PUSTULAR PSORIASIS OF PREGNANCY

Pustular psoriasis of pregnancy is rare, but the condition is serious owing to its metabolic complications and extent of involvement. The more severe and longstanding the disease, the greater is the risk to the baby. This may lead on to placental insufficiency, stillbirth, neonatal death or fetal abnormalities.

Impetigo Herpetiformis or Gestational Pustular Psoriasis

Impetigo herpetiformis (IH) was first described by Hebra and an endocrine cause was suspected. The claims that impetigo herpetiformis stands as an entity separate from generalized pustular psoriasis (GPP) have been restated. IH or gestational pustular psoriasis is a rare form of pustular psoriasis related to pregnancy which normally occurs during the third trimester. However, there are reports of cases, occurring earlier and has been recorded in the first month of pregnancy and in the first day of the puerperium. The disease tends to persist until the child is born, and occasionally long afterward. Familial occurrence has been reported.

Pathogenesis

Primiparous women are at the highest risk, though severity increases in subsequent pregnancies. The worsening of pustular psoriasis just before menstruation is well recognized and challenge with progesterone or clomifene has produced pustular exacerbations in such patients. Maternal hypocalcemia, stress, and infection are considered as triggering factors.

Clinical Features

Impetigo herpetiformis is characterized by an acute eruption of erythematous patches studded with pustules at the margins, occurring usually in the last trimester of pregnancy and has been recorded in the first month of pregnancy. It presents superficial pustules with a tendency for grouping in a herpetiform distribution. The pustular eruption typically starts symmetrically over the inguinogenital region and other the flexural skin of axillae, groin, inframammary, and the periumbilical area. Pustules are sometimes seen over the abdominal striae. The lesions start as minute pustules arising on an acutely inflamed area of skin which extend centrifugally, drying in the center, or form plaques in which eroded greenish yellow pustules become fetid. Crusted or vegetating condyloma like lesions may form in the flexures. The eruption soon spreads to become generalized with desquamation. The pustules heal, leaving behind reddish-brown pigmentation. The tongue, buccal mucosa, and even the esophagus may be involved, with circinate or erosive lesions following short-lived pustules.

Occasionally, there may be painful oral erosions and involvement of subungual areas leading to onycholysis. The face, palms, and soles are commonly spared. The rashes may be pruritic or painful. Constitutional disturbance is characteristically severe with fever, and death may occur, attributable to cardiac or renal failure. Delirium, diarrhea, vomiting, and tetany has been described. The disease tends to persist until the child is born and occasionally long afterward. Recurrences are not uncommon with subsequent pregnancies, and on subsequent use of oral contraceptive.

Differentiation between acute generalized exanthematous pustulosis (AGEP) and pustular psoriasis is very difficult during the first episode in the absence of history or evidence of psoriasis. The duration of pustules is shorter lived in AGEP as against IH. Histology will be the most important diagnostic tool under such situations where in AGEP, there is eosinophilic exocytosis and necrotic keratinocytes in the epidermis with marked dermal edema and evidence of vasculitis. Whereas, IH will show acanthosis and papillomatosis with neutrophilic pustules. Other differential diagnosis includes pustular drug eruption, subcorneal pustular dermatoses, pemphigoid gestationis, pemphigus vulgaris, and dermatitis herpetiformis. Pustular drug eruption will have a definite drug-intake history.

Subcorneal pustular dermatoses lesions also have flexural predilection, presence of hypopyon gives a clue to the diagnosis.

Pemphigoid gestation usually occurs at the twenty-first week of pregnancy characterized by pruritic urticarial papules and plaques, target lesions, and annular wheals and may flare up immediately postpartum, unlike IH, which generally resolves postpartum.

Pemphigus vulgaris starts with oral involvement and the skin lesions are tense vesicles which later turn into pustules that grow organism on culture. Tzanck smear can demonstrate acantholytic cells which is almost diagnostic of pemphigus vulgaris.

Dermatitis herpetiformis is characterized by grouped itchy vesicular lesions, predominantly on the extensors. Positive iodine challenge test will prove the diagnosis.

Course and Prognosis

Impetigo herpetiformis is a medical emergency involving the mother as well as the fetus. Apart from the complications of hypocalcemia, the other complications include fluid and electrolyte imbalance and maternal secondary infection and sepsis. The more severe and long-standing the disease, the greater are the risks of placental insufficiency leading to stillbirth, neonatal death or fetal abnormalities (Figs 6.2 and 6.3). In many cases, there is derangement of liver enzymes. Even when the disease is controlled in the mother, an increased stillbirth risk and fetal abnormalities are noted.

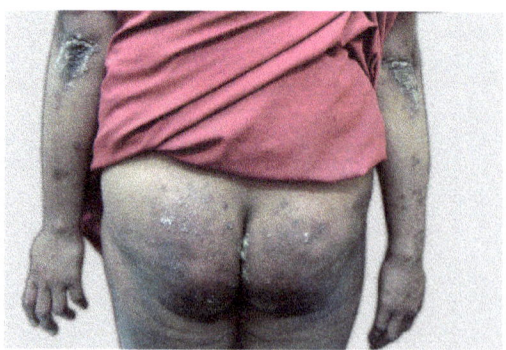

Fig. 6.2: Impetigo herpetiformis in a pregnant woman

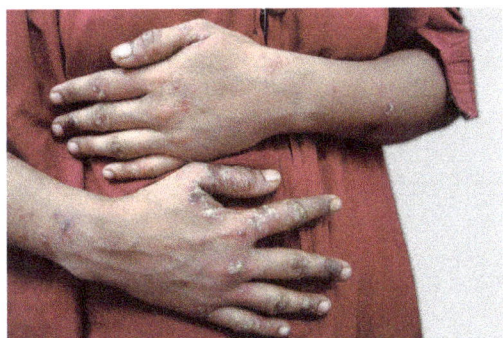

Fig. 6.3: Same patient as in Fig 6.2. Pustules persisting after termination of pregnancy; impetigo herpetiformis resulted in fetal loss

Lesions are expected to regress after delivery, but invariably reoccur at times of stress and at an earlier gestational age in further pregnancies, as a characteristic eruption of erythematosquamous plaques with or without pustules. Characteristically, the disease recurs in subsequent pregnancies and on subsequent use of oral contraceptives. There is one report where the disease continued unabated despite termination of the pregnancy.

Investigations

Blood investigations should be carried out to look for leukocytosis, neutrophilia, elevated erythrocyte sedimentation rate, anemia, hypoalbuminemia, hypocalcemia, electrolyte imbalance, low vitamin D levels, altered liver and renal functions. Blood and pus cultures are negative. Biopsy should be performed to confirm diagnosis in patients who present with IH for the first time in the absence of a history of psoriasis.

Treatment

Oral corticosteroid remains the mainstay of treatment in the management of pustular psoriasis of pregnancy. IH can be successfully treated with topical and systemic corticosteroids. Antibiotics may be indicated for secondary bacterial infection. Fluid and electrolytes, especially calcium should be monitored and normalized. Unresponsive cases can be given cyclosporine, narrowband ultraviolet B (NBUVB), psoralen ultraviolet A (PUVA), clofazimine or induction of early delivery. During the postpartum period, oral retinoid can be given. Treatment is imperative due to the life, threatening nature of the disease. The treatment of choice in pregnancy is prednisolone 15–30 mg/day. Cyclosporine is used only if the potential benefits justify the potential risk to the fetus. As the fetal mortality is high, even when the disease appears well controlled with corticosteroids, fetal well-being should be monitored using biophysical profile and umbilical artery Doppler studies. If fetal or maternal conditions deteriorate, pregnancy should be terminated by induction of labor or cesarean section, as indicated. Though maternal mortality is less with the advent of treatment options available, stillbirth and intrauterine growth retardation may occur even when the disease appears to be controlled with corticosteroids. Low-dose methotrexate can be substituted in the postpartum period to prevent rebound of rashes, but is contraindicated in pregnancy and lactation. The disease remits after delivery but may recur in successive pregnancies. Of late, cyclosporine as well as methotrexate has been found to be useful in this condition.[4,5]

Cyclosporine, which is categorized as pregnancy category "C", has been successfully used at doses between 5 mg/kg and 10 mg/kg weight daily, to treat cases that are refractory to a high dose of systemic corticosteroids. Cyclosporine is a natural cyclic peptide compound of 11 amino acids, metabolized in the liver by P450, 34A cytochrome, and excreted primarily by way of bile, through feces. Only 6% of the total dose is excreted in urine and minimally through breast milk. Spontaneous regression observed after delivery will help to withdraw the drug quickly.

SAFETY OF DRUGS IN PREGNANCY WHILE TREATING PSORIASIS

The appropriate treatment for psoriasis in a woman who is pregnant, or who plans pregnancy, will depend on the extent and severity of the skin condition.

Topical therapy can be used with confidence, but using large quantities of salicylic acid, calcipotriol, topical steroids, and calcineurin inhibitors for long periods of time should be avoided.

Ultraviolet B (UVB) phototherapy is safe for pregnant women with more severe psoriasis. Cyclosporine can be prescribed when systemic therapy is essential, providing blood pressure and kidney function are very carefully monitored.

There is little research on the impact of psoriasis and psoriatic arthritis treatments on pregnant and nursing women. The National Psoriasis Foundation released guidelines in 2012 for treating psoriasis in pregnant or breastfeeding women. Topical treatments are the first choice of treatment, particularly moisturizers and emollients, such as petroleum jelly. Limited use of low-dose to moderate-dose topical steroids appears safe, but women should use caution when applying topical steroids to the breasts to avoid passing the medication to the baby while nursing. Read more about using topical treatments during pregnancy or nursing.

Narrow-band ultraviolet light B phototherapy should be the second-line treatment. If NBUVB is not available, then broad-band UVB may be used. Nursing women should avoid psoralen and ultraviolet light A because psoralen enters breast milk and could cause light sensitivity to infants.

For a better understanding of drug therapy in psoriasis, it is advisable that a clear knowledge of drug categories used in psoriasis is agreed.

Australian Drug Evaluation Committee pregnancy categories:

A Drugs which have been taken by a large number of pregnant women and women of childbearing age without an increase in the frequency of malformations or other direct or indirect harmful effects on the fetus having been observed

B1 Drugs which have been taken by only a limited number of pregnant women and women of childbearing age, without an increase in the frequency of malformation or other direct or indirect harmful effects on the human fetus having been observed. Studies in animals have not shown evidence of an increased occurrence of fetal damage

B2 Drugs which have been taken by only a limited number of pregnant women and women of childbearing age, without an increase in the frequency of malformation or other direct or indirect harmful effects on the human fetus having been observed. Studies in animals are inadequate or may be lacking, but available data show no evidence of an increased occurrence of fetal damage

B3 Drugs which have been taken by only a limited number of pregnant women and women of childbearing age, without an increase in the frequency of malformation or other direct or indirect harmful effects on the human fetus having been observed. Studies in animals have shown evidence of an increased occurrence of fetal damage, the significance of which is considered uncertain in humans

C Drugs which, owing to their pharmaceutical effects, have caused or may be suspected of causing harmful effects on the human fetus or neonate without causing malformations. These effects may be reversible
D Drugs which have caused, are suspected to have caused or may be expected to cause, an increased incidence of human fetal malformations or irreversible damage. These drugs may also have adverse pharmacological effects
X Drugs that have such a high risk of causing permanent damage to the fetus that they should not be used in pregnancy or when there is a possibility of pregnancy.

MANAGEMENT OF PSORIASIS IN PREGNANCY AND LACTATION

Psoriasis is known to be associated with metabolic syndrome. Comorbidities, such as diabetes, obesity or hypertension in pregnancy may worsen psoriasis and vice versa. Therefore, the management of psoriasis in such patients means medical, dermatological, and obstetric challenge which has to be born in mind while treating a pregnant woman with psoriasis. It is also possible that some women experience spontaneous improvement of psoriasis during pregnancy.

Safety of different therapeutic modalities during gestation and lactation should be taken into account while treating pregnant and lactating women. Teratogenicity and other adverse effects on the fetus or child must be balanced with the risk from uncontrolled skin inflammation affecting the course of pregnancy and postpartum period. Similarly, in a patient planning for pregnancy, adequate precaution should be taken while prescribing drugs. Patient counseling before conception is invaluable and must be given to all married women who have not completed their family.

It is noteworthy that about half of patients with psoriasis experience improvement or remission during pregnancy.

First-line therapy for pregnant or breastfeeding psoriasis patients, with limited disease will include topical mid potent steroid and UVB phototherapy.

In women with active, moderate-to-severe psoriasis, systemic treatment therapy may be needed. Those systemic medications with teratogenic and mutagenic potential must be avoided.

Topical Therapies for Psoriasis in Pregnancy and Lactation

Simple emollients appear safe to use in pregnancy. Salicylic acid is absorbed through the skin (10–25%). It is proved that oral salicylates are associated with bleeding and are harmful to the baby; it is better to avoid topical salicylic acid over large areas of the body for prolonged periods.

Coal tar products are considered safe, if used for short periods or on localized areas, such as the scalp. Though the risk of coal tar and injury to the baby is unknown, it is better to avoid their use over large areas of the body for prolonged periods as they contain potentially hazardous polycyclic aromatic hydrocarbons.

Since dithranol or anthralin are not absorbed through skin, the risk in pregnancy is unknown, but the drug is not frequently advised due to its irritant nature.

Topical corticosteroids appear to be safe during pregnancy, if used judiciously. Mild-potency to moderate-potency topical corticosteroids should be preferred to more potent corticosteroids during pregnancy. Potent-to-very potent topical corticosteroids should be used only as second-line therapy for as short a time as possible. They are better avoided over high-absorption areas like the eyelids, genitals, and flexures. Whether the newer potent lipophilic topical corticosteroids (e.g., mometasone, fluticasone, and methylprednisolone) are associated with less risk to fetus is not fully determined.

Mild, moderate, and potent topical corticosteroids are also considered safe to use when breastfeeding. Patient should be instructed to wash off any steroid cream applied on breasts before feeding. It is advisable that very potent topical corticosteroids are not recommended to use over the chest while breastfeeding.

Calcipotriol, a category B drug, with 6% systemic absorption, should be used with caution though the risk in pregnancy is unknown. Dose should not exceed 100 g/week, and should not be applied over the chest area, if the mother is breastfeeding.

Calcineurin inhibitors tacrolimus, pimecrolimus belong to category C and their risk in pregnancy is unknown.

Tazarotene, although topical, is a category X medication, therefore, is to be strictly avoided in pregnancy.

Phototherapy for Psoriasis in Pregnancy and Lactation

Phototherapy with broadband UVB and NBUVB appears as safe in pregnancy as at other times. The risk of topical PUVA in pregnancy is considered very low, but oral PUVA should be avoided during pregnancy.

Systemic Therapies for Psoriasis in Pregnancy and Lactation

It is always better to avoid systemic therapy in pregnancy. Most of the systemic drugs used in the treatment of psoriasis are unsafe in pregnancy and lactation. Systemic drugs and the pregnancy category are mentioned in Box 6.1. Cyclosporine and biologics are the only drugs relatively safe in pregnancy coming under category C.

> **BOX 6.1: Systemic drugs in pregnancy**
> - Methotrexate; Category D
> - Cyclosporine; Category C
> - Acitretin; Category X
> - Biologics; Category C
> - Hydroxyurea; Category D
> - Mycophenolate mofetil; Category D

Methotrexate

Methotrexate is a systemic treatment for moderate-to-severe psoriasis since 1958. It is a widely accepted drug due to its efficacy, extensive clinical experience, and low cost. It is also a well-known abortifacient. It inhibits the synthesis of deoxyribonucleic acid (DNA) by competitive binding to dihydrofolate reductase and has been known as a mutagen and teratogen. It is absolutely contraindicated during pregnancy and belongs to Food and Drug Administration (FDA) category X. The sensitive period for the occurrence of malformations is between 6 and 8 weeks after conception and the dose required to produce defects is greater than 10 mg/week.

The abnormalities can occur even in doses lower than 10 mg weekly.[6] Methotrexate increases the risk of abortion and birth defects, such as central nervous system, craniofacial, limb, gastrointestinal, and cardiopulmonary malformations as well as growth delay. Because 6–8 weeks after conception is the critical period for abnormalities, a "washout" period of at least 3 months is advisable before conceiving, and supplementation with folic acid during this period and throughout pregnancy is recommended.[7] Methotrexate has been linked to disturbances in spermatogenesis, such as chromosomal abnormalities and alterations in the sperm mobility. However, a prospective study of 42 fetuses whose fathers were exposed to weekly doses between 7.5 and 30 mg 3 months before or until conception reported no birth abnormalities. Methotrexate is transferred into breast milk in significantly lower concentrations compared to maternal serum. It could be present in child tissues for months and therefore, it is contraindicated during lactation.[8]

Cyclosporine

Cyclosporine, a selective immunomodulator by acting as a calcineurin inhibitor has been classified as a traditional systemic agent for psoriasis treatment and has been approved for this indication since 1993. It is usually given as a crisis buster for a short-term therapy for 2-4 months. The drug passively crosses the placental blood barrier to achieve 10-50% of the maternal plasma concentration. It is not teratogenic in animals or humans and comes under FDA category C. The drug is found to have no mutagenic properties. However, there was an increased risk of premature delivery and low birth weight recorded in pregnant women treated with cyclosporine.[9] Cyclosporine is not absolutely contraindicated in pregnancy and has been used successfully in pregnant women and is considered as a possible rescue therapy for pregnant psoriasis patients in the case of severe disease. Cyclosporine is excreted in breast milk at variable levels. Although there are reports of safe infant exposure during lactation with normal development and growth, the current recommendation is that breastfeeding should be avoided while taking cyclosporine due to concerns of immunosuppression in the infant.

Acitretin

Acitretin belongs to the group of retinoids. It affects cellular differentiation and proliferation resulting in good control over the disease like psoriasis where there is proliferation of keratinocytes. All the more, it acts a teratogen probably acting by affecting cellular differentiation and proliferation. It is absolutely contraindicated during pregnancy as it is category X drug. Acitretin administered in the first trimester of pregnancy increases the risk of spontaneous abortion and congenital defects, such as central nervous system, craniofacial, limb, thymic, and cardiovascular malformations.[10] Therefore, pregnancy should be avoided during and up to 2 years after the end of therapy, which makes acitretin an impractical and unsuitable therapy for women in their reproductive years unless they no longer have to bear children. Despite the short elimination half-life of acitretin of only 2 days, it can be converted in small amounts to etretinate with a much longer half-life of 100 days, especially by concomitant intake of ethanol. Therefore, women of childbearing age should be discouraged from taking acitretin, and strict contraception should be followed during and two years after acitretin therapy. The drug should be introduced on the second or third day of the menstrual cycle, after at least 1 month of satisfactory double contraception. Monthly pregnancy tests are recommended in order to check possibility of pregnancy. Though there is only minimal excretion of acitretin into breast milk, breastfeeding should be avoided due to the potential for cumulative neonatal toxicity.[11]

Biologics

Biologic therapy is also known as protein therapeutics. Biological agents are a group of pharmacologically active protein (or peptide)-based molecules produced by living organisms that are designed to alleviate disease by inhibiting or imitating naturally occurring proteins in the body. Biological agents are approved for moderate-to-severe psoriasis treatment, which is inadequately controlled with conventional systemic agents or if these agents are contraindicated. Etanercept, infliximab, adalimumab, and ustekinumab are biologics approved for the treatment of moderate-to-severe psoriasis, but not currently recommended in pregnancy.[12]

However, the existing evidence implies that the risk of biologics in pregnancy is relatively low. Etanercept, infliximab, adalimumab, and ustekinumab, the biologics approved for psoriasis treatment are classified as pregnancy FDA category B drugs, which means that there is no risk from animal studies; however, there are no adequate and controlled studies in women receiving biologic agents during pregnancy. Of these, etanercept, infliximab, and adalimumab belong to the tumor necrosis factor (TNF) inhibitors, which prevent the activation of TNF-α receptor by binding to circulating TNF-α. Ustekinumab is an interleukin (IL)-12/23 inhibitor that blocks the activity of IL12 and IL23 by binding to their p40 subunit.

Biologics should be discontinued in women planning for pregnancy. The period may range from 1–6 months depending on the drug used. Etanercept should be discontinued 1 month prior to conception. Similarly, infliximab, adalimumab, and ustekinumab are to be withheld at least 4–6 months, before pregnancy. Despite some isolated reports of congenital malformations in children exposed to biologics during pregnancy, data on major congenital malformations after exposure to biologics prior to conception or during the first 3 months of pregnancy occur at rates that are lower than the estimated population rate, which is approximately 3%. No specific or consistent pattern of malformations connected to exposure to biologics has been reported so far. However, these studies were undertaken with patients using biologics for indications other than psoriasis. The Organization for Teratology Information Specialists registry reported 100 pregnancies exposed to etanercept, which had similar live birth rates and similar rates of major congenital malformations compared to a control group of pregnant patients with inflammatory arthritis not exposed to etanercept. The same registry reported 66 pregnancies exposed to adalimumab for rheumatoid arthritis during the first trimester, comparing them to non-adalimumab treated patients and healthy controls. There was no increased risk or evidence of a specific pattern of major or minor birth defects connected with adalimumab exposure. Ustekinumab is a relatively new biologic drug and experience during pregnancy is extremely limited. One reported case of its use during pregnancy in a psoriasis patient reported an uncomplicated pregnancy and a healthy infant delivered at term. From the above studies, it may be viewed that termination of pregnancy is not necessary for women that inadvertently become pregnant while taking biologics. An exposure to biologics during the first trimester does not seem to hold an increased risk of congenital defects or other unfavorable outcomes of pregnancy.

Effect of biologics on fetus may to some extent depend on the structure of the molecule and transplacental transfer. The structure of infliximab, adalimumab, and ustekinumab is an immunoglobulin G1 (IgG1) monoclonal antibody, whereas etanercept is a fusion protein. It is well-known that maternal IgG antibodies are large hydrophilic proteins of more than 100 kDa and cannot cross the placenta by simple diffusion, but are actively transported via Fc receptors on the syncytiotrophoblast. These receptors have not been observed before week 14 of gestation; however, the active transport of IgG immunoglobulins begins during the second trimester and rapidly increases over the third trimester, leading to higher fetal levels of IgG in comparison to those in maternal circulation. The half-life of immunoglobulins in an infant is considerably longer than in adults. Infliximab and adalimumab have been found in newborns in much higher concentrations than in their mothers' peripheral blood, and they remain detectable from 2 to 7 months after birth. The median concentration of infliximab, adalimumab measured in cord blood at delivery was 160 and 153% of maternal, respectively. Etanercept, on the other hand, shows considerably less transplacental transport than the IgG immunoglobulins. The concentration of etanercept in cord blood after treatment in the second and third trimester was 4–7% of that in maternal blood.[13] The use of biologics that actively cross the placenta could lead to immunosuppression in the newborn increasing the risk of infection. Fatal disseminated Bacillus Calmette-Guérin infection was reported in an infant after regular vaccination who was delivered to a mother treated with infliximab during pregnancy. Infliximab, adalimumab and ustekinumab, the IgG antibodies, should be discontinued as soon as pregnancy is confirmed. This would probably limit significant intrauterine and postnatal drug exposure of an infant and, likewise, the risk of infection.

The administration of live vaccines in a newborn that was exposed to biologic medication during the late second and third trimester should be postponed until 6–7 months of age or until the biological agent is no longer detectable in the infant circulation. Routine vaccinations with nonlive vaccines appear to be safe and responses appear to be appropriate.

Breastfeeding During Therapy with Biologics

Breastfeeding during therapy with biologics is not generally recommended, although the levels of the drugs detectable in breast milk are significantly lower than those in maternal circulation.

Two to three days after the infusion of infliximab, the milk concentration was 1/200 of that in maternal serum.[14] 6 days after injection of adalimumab, the level of drug detected in milk was 1/100 of that in maternal serum.[15]

Etanercept was detected in milk in extremely small concentrations; namely, 1/800 of that in maternal serum. Absorption of a biologic drug from milk is probably minimal because of protein structure degradation in the infant's digestive system. Therefore, biologic medications could be considered compatible during breastfeeding.[16]

There are limited data on men exposed to biologic drugs at the time of conception. So far, there are no specific reports on adverse pregnancy outcomes.[17]

PREGNANCY OUTCOMES IN WOMEN WITH PSORIASIS

Psoriasis in pregnancy affects both the mother's health and the fetal outcome. The more severe the disease, the worse is the affection.

The disease fortunately does not affect the reproductive system. However, there is higher incidence of infertility in psoriatics than the normal females (Figs 6.4 and 6.5).

Moderate-to-severe psoriasis is associated with spontaneous and induced abortions, pregnancy-induced hypertensive diseases, and premature rupture of membranes, large-for-gestational age newborns, and macrosomia.[3]

Lima XT et al., have evaluated cesarean delivery, pre-eclampsia or eclampsia and spontaneous abortion in pregnant women.[18] For women with psoriasis, there was a 1.89 fold increase in odds of POC (95% confidence interval 1.06–3.39) in the analysis. This

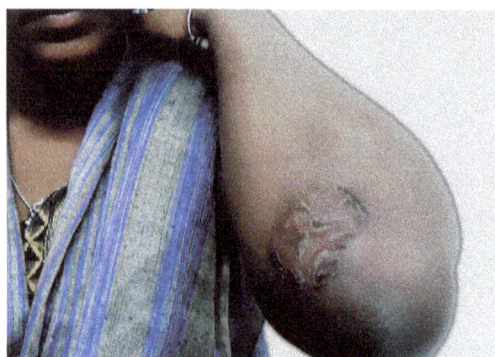

Fig. 6.4: Woman on treatment for primary infertility

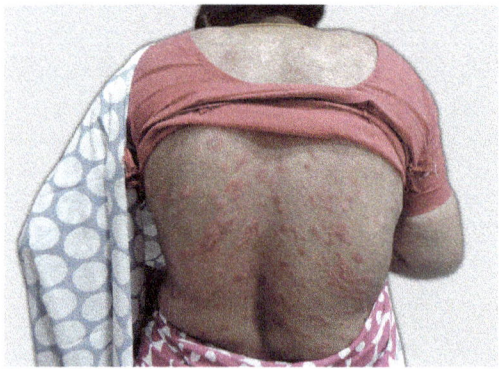

Fig. 6.5: Woman with psoriasis since childhood with infertility

effect remained statistically significant in the multivariable analyses. Psoriasis was not associated with cesarean delivery, pre-eclampsia or eclampsia, and spontaneous abortion. This study has shown higher odds of poor outcome composite in patients with psoriasis.

Therapy of pregnant woman with psoriasis when administered judiciously does not harm the mother or fetus. Drugs which are contraindicated during pregnancy should be avoided.

PSORIASIS AND LACTATION[12]

Lactating women are best treated with topical agents and phototherapy. When there is involvement of the skin over the breast, milk may be expressed and fed to the baby.

Breastfeeding during therapy with biologics is not generally recommended, although the levels of the drugs detectable in breast milk are significantly lower than those in maternal circulation. Infliximab, adalimumab, etanercept were detected in milk in extremely small concentrations; absorption of a biologic drug from milk is probably minimal because of protein structure degradation in the infant's digestive system. Therefore, biologic medications could be compatible during breastfeeding.

Pregnant and lactating women with psoriasis should be managed with caution. Topical therapy including emollients and topical steroids as well as UVB phototherapy is regarded as a safe option for these patients. In the case of uncontrollable psoriasis and a need for more potent systemic treatment, methotrexate and acitretin must be strictly avoided. However, cyclosporine may be considered as an option for controlling the disease. Newer biologic agents are currently not recommended due to a lack of controlled studies in pregnant women. Information regarding their use during pregnancy and lactation is slowly accumulating, mostly from pregnant patients with inflammatory arthritis and inflammatory bowel disease. Biologics may be considered as a possible therapy for pregnant psoriasis patients. Data collected so far show that biologics currently marketed for psoriasis treatment are not connected with higher incidence of unfavorable pregnancy outcomes and congenital malformations. There are concerns about immunosuppression in infants exposed to biologics in the late second and third trimesters of pregnancy, especially to monoclonal IgG antibodies, such as infliximab, adalimumab, and ustekinumab. These drugs actively cross the placenta similarly to natural antibodies, leading to higher infant drug levels at delivery compared to the levels in maternal circulation, and they should be discontinued at least in the second trimester to limit significant intrauterine and postnatal drug exposure of an infant and the risk of infection. The administration of live vaccines in a newborn exposed to biologic medication during the late second and third trimesters should be postponed at least until 6–7 months of age. Breastfeeding during therapy with biologics is currently not recommended; however, it could be considered reasonable in the future because only negligible amounts of drug pass into the milk. The decision to use biological therapy during pregnancy should take into account benefits and risks and should be made on a case-by-case basis after careful discussion with the patient.

CONCLUSION

Psoriasis in pregnancy does affect both the mother's health and the fetal outcome, more so, when the disease is severe.

Topical therapies including emollients and low-to-moderate-potency topical steroids are first-line therapy for patients with limited psoriasis who are pregnant or breast-feeding.

The second-line treatment for pregnant women is NBUVB phototherapy or broadband UVB, if NBUVB is not available.

Lastly, TNF-α inhibitors including adalimumab, etanercept, and infliximab may be used with caution as may cyclosporine and systemic steroids (in second and third trimesters). Some specific strategies may be used to minimize risk and exposure.[8]

Impetigo herpetiformis is a medical emergency requiring multidisciplinary approach. Even if the disease is controlled in the mother, there can still be adverse effect on the fetus which should be born in mid while following up the patient. IH is known to recur during subsequent pregnancy about which the patient and the family should be kept aware of FDA-approved psoriasis treatments and their category for use by pregnant and nursing women are shown in Table 6.1.[19]

TABLE 6.1: Food and Drug Administration categories of drugs

Generic name	FDA category	Comments
Acitretin	X	Causes birth defects. Absolutely avoid
Adalimumab	B	Long-term animal studies showed no harm. No human studies conducted. Avoid unless necessary
Alefacept	B	Long-term animal studies showed no harm. No human studies conducted. Avoid unless necessary
Anthralin	C	No clear evidence of birth defects. Avoid unless necessary
Calcipotriene	C	No clear evidence of birth defects. Avoid unless necessary
Calcipotriene and betamethasone dipropionate	C	No clear evidence of birth defects. Avoid unless necessary
Calcitriol	C	No clear evidence of birth defects. Avoid unless necessary
Cyclosporine	C	No clear evidence of birth defects. Avoid unless necessary
Efalizumab	C	No clear evidence of birth defects. Avoid unless necessary
Etanercept	B	Long-term animal studies showed no harm. No human studies conducted. Avoid unless necessary

Continued

Continued

Generic name	FDA category	Comments
Infliximab	B	Long-term animal studies showed no harm. No human studies conducted. Avoid unless necessary
Methotrexate	X	Even small doses can cause defects in first trimester. Absolutely avoid
PUVA	C	No clear evidence of birth defects, although PUVA affects DNA. Avoid unless necessary
Tazarotene	X	Risk of internal absorption. Absolutely avoid
Topical steroids	C	No clear evidence of birth defects. Avoid unless necessary
UVB	—	Safe during pregnancy. May cause skin discoloration

PUVA, psoralen ultraviolet A; UVB, ultraviolet B; FDA, Food and Drug Administration.

Key: B. Studies with animals have not found risk to the fetus but no studies have been done in humans
C. Safety is not substantiated by animal or human studies
X. Risk in pregnancy outweighs any benefits

REFERENCES

1. Murasse JE, Chan KK, Garite TJ, Cooper DM, Weinstein GD. Hormonal effect on psoriasis in pregnancy and postpartum. Arch Dermatol. 2005;141(5):601-6.
2. Raychaudhuri SP, Navare T, Gross J, Raychaudhuri SK. Clinical course of psoriasis during pregnancy. Int J Dermatol. 2003;42(7):518-20.
3. Cohen-Barak E, Nachum Z, Rozenman D, Ziv M. Pregnancy outcomes in women with moderate-to-severe psoriasis. J Eur Acad Dermatol Venereol. 2011;25:1041-47.
4. Brightman L, Stefanato CM, Bhawan J, Phillips TJ. Third trimester impetigo herpetiformis treated with cyclosporine. J Am Acad Dermatol. 2007;56:S62-4.
5. Cravo M, Vieira R, Telle O, Figueiredo A. Recurrent impetigo herpetiformis successfully treated with methotrexate. J EurAcad Dermatol Venereol. 2009;23:336.
6. Kozlowski RD, Steinbrunner JV, MacKenzie AH, Clough JD, Wilke WS, Segal AM. Outcome of first-trimester exposure to low-dose methotrexate in eight patients with rheumatic disease. Am J Med. 1990;88:589-92.
7. Nguyen C, Duhl AJ, Escallon CS, Blakemore KJ. Multiple anomalies in a fetus exposed to low-dose methotrexate in the first trimester. Obstet Gynecol. 2002;99:599-602.
8. Bae YS, Van Voorhees AS, Hsu S, Korman NJ, Lebwohl MG, Young M, et al. Review of treatment options for psoriasis in pregnant or lactating women: from the Medical Board of the National Psoriasis Foundation. J Am Acad Dermatol. 2012;67(3):459-77.
9. Bar-Oz B, Janice, Hackman R, Tsao S, Zamin M, Tom R, et al. The effects of cyclosporine therapy on pregnancy outcome in organ transplanted women: a meta-analytical review. Pediatric Research. 1999;45:73A-73A.
10. Geiger JM, Baudin M, Saurat JH. Teratogenic risk with etretinate and acitretin treatment. Dermatology. 1994;189:109-16.
11. Rollman O, Pihl-Lundin I. Acitretin excretion into human breast milk. Acta Derm Venereol. 1990;70:487-90.
12. Mervic L. Management of moderate to severe plaque psoriasis in pregnancy and lactation in the era of biologics. Acta Dermatovenerol APA. 2014;23:27-31.
13. Berthelsen BG, Fjeldsoe-Nielsen H, Christoffer T, Nielsen CT, Hellmut E. Etanercept concentrations in maternal serum, umbilical cord serum, breast milk and child serum during breastfeeding. Rheumatology. 2010;49:2225-7.
14. Ben-Horin S, Yavzori M, Kopylov U, Picard O, Fudim E, Eliakim R, et al. Detection of infliximab in breast milk of nursing mothers with inflammatory bowel disease. J Crohns Colitis. 2011;5:555-8.
15. Ben-Horin S, Yavzori M, Katz L, Picard O, Fudim E, Chowers Y, et al. Adalimumab level in breast milk of a nursing mother. Clin Gastroenterol Hepatol. 2010;8:475-6.
16. Hyrich KL, Verstappen SM. Biologic therapies and pregnancy: the story so far. Rheumatology (Oxford). 2014;53(8):1377-85.
17. Saougou I, Markatseli TE, Papagoras C, Kaltsonoudis E, Voulgari PV, Drosos AA. Fertility in male patients with seronegative spondylo arthropathies treated with infliximab. Joint Bone Spine. 2013;80:34-7.
18. Lima XT, Janakiraman V, Hughes MD, Kimbal AB. The impact of psoriasis on pregnancy outcomes. J Investigative Dermatol. 2012;132:85-91.
19. Food Drug Administration determinations for pregnant and nursing women. National psoriasis foundation. [online] Available from https://www.psoriasis.org/pregnancy/fda-determinations [Accessed August, 2015].

CHAPTER 7

Psoriasis and Human Immunodeficiency Virus

INTRODUCTION

Psoriasis and human immunodeficiency virus (HIV) infection do not influence each other with reference to predisposition and prevalence. However, the manifestation, severity, and response to treatment may vary significantly between psoriatic with and without HIV infection. The challenge lies is in the treatment of a patient with HIV infection having severe psoriasis with metabolic comorbidities where most of the drugs otherwise useful in the management of psoriasis are not advisable. This chapter will also mention a few lines about HIV-associated Reiter's disease and pityriasis rubra pilaris (PRP) both having psoriasis form skin lesions and follicular involvement, respectively.

PSORIASIS AND HUMAN IMMUNODEFICIENCY VIRUS

Unlike some dermatoses that have a higher frequency in patients infected with HIV, psoriasis presents a similar prevalence in these patients, to that of the general population. Psoriasis in these patients, however, presents certain clinical and therapeutic characteristics (Figs 7.1A to G). The main features of HIV-associated psoriasis are: sudden onset of the disease, with increased frequency of joint involvement. Pustular forms of psoriasis and severe nail involvement are other manifestations frequently observed with HIV-positive patients. Patients with severe psoriasis with a positive HIV test show severe involvement of the flexural areas. Similarly, palmoplantar psoriasis in HIV-positive persons manifest with diffuse involvement and keratoderma. Features of HIV-associated psoriasis are given in Box 7.1.

Sudden exacerbation of extensive and severe inflammatory psoriasis should indicatesuspected HIV inspection and requires a serological analysis. In patients already diagnosed with HIV, the considerable efficacy of the new antiretroviral drugs has meant that the classical clinical forms predominate due to the improved immune status of these patients. HIV-positive patients present different types of spondyloarthropathy in which severe joint involvement is observed,

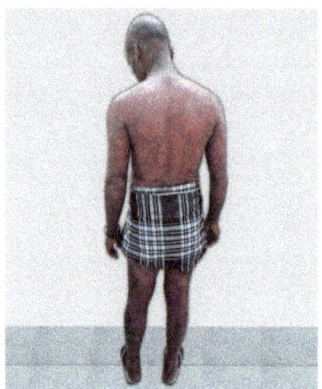

Fig. 7.1A: Human immunodeficiency virus positive man with sudden onset of psoriasis

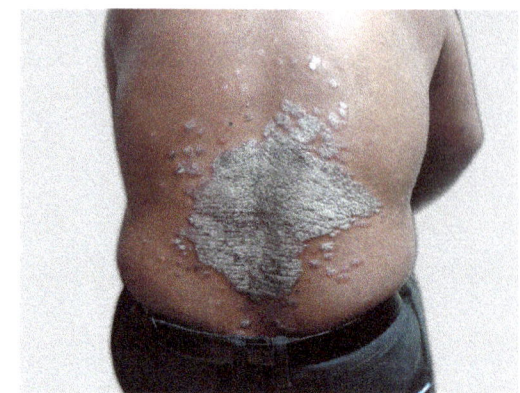

Fig. 7.1B: Severe form of psoriasis in Human immunodeficiency virus positive man resistant to treatment

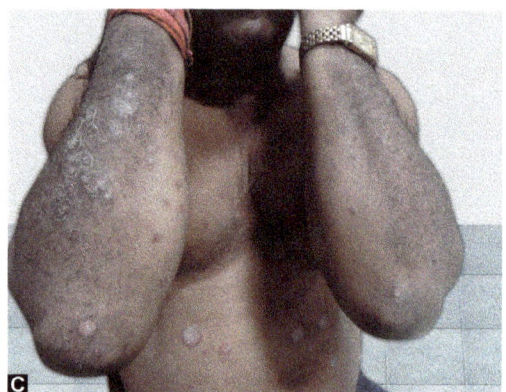

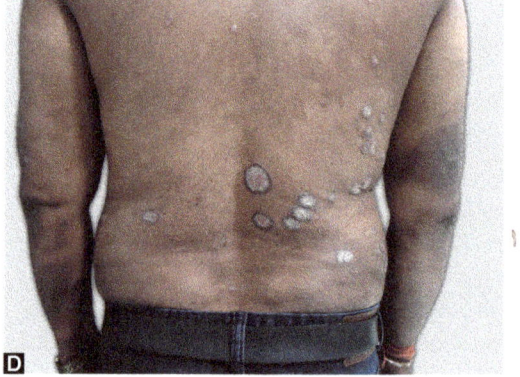

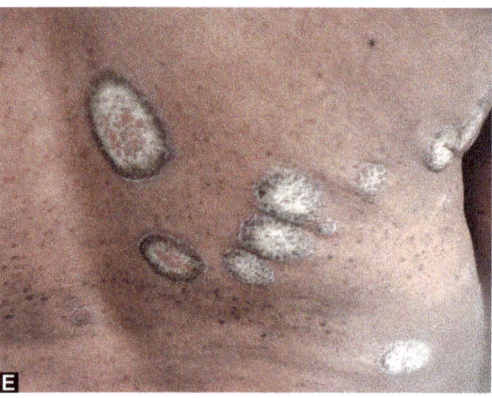

Figs 7.1C to E: Patient on zidovudine showing improvement with acitretin

with joint destruction; they also present nail involvement and associated palmoplantar lesions. Joint involvement in patients with psoriasis and HIV infection is aggressive and is more prevalent and clinically more florid than in HIV-negative patients. Unlike in

REITER'S DISEASE

Reiter's syndrome illustrates the difficulty of differential diagnosis in HIV-positive patients, due to the severe joint involvement and the varied morphology of the lesions that may develop in patients with psoriasis (Figs 7.2A to C). Diagnosis of Reiter's disease is indicated by the characteristic triad of polyarthritis, urethritis, and conjunctivitis, together with the typical psoriasis form skin lesions. CUSP syndrome is an acronym used for the manifestation of Reiter's

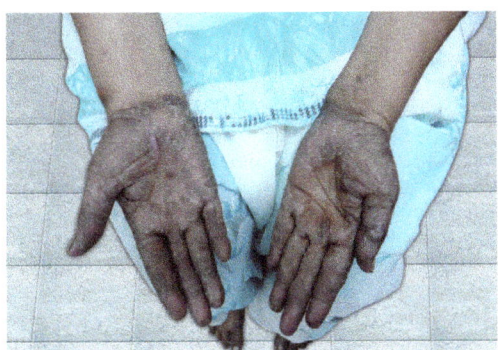

Fig. 7.1F: Severe involvement of palm as keratoderma in human immunodeficiency virus positive woman

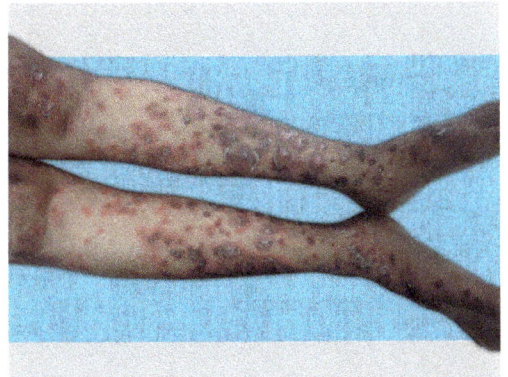

Fig. 7.1G: Pustular lesions in human immunodeficiency virus positive psoriasis patient

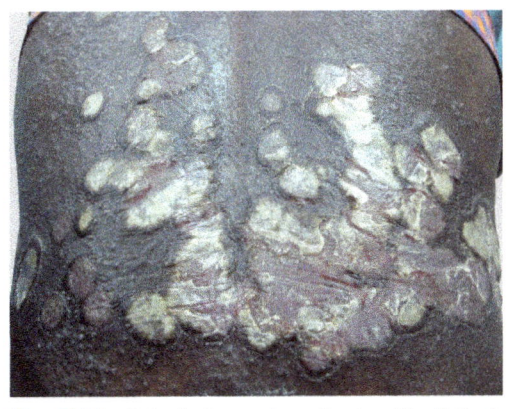

Fig. 7.2A: Skin lesions of patient with Reiter's syndrome

BOX 7.1: Features of HIV-associated psoriasis

- Sudden onset
- Palmoplantar keratoderma
- Severe nail dystrophy
- Involvement of skinfolds
- Pustular forms
- High frequency of arthritis

Reiter's disease, sacroiliac involvement is rare in these patients. The prevalence of Reiter, disease is, therefore, higher in HIV-positive patients than in the general population.[1]

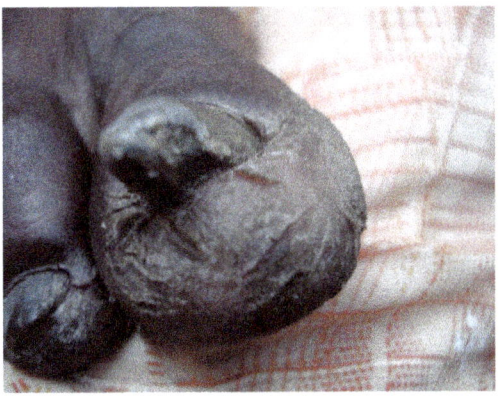

Fig. 7.2B: human immunodeficiency virus positive patient with Rieter's syndrome having nail change

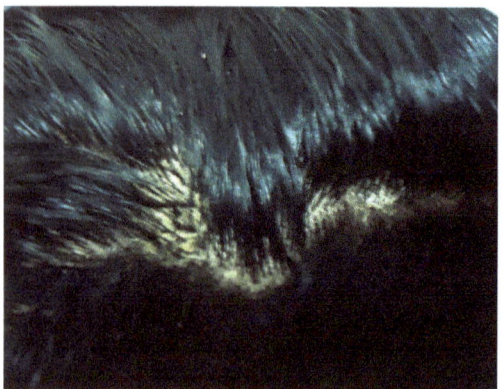

Fig. 7.2C: Thick scales on the scalp in Reiter's syndrome in a patient on zidovudine

disease, having conjunctivitis, urethritis, seronegative arthritis, and psoriasiform skin lesions. It is worth testing these patients for HIV status.

The disease is most frequent among young men and the association with human leukocyte antigen B27 is a characteristic finding, which is present in between approximately 80% and 90% of patients. Patients with this association typically have more serious disease.

Typical of the disease are episodes of vesicular-pustular lesions on the palms and soles; over the course of the episode, the lesions coalesce, progressing to scabs, and hyperkeratosis.

Also, typical are genital involvement in the form of circinate balanitis and involvement of the nails. The extensor surface of the limbs and the scalp may also be affected, though to a lesser extent. Due to the clinical similarity to psoriasis lesions, diagnosis requires the presence of more elements of the triad. There seems to be an intimate link between "psoriatic arthritis" (PsA) and "Reiter's syndrome".[2] The association with HIV is higher in these patients than those with psoriasis.

PITYRIASIS RUBRA PILARIS

Pityriasis rubra pilaris also called follicular psoriasis, from which it differs histologically, is a rare disease that is clinically characterized by the appearance of follicular hyperkeratotic papules on an erythematous base. The lesions show a marked tendency to coalesce, extending in a caudal direction and leaving islands of sparing. Involvement of the palms and soles also often occurs in the form of reddish orange keratoderma with a waxy appearance. Development of varying degrees of erythroderma is characteristic of the disease. Most cases of PRP are acquired, though occasional familial cases occur. Different environmental factors have been suggested as triggers including infections, particularly HIV. PRP is divided into five categories, depending on age, duration, and type of skin involvement. A sixth category has been proposed for the form of PRP-associated with HIV infection (Figs 7.3A and B).

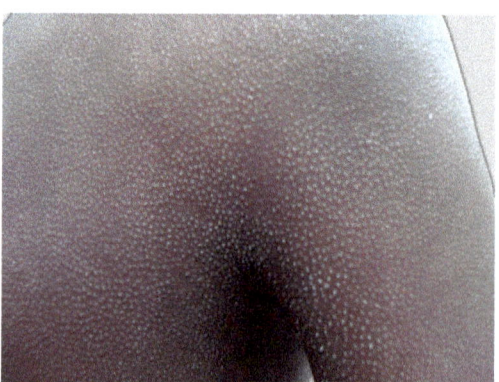

Fig. 7.3A: Classical grouped follicular papules of pityriasis rubra pilaris

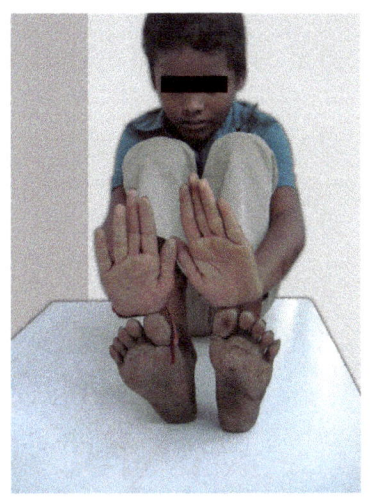

Fig. 7.3B: Palmoplantar keratoderma of pityriasis rubra pilaris. This child was seronegative

TREATMENT OF PSORIASIS IN HUMAN IMMUNODEFICIENCY SYNDROME AFFECTED PATIENTS

Psoriasis occurs with at least undiminished frequency in HIV-infected individuals. The behavior of psoriasis in HIV disease is of interest, in terms of pathogenesis and therapy because of the background of profound immune dysregulation. It is paradoxical that, while drugs that target T lymphocytes are effective in psoriasis, the condition should be exacerbated by HIV infection.

HIV-associated psoriasis is often refractory to traditional treatments. Treatment is challenging and requires careful consideration. Selection of drugs should be tailored to suit individual patient based on disease severity and the input from an infectious disease specialist. Close monitoring for potential adverse events is necessary.[3]

Psoriasis in the setting of HIV disease may be mild, moderate or severe. Standard therapies and zidovudine are effective in the management. Survival does not seem to be adversely affected by the presence of psoriasis or its therapy. Zidovudine therapy, at a dosage of 1200 mg/d, appears to be beneficial in the treatment of HIV-associated psoriasis, although long-term relapses occurred and the associated arthritis did not seem to improve.[4]

Oral gold was found to be safe and useful in a woman in the treatment of disabling PsA with HIV infection, in whom CD4 count during oral gold therapy showed a significant, sustained increase in CD4 cells.[5]

According to Chiricozzi A et al., psoriasis is a chronic, inflammatory disease affecting 2-3% of the worldwide population, may worsen with HIV or be detected as HIV cutaneous manifestation. However, according to the authors, there does not seem to an increase in the prevalence of HIV positivity in psoriasis or vice versa. HIV-related psoriasis shows a severe and prolonged clinical course with more frequent exacerbations. The management of this condition is challenging because immune modulating and immune suppressant agents may have variable and partial efficacy, and therefore, antiretroviral treatment represents a potential adjunctive therapeutic option. The HIV test should be considered in high-risk patients affected by severe psoriasis and resistant to conventional and biological treatments.[6]

Following will be the summary of treatment options in HIV-associated psoriasis:
- Mild-to-moderate disease
  o Topical therapy is the first-line recommended treatment
  o UVB can be considered as second-line therapy
- Moderate-to-severe disease
  o Phototherapy is the recommended first-line therapeutic agents
  o Oral retinoids may be used as second-line treatment
- Refractory, severe disease
  o Cyclosporine

- o Methotrexate
- o Hydroxyurea

Tumor necrosis factor-α inhibitors may be considered and used with extreme caution.

Since skin lesions of patients with therapy-resistant, acquired immunodeficiency syndrome (AIDS)-associated psoriasis have been reported to clear with oral zidovudine, this drug may be considered in retinoid-resistant AIDS-associated psoriasis, where methotrexate, cyclosporine, and photochemotherapy psoralen and ultraviolet A may be contraindicated.

CONCLUSION

The incidence and prevalence of psoriasis in HIV-positive patients is not much different from those with a negative serology. Possible epidermal proliferative effect and increased production of nitic oxide driven by the virus along with the altered CD8/CD4 ratio account for the pathogenesis of psoriasis in HIV-infected patients. Sudden onset, inverse and pustular forms, palmoplantar keratoderma, severe nail dystrophy, and high frequency of arthritis are features of HIV-associated psoriasis. Phototherapy and antiretroviral therapy are the best ways to manage these patients.

REFERENCES

1. Leal L, Ribera M, Daudénb E. Psoriasis and HIV infection. Actas Dermosifiliogr. 2008;99:753-63.
2. Wright V, Reed WB. The link between Reiter's syndrome and psoriatic arthritis. Ann Rheum Dis. 1964;23:12.
3. Menon K, Van Voorhees AS, Bebo BF, Gladman DD, Hsu S, Kalb RE, et.al. Psoriasis in patients with HIV infection: from the medical board of the National Psoriasis Foundation. J Am Acad Dermatol. 2010;62:291-9.
4. Duvic M, Crane MM, Conant M, Mahoney SE, Reveille JD, Lehrman SN. Zidovudine improves psoriasis in human immunodeficiency virus-positive males. Arch Dermatol. 1994;130:447-51.
5. Shapiro DL, Masci JR. Treatment of HIV associated psoriatic arthritis with oral gold. J Rheumatol. 1996;23:1818-20.
6. Chiricozzi A, Saraceno R, Cannizzaro MV, Nisticò SP, Chimenti S, Giunta A. Complete resolution of erythrodermic psoriasis in an HIV and HCV patient unresponsive to antipsoriatic treatments after highly active antiretroviral therapy (Ritonavir, Atazanavir, Emtricitabine, Tenofovir). Dermatology. 2012;225(4):333-7.

CHAPTER 8

Psoriasis as a Systemic Disease

INTRODUCTION

Psoriasis is now classified as an immune-mediated inflammatory disease (IMID) of the skin. Patients with various IMIDs are at higher risk of developing "systemic" comorbidities. IMIDs may impact these comorbid conditions through shared genetic, environmental factors, or common inflammatory pathways that are coexpressed in IMIDs and target organs (Fig. 8.1). The presence of a higher than expected prevalence of an entity in combination with another disorder, among psoriasis patients, has been known for decades.

Psoriasis patients are frequently obese, unknowingly at greater risk than general population for myocardial infarction (MI), metabolic syndrome (MBS), and other comorbidities. There is strong evidence to suggest that psoriasis is an independent risk factor for the development of metabolic and cardiovascular comorbidities. Having observed these findings consistently by many authors, the questions that arise are:

- Is psoriasis a cutaneous disease or systemic disease?

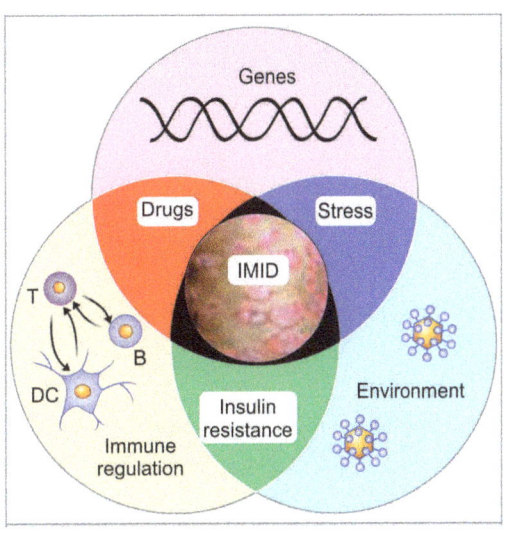

B, B-lymphocyte; DC, Dendritic Cell; T, T-lymphocyte; IMID, immune-mediated inflammatory disease.

Fig. 8.1: Psoriasis: a systemic disease—the missing link: picture depicting the interplay of various factors involved in the genesis of psoriasis

- Is psoriasis a marker of underlying systemic disease?
- Is psoriasis a risk factor for systemic disease?
- What are the potential mechanistic links between psoriasis and systemic comorbid conditions?

With the advancing research that is going on, it is proved beyond doubt that psoriasis can now be considered as a systemic disease. Psoriasis, by itself, predisposes an individual to other systemic diseases and therefore, is viewed as a marker of such systemic illness. There is strong evidence to suggest that psoriasis is an independent risk factor for the development of metabolic and cardiovascular comorbidities. Probably, the connecting link is the persistent inflammation that triggers off, and perpetuates the comorbid manifestations.

Mediators of inflammation produced in the skin are released into the systemic circulation and thus, may contribute to the increased risk of inflammation in additional organs or tissues (Fig. 8.2). Psoriasis being an IMID, is capable of injuring the other organ system through a cascade of events. Insulin resistance and endothelial damage lead to organ dysfunction either directly or indirectly. There seems to exist a common pathway driven by many of the proinflammatory cytokines, such as tumor necrosis factor-α (TNF-α), T helper (Th) 1 and interleukin-6 (IL-6) in the pathogenesis of psoriasis and its comorbidities.[1]

The systemic disease that are more common in patients with psoriasis (Fig. 8.3)

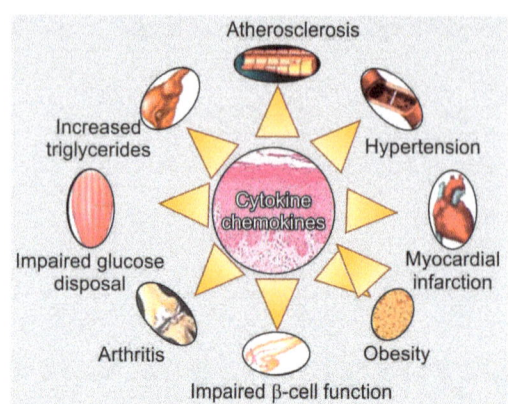

Fig. 8.2: Inflammatory mediators of psoriasis leading to organ damage

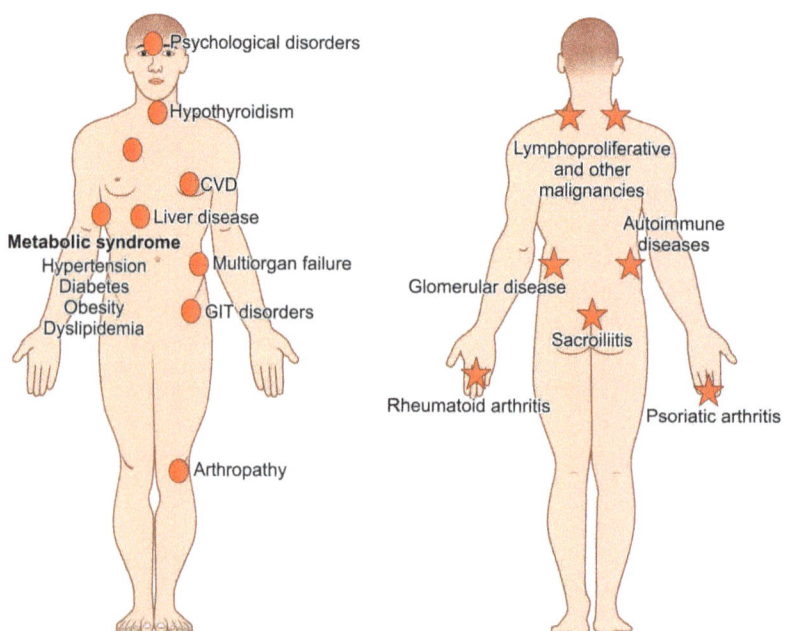

COPD, chronic obstructive pulmonary disease; GIT, gastrointestinal tract; CVD, cardiovascular disease.

Fig. 8.3: Systemic diseases in psoriasis

Psoriasis as a Systemic Disease

> **BOX 8.1: Psoriasis and systemic disease**
>
> - Arthropathy/arthritis
> - Psychological disorders
> - Hypertension
> - Cardiovascular disease
> - Metabolic syndrome
> - Insulin resistance and diabetes
> - Pulmonary Disease
> - Gastrointestinal tract and liver disease
> - Autoimmune and collagen vascular diseases
> - Renal disease
> - Multiorgan failure
> - Malignancy

are, arthropathy or arthritis, psychological disorders, hypertension, cardiovascular disease, chronic obstructive pulmonary disease, MBS, insulin resistance, diabetes, celiac disease, autoimmune and collagen vascular diseases, malignancy. The following section will deal with psoriasis and associated diseases of various systems.

Various systemic diseases seen in psoriasis are listed in Box 8.1.

PSORIATIC ARTHROPATHY AND ARTHRITIS

When genetically primed individual is exposed to a bacterial, stress, or entheseal-related peptide, the innate immune response, gets activated resulting in CD8 infiltration and chemokine or cytokine release. The process is amplified with angiogenesis and cellular infiltration of involved tissues. Human leukocyte antigen and other genes expressed may determine the exact pattern of tissue involvement. In as many as 15–20% of patients, arthritis appears before the skin involvement in psoriasis.[2] 40–57% have deforming arthritis. Nearly one-fifth of them have more than five joints involved. Spine is involved in as high as 40%. Psoriatic arthritis (PsA) leads to disability in nearly one-fifth of the affected individuals. The mortality is increased than the general population. The morbidity and mortality can be reduced if the inflammation can be controlled at an early stage. For a detailed description of (PsA) the reader is suggested to refer to chapter 4.

Psychological aspects of psoriasis will be discussed separately in chapter 12.

HYPERTENSION

There are many reports supporting the fact that patients with psoriasis are more prone to develop hypertension (Figs 8.4A to C). Drugs like β-blockers used in the management of hypertension can precipitate, sustain or perpetuate psoriasis. In a large study with multivariate analysis, hypertension was found to be more frequently associated with psoriasis after controlling for age, sex, smoking status, obesity, diabetes, non-steroidal anti-inflammatory drugs (NSAIDs), and use of cyclooxygenase-2 (COX-2) COX-2 inhibitors supporting the previously noted association between psoriasis and hypertension.[3] Association between psoriasis and hypertension may be attributed to

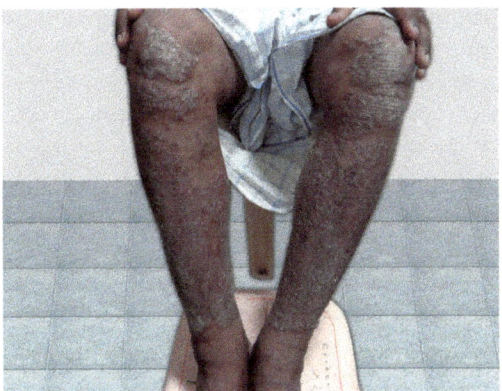

Fig. 8.4A: Patient with psoriasis detected to have systemic hypertension on screening

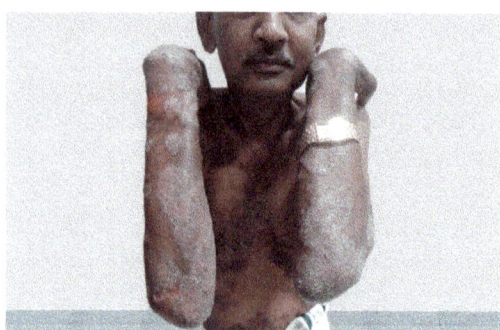

Fig. 8.4B: Patient with hypertension

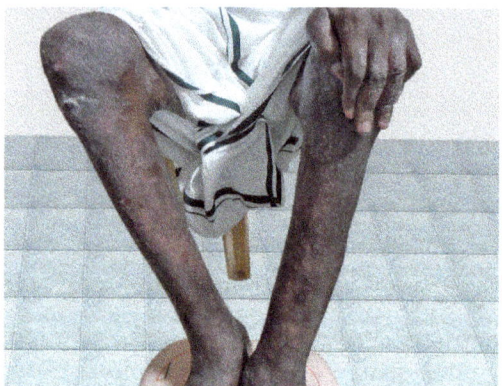

Fig. 8.4C: Patient with systemic hypertension on long-term β-blockers

angiotensin II, a product of angiotensin-converting enzyme that regulates vascular tone and stimulates the release of proinflammatory cytokines. Elevated plasma renin activity and endothelin-1 seen in both sera and lesional skin of patients with psoriasis may contribute to the pathogenesis of hypertension in psoriasis patients. Endothelial damage due to oxidative stress present in patients with psoriasis, may further add to the development of hypertension by destructive effects of reactive oxygen species, damaging endothelium-dependent vasodilatation. NSAIDs and COX-2 inhibitors used for PsA could also contribute to increased blood pressure. Similarly, β-blockers used for control of hypertension can further worsen psoriasis thus, inducing a vicious cycle. When adjusted for age and sex, the association between psoriasis and hypertension appears to be significant mainly above the age of 40 years. Therefore, it is mandatory that all psoriatics above 40 years of age are screened for hypertension.

PSORIASIS AND CARDIOVASCULAR DISEASE OR ATHEROTHROMBOTIC DISEASES

Of emerging significance is the relationship between cardiovascular disease and severe psoriasis, as this may explain the increased mortality of the latter.[4] Severe psoriasis is a chronic systemic inflammatory disorder. It increases the inflammatory burden of the patient and causes a state of insulin resistance, resulting in endothelial cell dysfunction and atherosclerosis. At the level of coronary arteries, such changes result in MI. Atherosclerosis involving the carotid and cerebral arteries may result in stroke. Psoriasis and PsA are associated with increased atherothrombotic diseases, including myocardial infarction, deep venous thrombosis, and reduced life span (Figs 8.5A and B).

Comorbidity of psoriasis includes cardiovascular diseases, among others like obesity, lymphomas, and depression. The relationship between cardiovascular diseases and psoriasis is of particular importance, as it explains in part, the increased mortality of patients with severe psoriasis.

There is increasing epidemiologic evidence to suggest that severe psoriasis is a relevant and independent cardiovascular risk factor.

All physicians should be aware that severe psoriasis may increase cardiovascular morbidity and the risk of death, and preventive strategies for patients with severe disease should be considered.[5]

Psoriasis as a Systemic Disease

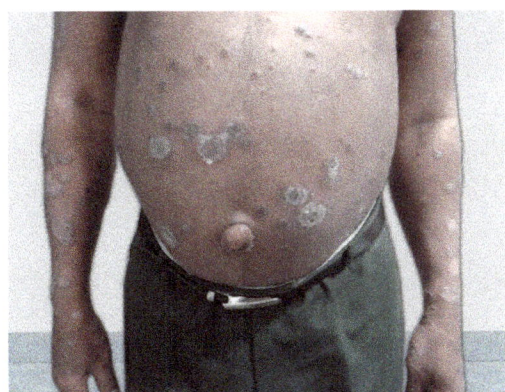

Fig. 8.5A: Man developed myocardial infarction who was having psoriasis for 5 years before the infarct

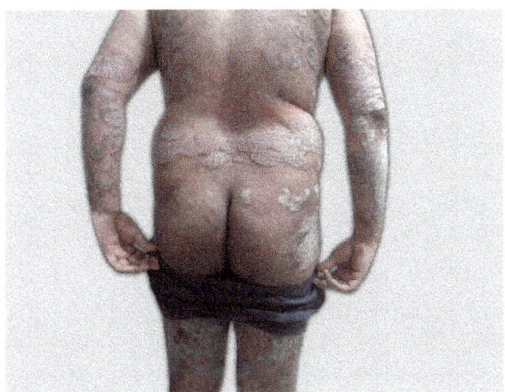

Fig. 8.5B: Patient had myocardial infarction 1 year after the onset of psoriasis

Several of the epidemiological studies confirm that the cardiovascular risk of psoriasis patients depends on the severity of their disease which is evident from the fact that in patients suffering from severe psoriasis exhibit increased mortality when compared to the outpatients with mild psoriasis.

This segment will look into the following aspects:
- How inflammation can lead to MI
- MI and other cardiovascular changes in psoriasis.

Role of Inflammation in the Development of Atherosclerosis

Endothelial cell dysfunction is an imbalance in release of vasodilating factors, such as nitric oxide and prostacyclin, and vasoconstricting factors, such as endothelin-1 and angiotensin-II. It has been proved that endothelin appears to be produced by keratinocytes and endothelin-1 levels are significantly elevated in psoriasis. Therefore, an imbalance between the vasoconstriction and vasodilating factors predisposes the endothelium toward an atherogenic milieu. Adhesion-mediated leukocyte extravasation, which is facilitated by activated platelets and followed by infiltrating macrophages, releasing cytokines, and enzymes, such as matrix metalloproteinases, thus degrading the connective tissue matrix. Once the connective tissue matrix is degraded, there are accumulation of lipid-rich necrotic debris leading to the formation of a more advanced fibrous lesion. This fibrous plaque due to the continued effect of inflammation develops into an unstable plaque which can easily get dislodged and cause thromboembolic complication. Depending on the vessel involved, such thromboembolic phenomenon can result in major catastrophe, such as MI or stroke.

Role of Inflammation in Inducing Myocardial Infarction

Several biomarkers and adipokines like C-reactive protein (CRP) vascular endothelial growth factor (VEGF), P-selectin, resistin, and leptin have been observed to be elevated in the blood of psoriasis patients, indicating a state of systemic inflammation.

It is of interest to note that the adipokine milieu in the blood of psoriasis patients is strikingly similar of that in prediabetic individuals, the latter exhibiting signs of insulin resistance.

Hence, it can be concluded that it is the smoldering inflammation that probably leads to insulin resistance, which in turn triggers endothelial cell dysfunction, subsequently leading to atherosclerosis and finally, MI. Continuous effective systemic therapy may interfere with insulin resistance and endothelial dysfunction, thereby preventing major catastrophe like MI. A simple diagrammatic representation of cascade of events is depicted in the Figure 8.5C.

Among the various risk factors, some are considered disease specific while others are disease nonspecific. Disease specific risk factors are those that are a direct consequence of psoriasis inflammation:
- Hyperhomocysteinemia
- Elevated CRP
- Elevated blood inflammatory cytokines
- Platelet hyperactivity.

Psoriasis non-disease specific risk factors include:
- Insulin resistance or diabetes

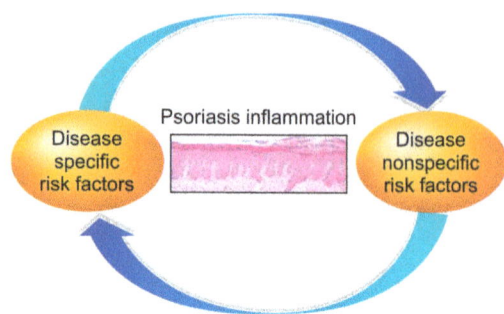

Fig. 8.6: Risk factors involved in perpetuation of cardiac disease

- Obesity
- Dyslipidemia
- Hypertension
- MBS
- Habitual tobacco smoking.

Both disease specific and non-disease specific risk factors are likely to fuel one another in deleterious vicious circles. Patients with psoriasis should be treated effectively and encouraged to aggressively correct their modifiable cardiovascular risk factors (Fig. 8.6).

Cytokine activated leukocytes in the skin enter circulation after rolling on inflamed endothelial cells in psoriatic plaques. The inflammatory chemokines released into the systemic circulation, like TNF, IL-1 or IL-6, may alter the function of hepatocytes, vascular cells, leukocyte physiology, and increase cardiovascular risk factors or overt pathological pathways.

Myocardial Infarction and Other Cardiovascular Changes in Psoriasis

There is an age-dependent increase in MI among psoriatic patients compared with control population. Young patients with severe disease have the greatest risks, which is still worse in females. Psoriasis was found to be an independent risk factor for MI,

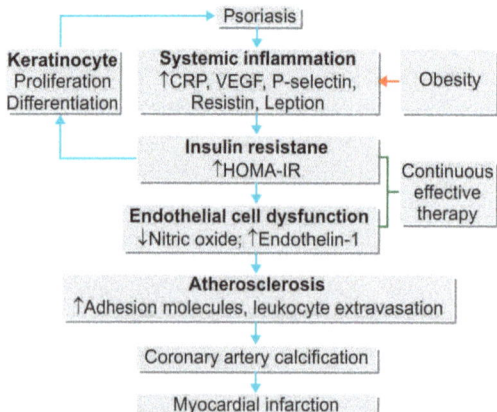

CRP, C-reactive protein; VEGF, vascular endothelial growth factor; HOMA-IR, homeostatic model assessment-insulin resistance.

Fig. 8.5C: Cascade of events to show how inflammation leads to myocardial infarction in psoriasis, if left untreated

after adjustment for other confounding conditions for cardiovascular disease, such as hypertension, diabetes, history of MI, hyperlipidemia, age, sex, smoking, and body mass index (BMI). According to Gelfand JM, psoriasis may confer an independent risk of MI. The relative risk was greatest in young patients with severe psoriasis.[6]

Psoriasis is associated with increased risk of atrial fibrillation (AF) and ischemic stroke. These novel results add to a growing body of evidence, suggesting that patients with psoriasis could be considered at increased cardiovascular risk.[7] A Cohort study of the entire Danish population including all individuals who experienced first-time MI conducted by Ahlehoff O et al. on the impact of psoriasis on prognosis after first-time MI indicated a significantly impaired prognosis in patients with psoriasis. This study included 462 patients with psoriasis and 48935 controls who were identified with first-time MI during the study period.[8] According to Mehta NN et al., severe psoriasis confers an additional 6.2% absolute risk of a 10-year rate of major adverse cardiac events compared with the general population. This potentially has important therapeutic implications for cardiovascular risk stratification and prevention in patients with severe psoriasis. Future prospective studies are needed to validate these findings.[9] It has been shown that cardiovascular biomarkers are altered in patients with psoriasis.

METABOLIC SYNDROME

Metabolic syndrome is defined as the presence of three or more of the following components:
- Abdominal obesity
- Increased insulin resistance or elevated fasting glucose level
- Decreased high-density lipoprotein cholesterol
- Hypertriglyceridemia
- Hypertension.

The factors defining MBS go hand in hand with an increased risk for diabetes and atherosclerotic cardiovascular disease. Emerging data clearly indicate that psoriasis might be an independent risk factor for cardiovascular disease even after correcting for components of the MBS. The incidence of one or more of the components of MBS is much higher in female patients over 40 years of age.[10] The incidence of one or more of the components in females is as high as 88.5% whereas it ranges from 52%–56%, if both genders are taken into consideration.

Obesity and Psoriasis

Adipocytes produce CRP and proinflammatory cytokines under the influence of inflammatory mediators, such as TNF-α suggesting that that an interplay may exist between adipocytes and the inflammation that drives psoriasis. There is distinct interaction between adipokines and Th17 cytokines is involved in the pathogenesis of psoriasis. As systemic inflammation drives the development of disease, adiponectin is down-regulated while leptin and resistin are simultaneously upregulated. Leptin plays a key role in metabolism and enhances macrophage activity, upregulating TNF-α and IL-6, the latter of which promotes CRP production. Resistin, being a secretory factor linked to inflammation that drives insulin resistance, favors the development of atherosclerosis. Overall, compared with the general population, psoriasis patients have higher prevalence and incidence of obesity. Patients with severe psoriasis have greater odds of obesity than those with mild psoriasis. Whether obesity is a contributing factor to or a manifestation of psoriasis is still under debate. Recent data suggest that obesity is a

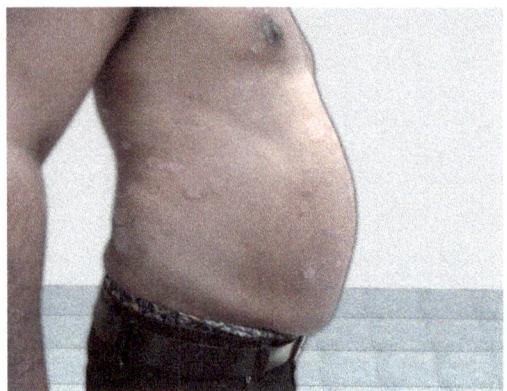

Fig. 8.7A: Psoriasis and obesity a potential risk factor

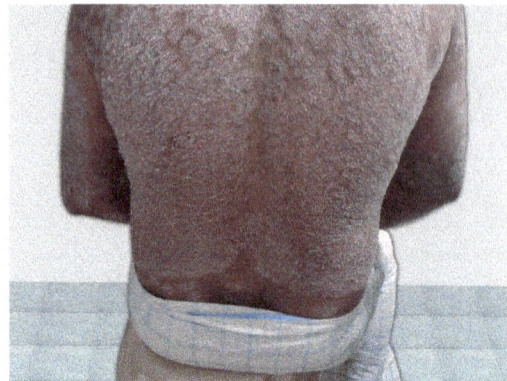

Fig. 8.7C: Patient on statin for dyslipidemia needs strict control of both skin disease and lipid profile

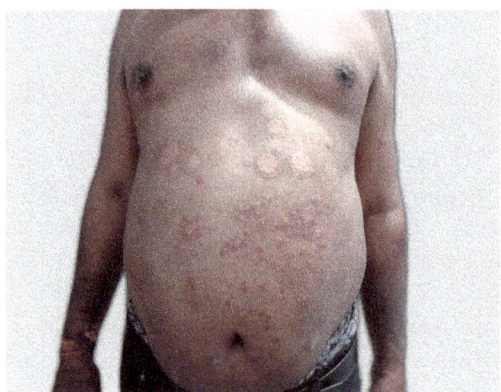

Fig. 8.7B: Same patient as in Fig. 8.7A

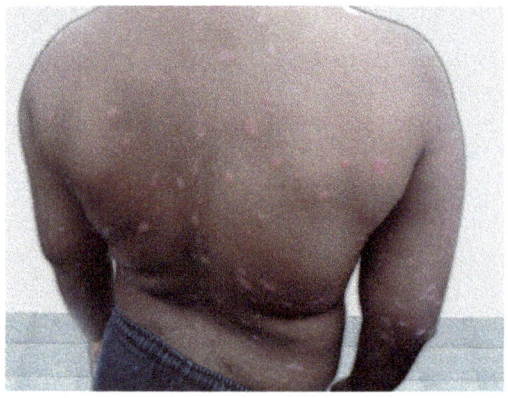

Fig. 8.7D: Same patient as in Fig. 8.7C

risk factor for the development of psoriasis (Figs 8.7A to D). Those data which indicate that BMI increased in patients after psoriasis diagnosis, suggest that obesity is secondary to psoriasis. Irrespective of whether obesity is cause or consequence of psoriasis, it has been noted that increased BMI coincides with a greater degree of psoriasis disease severity.

Defining risk factors leading to comorbidities is important in psoriasis. Eating disorders (EDs) seem to have an impact on the development of MBS in psoriasis. Establishment and treatment of EDs in patients with psoriasis may prevent the onset of MBS and other comorbidities due to MBS.[11]

INSULIN RESISTANCE OR DIABETES

There is significant association between psoriasis, diabetes, and insulin resistance.

Psoriasis is chronic systemic inflammatory disorder characterized by remission and exacerbation. It is documented that chronic and severe disease will increase the inflammatory burden. This increased and prolonged inflammatory burden leads to a state of insulin resistance, resulting in endothelial cell dysfunction. This can further result in atherosclerosis leading to MI or stroke depending on the level of damage and the involved vessel, be it coronary, carotid or the cerebral arteries (Fig. 8.8).

Patients with psoriasis were more insulin resistant compared with healthy control subjects. This supports that psoriasis may be a prediabetic condition.[12] Insulin has dual effects on endothelial cells. On one hand, insulin can induce nitric oxide-dependent vasodilation. On the other hand, insulin can activate the proatherogenic mitogen-activated protein (MAP) kinase pathway.[13] Several measurements indicative of insulin resistance were found to be significantly correlated with the psoriasis area and severity index (PASI) score. The concept of insulin resistance as a consequence of chronic inflammation and possible pathogenetic cause for comorbidities known to be associated with psoriasis is supported by these data.[14] Systemic inflammation causing insulin resistance, in turn, triggers endothelial cell dysfunction, subsequently leading to atherosclerosis and finally MI or stroke. Obesity, being a known risk factor for psoriasis, may induce the phenotype through systemic inflammation further leading to insulin resistance which increases keratinocyte proliferation and reduce differentiation. This further perpetuates the skin disease, thus keeping the vicious cycle on. There is increased prevalence and incidence of diabetes in psoriatics, the association being strongest among patients with severe psoriasis. According to a research data, those with severe psoriasis were 46% more likely to get diabetes than people without the condition, after weight and other health measures were taken into account.

Pathogenesis of insulin resistance is complex and the effect of insulin resistance on patients with psoriasis is still more complex with reference to both the skin disease and the systemic complications of psoriasis. It is probably the constant interplay between adipokines and cytokines associated with psoriasis that leads to a state of insulin resistance.

In obese individuals, adipose tissue macrophages constitute 40% of adipose tissue and produce various adipokines. These adipokines are capable of influencing glucose metabolism. Visceral adipose tissue, thus can act as an endocrine organ and play a role in the development of the MBS and type 2 diabetes mellitus (T2DM). It is documented that prevalence of obesity is more in psoriatics; these adipose tissue may contribute to the development of insulin resistance in such patients by secreting such adipokines.

Resistin, leptin, and adiponectin are secreted by the adipocytes and the first two are responsible for the development of insulin resistance, while adiponectin is negatively associated. Resistin is a polypeptide synthesized by monocytes and macrophages in fat tissue, capable of promoting synthesis of TNF-α which is involved in the pathogenesis of psoriasis. A

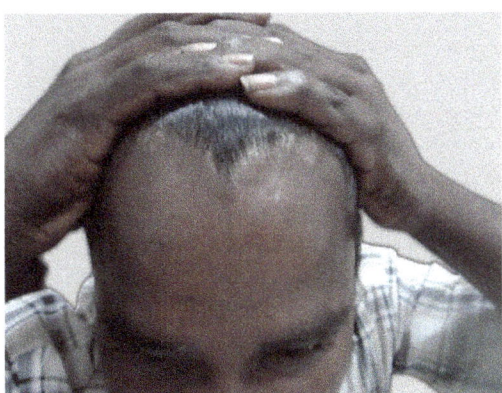

Fig. 8.8: Obese man with patterned hair loss, obesity, dyslipidemia whose father a known case of psoriasis died of myocardial infarction

link between resistin and insulin resistance has been demonstrated.

Psoriasis severity and PASI scores are associated with elevated levels of resistin, and indeed, levels of resistin fall with therapy. Leptin, a polypeptide also produced by adipocytes, acts as a neuropeptide to reduce appetite and therefore, regulate food consumption. Leptin deficiency is a pathological cause of obesity, however, in patients who are obese due to excess food consumption and insufficient exertion, leptin levels are high, and this hyper leptinemia is a risk factor for T2DM. It is also postulated that leptin may in fact contribute to the development of psoriasis by promoting Th1 cytokine synthesis.

Adiponectin, produced by the abdominal adipose tissue is a polypeptide that has both anti-inflammatory and antiatherogenic effects. However, both patients with T2DM and psoriasis have lower levels of adiponectin than controls, and interestingly, adiponectin levels are negatively correlated with both disease severity, as indicated by PASI scores, and plasma concentration of TNF-α.

Inflammatory molecules associated with psoriasis may not only antagonize the effects of insulin, but also contribute to the downstream effects of insulin resistance. TNF-α is a proinflammatory cytokine produced by various cells that influences the production of other cytokines as well as the proliferation and activation of cells involved in inflammation. The key role of TNF-α in psoriasis has been demonstrated by the fact that levels are elevated in patients with psoriasis and correlate with disease severity. It was also found that TNF-α may contribute to the development of insulin resistance in patients with psoriasis evidenced by the finding that obese individuals also have higher levels of TNF-α, which fall with weight loss. TNF-α may act by reducing tyrosine kinase activity of the insulin receptor.

It is also found that IL-6, 8, 17, and 18 may also contribute to the development of insulin resistance. IL-6 is a proinflammatory cytokine, levels of which are significantly increased, particularly in obese patients with psoriasis and increase with disease severity. Higher levels of IL-6 are having been found to positively correlate with poor glucose tolerance, blood pressure, and levels of triglycerides, suggesting a role in the development of insulin resistance and the MBS. IL-1-β, a proinflammatory cytokine, may act in conjunction with IL-6, thereby increasing the risk of diabetes in patients with higher levels of both IL-6 and 1β compared with patients with elevated IL-6 only. IL-8, a chemokine, may inhibit the action of insulin through MAP kinase. Levels of this chemokine are also elevated in psoriasis and fall with successful treatment.

Plasminogen-activator-inhibitor 1 (PAI-1) is a serine protease inhibitor considered a risk factor for the development of diabetes. Elevated levels of PAI-1 correlate with insulin resistance. Levels of this glycoprotein are also noted to be elevated in patients with psoriasis and decrease with successful treatment.

Similarly, serum lipocalin-2 levels, also related to insulin resistance, are significantly higher in patients with psoriasis. It is thought that the development of islet amyloid in the pancreas may contribute to the pathogenesis of T2DM and serum amyloid A may be elevated in patients with psoriasis, particularly in those with psoriatic arthropathy.

Study results indicate increased oxidative stress in psoriasis, increased protein Glycation and stimulation of the immune system. Increased protein glyco–oxidation is considered as a link between psoriasis and increased prevalence of atherosclerosis, cardiovascular incidents and vascular complications of diabetes.[15]

PULMONARY DISEASE AND PSORIASIS

It has been observed that chronic obstructive pulmonary disease (COPD), which is mainly caused by smoking, is significantly more common among psoriasis patients than the general population[16] (Figs 8.9A and B). About 5.7% of psoriasis patients had been diagnosed with COPD compared with just 3.6% of those without the skin condition. Even though the difference is small, this has to be born in mind while treating patients with psoriasis. Methotrexate (MTX) and other immunosuppressive agents, biologics may lead to development of tuberculosis. Lung fibrosis can be precipitated by long-term use of MTX. Increased incidence of malignancy has also been noted. The cyclical triad of stress-smoking–worsening of disease should be broken, lest may further lead to more severe consequences.

GASTROINTESTINAL AND HEPATOBILIARY SYSTEM AND PSORIASIS

The impact of psoriasis on gastrointestinal system can be either directly due to the disease or from the drugs used in the treatment of psoriasis. It has been documented that there is a decrease in the small bowel surface area in patients with severe psoriasis. Smoothing of the intestinal wall in the jejunal area of the bowel was demonstrated as a feature of severe psoriasis. There is an increased prevalence of psoriasis in Crohn's disease and ulcerative colitis and their first degree relatives than control.[17] There is an increase in mast cells, eosinophils, duodenal intra-epithelial lymphocytes, immunoglobulin (Ig) A antibodies to gliadin, serum eosinophil cationic protein, and numbers of EG2 positive eosinophils in the duodenal mucosa of psoriasis patients. There are reports quoting that in psoriatic patients with celiac disease having gluten sensitivity, avoidance of gluten induces remission of psoriasis and re-introduction led to active skin disease. There are enough studies to show that psoriasis is associated with alcoholic liver disease and hepatitis C virus infection (Figs 8.10A and B).

This section will discuss the impact of psoriasis on gastrointestinal tract in detail which will include changes in the following order:

- Intraoral
- Esophagus

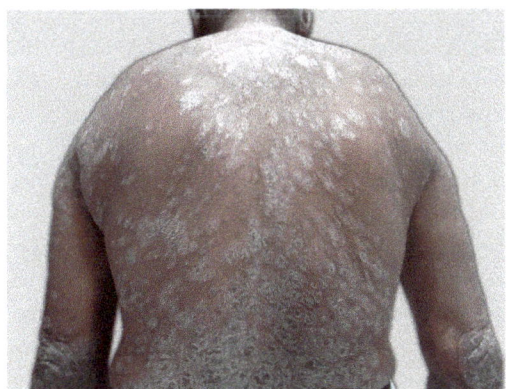

Fig. 8.9A: This man with psoriasis developed chronic obstructive pulmonary disease

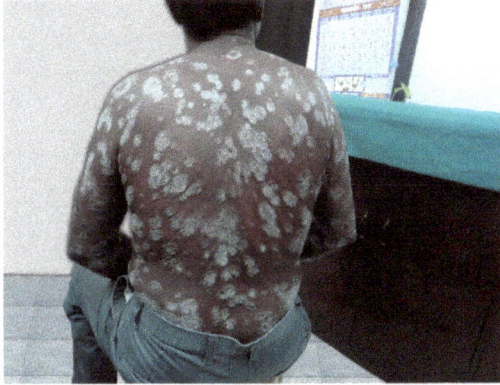

Fig. 8.9B: Man with psoriasis who is on treatment for chronic obstructive pulmonary disease

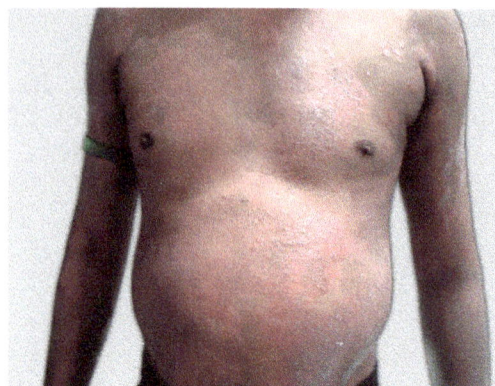

Fig. 8.10A: Man with alcoholic liver disease

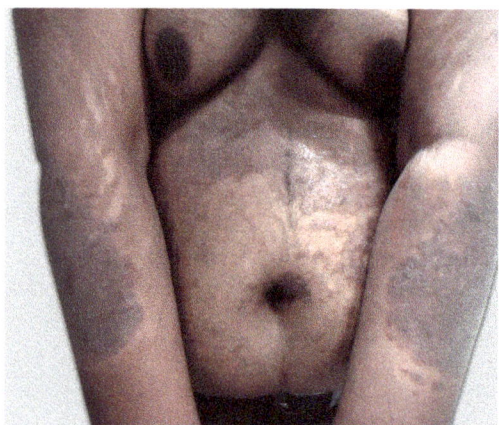

Fig. 8.10B: Patient with hepatitis C virus infection

- Gastric secretory function
- Duodenum
- Jejunum and small intestine
- Psoriatic gastrointestinopathy
- Inflammatory bowel disease (IBD)
- Secondary gastrointestinal amyloidosis due to psoriasis
- Drug-induced gastrointestinal disorders
- Liver and gall bladder.

Intraoral Manifestations of Psoriasis

Geographic tongue is the most common manifestation of psoriasis. This finding is seen in almost all cases of generalized pustular psoriasis (GPP). Erythema, ulcers, desquamative gingivitis, and pustules are other manifestation observed in psoriasis.

Psoriasis and Esophagus

Dysphagia can be a manifestation secondary to esophagial webs, though there are not many reports on this. Harty RF et al., have reported esophageal webs and rings with features of achalasia cardia in three cases of psoriasis. The real association, however, could not be proved beyond doubt.[18]

Gastric Secretory Function

There are not many reports to state the involvement of gastric mucosa and psoriasis. However, it was reported that gastric secretory function in psoriatic patients is characterized by reduced hydrochloric acid and pepsin outputs and it is more impaired in patients with mixed pathology, which necessitates antihelminthic therapy in this category of patients.[19] Valencak have reported complete remission of skin lesions in a 58-year-old woman with chronic plaque psoriasis with gastric marginal zone B-cell lymphoma of mucosa-associated lymphoid tissue (MALT) type after treatment with intravenous 2-chlorodeoxyadenosine. This leads to a reservation whether psoriasis can be considered as paraneoplastic condition.[20]

Psoriasis and Duodenum

Michaëlsson et al. have shown that the number of tryptase-positive mast cells in the duodenal mucosa in psoriasis is increased and that a subgroup of psoriasis patients showed elevated levels of antibodies to gliadin. They suggest that there are at least two types of abnormalities in the duodenal mucosa in psoriasis, one type is that present in most psoriasis patients and characterized by an increase in mast cells and eosinophils, and another is that present in a subgroup of patients with antibodies to gliadin and an increased number of duodenal intraepithelial lymphocytes. There were features of as diffuse duodenitis on gastroscopy of such patients. However, the mechanisms underlying the increase in the number of mast cells and its relevance are not yet known.[21]

Jejunum and Small Intestine

Clearly, psoriasis can cause a small bowel disorder and malabsorption. However, the exact mechanism has not been determined as to why patients with extensive psoriasis or other skin lesions develop a small bowel disorder and, at times, malabsorption. Several theories have been proposed, none of which is entirely satisfactory. Possible mechanism for skin gut relationship includes:
- Bacterial absorption through skin
- Shunting of blood
- Absence of essential metabolites
- Enzyme abnormalities
- Toxic byproducts of inflamed skin.

There will be a nonspecific inflammation with mild blunting of villi on biopsy.

According to O'Laughlin and Di Giovanni, extensive skin involvement can lead to blunting of villi due to nonspecific inflammation presenting as malabsorption. Bacterial absorption through skin, shunting of blood, absence of essential metabolites, enzyme abnormalities, and toxic by-products of inflamed skin may attribute to the pathology.

Severity of small bowel disease may be directly proportionate to the severity of psoriasis meaning, more extensive the skin involvement more severe would be the intestinal malfunction. Biopsy and other investigations must be carried out which will help rule out other causes of malabsorption.[22]

There seems to exist a link between psoriasis and chronic jejunitis with hyperpermeability of small intestine. Abnormalities in permeability of intestinal walls for carbohydrates and fats correlate with severity and duration of psoriasis. The architectural changes seen in the jejunal mucosa are also seen in other chronically ill debilitated patients.[23]

Psoriatic Gastrointestinopathy

Psoriatic gastrointestinopathy refers to the degenerate-dystrophic changes of cell populations of integumentary and glandular gastrointestinal epithelium with the destruction of important cytoplasmatic organelles of epithelial cell which leads to abnormality of secretion and absorption processes. Korotky et al. consider microbiocenosis as one of the most probable causes of the increased intestinal permeability emphasizing the interrelation between psoriasis and intestine microflora.[24]

There seems to exist an interrelation between psoriasis and intestinal microflora. Psoriasis is considered to be a consequence of incorporation of β-streptococci into the microbiocenosis of highly permeable intestines. This leads to a reservation whether malabsorption in psoriasis is a cause or consequence. Psoriatic gastrointestinopathy should be differentiated from dermatogenic enteropathy where the fecal fat excretion is as high as up to 24 g/day. Clearing of the skin manifestation improves the dermatogenic enteropathy which returns on recurrence of skin disease. It is important to note that dermatogenic enteropathy is not accompanied by an alteration in microscopic appearance of the small bowel mucosa. Dermatogenic enteropathy is not specific to psoriasis and is seen in erythroderma of other causes like eczema. It is important to differentiate dermatogenic enteropathy and Psoriatic gastrointestinopathy from gluten sensitive enteropathy as in the latter, a gluten-free diet is indicated.[25]

Inflammatory Bowel Diseases

The association between psoriasis and IBDs could be at least partially related to a common genetic background. Several regions on chromosomes including the IBD3 locus involved in Crohn's disease and ulcerative colitis, and the psoriasis susceptibility 1 locus involved in psoriasis. Psoriasis and Crohn's disease are inflammatory disorders primarily mediated by Th1 lymphocytes producing cytokines, such as TNF-α and interferon-γ. Increased levels of IL-17 and IL-23 in the intestinal lamina propria of patients with Crohn's disease, in the serum, and in the cutaneous lesions of psoriatic patients have been reported. Increased titres of antigliadin antibodies, antireticuline, anti-transglutaminase, and anti-smooth muscle endomysium antibodies were found also in patients with psoriasis. Celiac disease-associated antibodies have been found to be correlated with psoriasis severity. It has been suggested that there could be a common genetic predisposition to dermatitis herpetiformis, plaque psoriasis, and PsA as an increased frequency of the Ig heavy-chain DNase hypersensitive region enhancer 2 allele was found in all the three disorders. It was found that the prevalence of psoriasis in Crohn's disease and ulcerative colitis is 11.2% and 5.7%, respectively which is higher than the prevalence seen in patients without IBD.

Psoriasis in patients with IBD differed in certain aspects from those without IBD. Cases of psoriasis concurrent with IBD had a younger age of onset, longer duration of psoriasis and a higher PASI score, increased incidence of prostate-specific antigen, and had more than one autoimmune disease. They also had elevated levels of erythrocyte sedimentation rate and CRP, the exact pathogenesis of which remains unclear.[26]

Behçet's disease and psoriasis are chronic inflammatory diseases characterized by multisystemic vasculitis and epidermal hyperplasia, respectively. Although it has been found that the pathogenesis of Behcet's disease and psoriasis share common perspectives, reports of patients who have both diseases in concurrence are rare. According to Cho et al., psoriasis can occur in concurrence with Behcet's disease and both can influence each other. They observed that all the nine patients studied had psoriasis vulgaris out of which six were females.[27]

Secondary Gastrointestinal Amyloidosis due to Psoriasis

Secondary amyloidosis is associated with a variety of neoplastic and chronic inflammatory disorders, but has rarely been described as a complication of psoriatic arthropathy. The clinical manifestations of gastrointestinal amyloidosis include dysphagia, motility disturbances and bleeding, malabsorption, infarction with perforation, intestinal obstruction, and protein-losing enteropathy. Willoughby et al. have reported secondary amyloidosis in patient with long-standing psoriasis and a seronegative arthritis, who presented with a severe disturbance of gastrointestinal motility.[28]

Drug-induced Gastrointestinal Changes

Oral candidiasis and gastritis are common gastrointestinal manifestations seen in patients on immunosuppressive drugs. Gastrointestinal bleed in up to 3% is documented with use of mycophenolate mofetil (MMF). Severe life-threatening lower gastrointestinal tract bleed was reported in patient with psoriasis who was treated with MMF.

Liver and Gall Bladder

Nonalcoholic fatty liver disease (NAFLD) is now regarded as the hepatic manifestation of the MBS, as it is largely dependent on the underlying insulin resistance state. Considering that MBS is associated to psoriasis and NAFLD, it is likely that both entities could coexist in the same patients. The frequency of NAFLD in patients with psoriasis was found remarkably greater than in controls, and NAFLD was associated with the severity of psoriasis independently of potential confounders, such as age, gender, BMI, psoriasis duration, and alcohol consumption. Psoriatic patients with NAFLD were much more likely to have PsA. It was found that prevalence of NAFLD was found to be 48–59% in patients with psoriasis as against 20–30% in the general population. Psoriatic patients with NAFLD is significantly more likely than their nonpsoriatic counterparts to develop severe liver disease (steatohepatitis and fibrosis).[29] It could be speculated that proinflammatory cytokines which are overproduced in patients with psoriasis likely contribute to the development of insulin resistance and that psoriatic patients with the highest insulin resistance are the ones who get NAFLD. It was found that psoriatic patients with NAFLD were more likely to have the MBS and had significantly higher serum CRP and IL-6 levels and lower serum adiponectin than those with psoriasis alone.

It is suggested that routine work-up for NAFLD may be warranted in patients with psoriasis, having features of the MBS, PsA, and/or unexplained transaminase elevations. In the presence of NAFLD, the choice of potentially hepatotoxic drug therapy, as MTX, should be considered with caution.

Alcoholic and nonalcoholic liver diseases have both been found to be common in psoriatic patients. TNF-α, a key cytokine in psoriasis pathogenesis, has been found to have a crucial role in alcoholic hepatitis, and small preliminary studies have evaluated the effect of anti-TNF therapy in this condition. However, the use of anti-TNF-α drugs in alcoholic hepatitis is still controversial and needs to be further investigated.[30]

Generalized pustular psoriasis is invariably associated with liver abnormality during the active stage. About 90% of patients with GPP, show at least one abnormal biological liver parameter and 50% show pronounced abnormality with jaundice and elevated enzymes. These changes return to normal range at the time of remission. Histology of liver biopsy shows neutrophilic cholangitis. It was also found that 75% showed features of sclerosing cholangitis on persistent magnetic resonance cholangiopancreatography. These changes are attributable to psoriasis as no causal factor other than pustular psoriasis could be identified. Owing to the high frequency of liver abnormalities in GPP, and the other evidences of neutrophilic cholangitis seen in GPP, neutrophilic cholangitis should be added to the spectrum of extracutaneous manifestations of this disease and every physician should be aware of such complication.

Impact of Drugs on the Liver

Elevated liver enzymes are a common feature seen with most of the systemic drugs like MTX. The presence of comorbidities has important implications in the global approach to patients. In particular, traditional systemic antipsoriatic agents (e.g., MTX, cyclosporine) could negatively affect cardiometabolic comorbidities as well as NAFLD and may have dangerous interactions with drugs commonly used by psoriasis patients. Moreover, patients with psoriasis should be encouraged to drastically correct their modifiable cardiovascular and liver risk factors, in particular obesity, alcohol consumption, and smoking habit, because this could positively affect both psoriasis and their life expectancy.

Methotrexate Hepatotoxicity

Hepatotoxicity, especially liver fibrosis, is the major concern with long-term, "low-dose" oral MTX therapy for psoriasis. The histological features are nonspecific and resemble those of nonalcoholic steatohepatitis (NASH). Moreover, most of the risk factors of MTX-induced liver injury are also associated with NASH.

Non-steatohepatitis, probably aggravated by MTX, is an important cause of liver injury in patients on long-term, low-dose MTX treatment for psoriasis. In addition, MTX alone can cause a NASH-like pattern of injury that is at least, in part, caused by a higher cumulative dose.[31] Histologic changes of MTX-induced NAFLD include steatosis, stellate cell hypertrophy, anisonucleosis, and hepatic fibrosis. Histology of liver in MTX-induced NAFLD shows steatosis, stellate (Ito) cell hypertrophy, anisonucleosis, and hepatic fibrosis. The mechanism involved is due to the depletion of hepatic folate stores. It is advisable to perform liver biopsy after a cumulative dose of 1.5 g and after each additional 1 g. However, noninvasive tests like serial procollagen 3 N-terminal peptide, transient elastography, and fibroscan can be performed and liver biopsy contemplated, if two of the above three are found abnormal.

Cyclosporine Hepatotoxicity

In several large clinical trials, initiation of cyclosporine therapy was associated with mild elevations in serum bilirubin levels, often without significant increases in serum alanine transaminase or alkaline phosphatase. Elevations in serum enzymes were also described, but less commonly. Recently, these complications appear to be less frequent, perhaps because of more careful dosing and monitoring of cyclosporine levels. The proposed mechanism of injury is related to its interaction with cytochrome P450. Cyclosporine undergoes extensive hepatic metabolism, and because of its interaction with the cytochrome P450 system (CYP 3A4), is susceptible to severe drug interactions. In animal models, cyclosporine decreases bile flow which may account for the mild hyperbilirubinemia that occurs with high doses. There can be biliary sludge leading to cholelithiasis.

Acitretin Hepatotoxicity

With acitretin, clinically apparent acute severe fatal liver injury has been documented which typically arises during the first 3 months of therapy.

The gastrointestinal and hepatobiliary manifestations of psoriasis are summarized in Box 8.2.

AUTOIMMUNE DISEASES AND PSORIASIS

Psoriasis was positively associated with many autoimmune diseases, which are statistically significant. The strongest association was with rheumatoid arthritis. Patients with

Psoriasis as a Systemic Disease

BOX 8.2: Gastrointestinal tract and hepatobiliary manifestations in psoriasis

- Geographic tongue, erythema, ulcers, desquamative gingivitis, pustules
- Dysphagia, esophageal webs or rings
- Reduced HCl and pepsin
- Increased number of mast cells, eosinophils, lymphocytes
- Diffuse dudenitis
- Jejunitis
- Psoriatic gastrointestinopathy
- Dermatogenic enteropathy
- IBD associated with:
  - Early onset, longer duration, more severe psoriasis
  - Prostate-specific antigen, >one autoimmune disease, elevated ESR, CRP
- Behcet's Disease and psoriasis influence each other
- IBS
- Elevated liver enzymes:
  - Obese, diabetics, alcoholics
  - Subclinical inflammation: N LFT's
  - NAFLD/NASH
- Neutrophilic cholangitis
- Amyloidosis

IBD, inflammatory bowel disease; ESR, erythrocyte sedimentation rate; CRP, C-reactive protein; NAFLD, nonalcoholic fatty liver disease; NASH, nonalcoholic steatohepatitis; LFT, liver function test; IBS, irritable bowel syndrome; HCl, hydrochloric acid.

systemic lupus erythematosus, Graves' disease, Hashimoto's disease, chronic glomerulonephritis, pulmonary fibrosis, Sjogren syndrome, Addison disease, immune thrombocytopenia, celiac disease, and primary biliary sclerosis. Vitiligo, alopecia areata, and chronic urticaria are common dermatological diseases with autoimmune etiology known to be associated with psoriasis (Figs 8.11A and B). Autoimmune diseases associated with psoriasis are listed in Box 8.3.

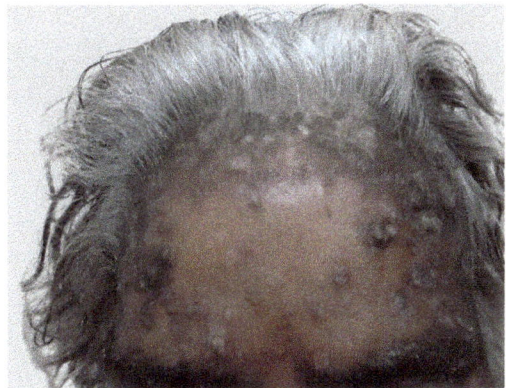

Fig. 8.11A: Lady with severe psoriasis having hypothyroidism, dyslipidemia

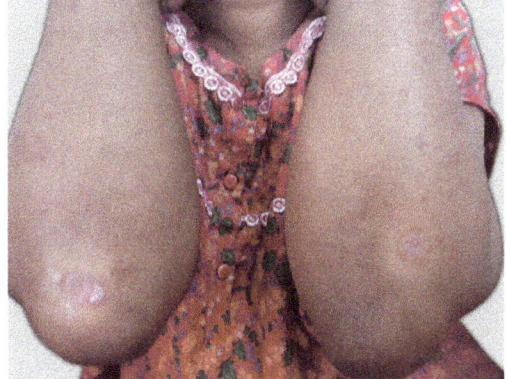

Fig. 8.11B: Psoriasis and hypothyroidism in a woman

psoriasis are more than 50% more likely than patients without psoriasis to have at least one other autoimmune disease and are nearly twice as likely to have at least two other autoimmune diseases.[32] The autoimmune diseases known to be associated with psoriasis include Crohn's disease, ulcerative colitis, type 1 diabetes mellitus, hemolytic anemia, giant cell arteritis, multiple sclerosis,

BOX 8.3: Autoimmune diseases in psoriasis

- Crohn's disease
- Ulcerative colitis
- Celiac disease
- Type 1 diabetes mellitus
- Hemolytic anemia
- Giant cell arteritis
- Multiple sclerosis
- Systemic lupus erythematosus
- Graves' disease
- Hashimoto's disease
- Chronic glomerulonephritis
- Pulmonary fibrosis
- Sjogren syndrome
- Addison disease
- Immune thrombocytopenia
- Primary biliary cirrhosis
- Alopecia areata
- Vitiligo
- Chronic urticaria

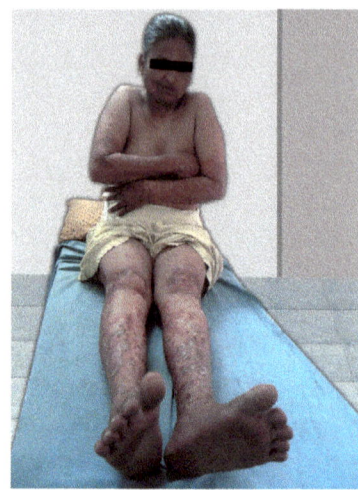

Fig. 8.12: Pustular psoriasis in a lady with chronic kidney disease

RENAL DISEASE AND PSORIASIS

While the existence of a "psoriatic nephropathy" having been proposed based on case reports of glomerulonephritis in patients with psoriasis, the association between psoriasis and kidney disease are now studied more widely. Studies found a fourfold increase in death from nephritic or non-hypertensive kidney disease among those with severe psoriasis. Multiple cross-sectional studies have also observed greater prevalence of microalbuminuria, a sign of subclinical glomerular dysfunction, in patients with psoriasis. Though some studies have detected no association between psoriasis and renal disease, it is now hypothesized that patients with psoriasis, especially if it is severe, have an increased risk of moderate-to-advanced (stage 3–5) chronic kidney disease (CKD) compared with patients without psoriasis (Fig. 8.12).

Moderate-to-severe psoriasis is associated with moderate-to-advanced CKD independent of traditional risk factors. Closer monitoring for renal insufficiency, such as routine screening with urine analysis for microalbuminuria, serum creatinine, and blood urea nitrogen testing, should be considered for patients with psoriasis affecting 3% or more of the body surface area. Increased screening efforts will allow earlier detection and intervention to reduce the substantial morbidity and mortality associated with CKD. Moderate-to-severe psoriasis is associated with an increased risk of CKD independent of traditional risk factors, such as diabetes and heart disease indicates a recent study.[33]

Secondary renal amyloidosis in psoriatic arthropathy and drug-induced renal lesions secondary to MTX or cyclosporine are accepted accompaniments of psoriasis. IgA nephropathy is also known to occur in psoriatics. Singh et al. have reported biopsy proven cases of mesangioproliferative glomerulonephritis with IgA nephropathy, focal proliferative glomerulonephritis, and membranous glomerulonephropathy in psoriatics. The authors propose that kidney disease may be a common accompaniment of psoriasis, which may be labeled as "psoriatic nephropathy" or "psoriatic kidney disease", the exact mechanism of which is yet to be elucidated.[34] The relative risk of CKD is especially increased in younger patients, similar to previous findings for MI in psoriasis. The absolute risk of CKD attributable to psoriasis increases with age. Additionally, the risk versus benefit of potentially nephrotoxic drugs in patients with moderate-to-severe psoriasis should be carefully considered.[35]

MULTIORGAN FAILURE DUE TO PSORIASIS

Multiorgan failure (multisystem organ failure) has been reported in patients with coronary artery bypass, high blood pressure, and rheumatoid arthritis. Now, there is emerging evidence documenting the occurrence of multi organ failure in patients with psoriasis (Figs 8.13A and B). Recent study involving 69 people who had psoriasis and multiorgan failure reflects an increase in the tendency for

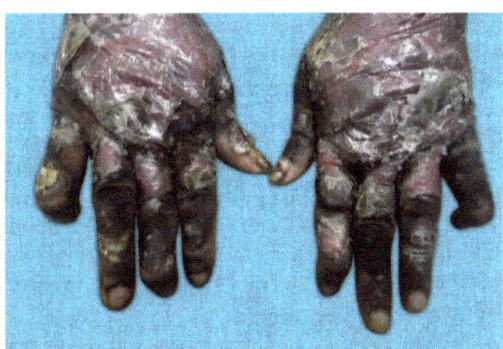

Fig. 8.13B: Severe psoriasis in a patient with multiorgan failure

multiorgan failure in patients with psoriasis in the recent years. Males seem to be more frequently affected than females. The gender difference in people who have psoriasis and experienced multiorgan failure was found to be 30.23% and 69.77% in females and males, respectively. The peak incidence was found in the 7th decade showing an incidence of 65.82%. Diabetes mellitus (18.84%), hyperlipidemia (17.39%), arthralgia (14.49%), gastritis (14.49%), iron deficiency anemia (14.49%), hypertension (7.25%), depression (4.35%) were found to be the associations. Ustekinumab (37.68%) and infliximab (30.43%) were the commonly used drugs in these patients.[36] In another report, a woman developed multiorgan failure as a result of erythrodermic psoriasis and shortly thereafter, developed bronchial pneumonia. There are reports where GPP appearing in patients after organ transplantation subsequently leading to multiorgan failure, while the European guidelines for renal transplantation reported by the European Best Practices Guidelines Expert Group in 2,000 do not include psoriasis in the exclusion criteria, with only two cases reported so far, whether psoriasis or a history of psoriasis in patients with chronic renal failure be considered as

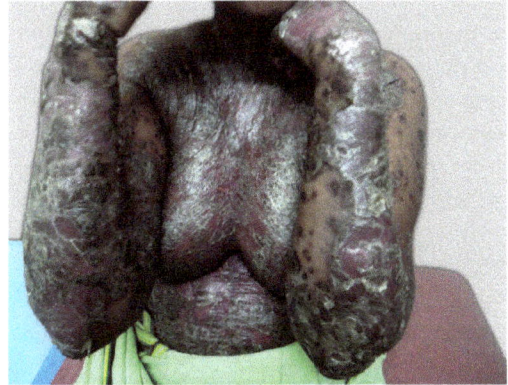

Fig. 8.13A: Lady with severe psoriasis, diabetes mellitus, hypertension, hypothyroid, dyslipidemia with multiorgan failure

a contraindication for transplantation or not is a question that remains unanswered.[37]

MALIGNANCY AND PSORIASIS

Patients with psoriasis are at an increased risk of developing malignancy, particularly non-melanoma skin cancer and lymphoproliferative cancers (Fig. 8.14). The fact that risk is greatest for those with severe disease probably is a reflection of treatment with systemic agents and phototherapy. The risk of psoriatic patients developing lymphoid malignancies may be attributable to the abnormal immune activation that has been demonstrated in them.

In addition to lymphoma, psoriatic patients have an increased risk for other malignancies, including those of the head and neck, solid organs (liver, pancreas, lung, breast, and kidney) and genitals.[38]

Lymphomas are a significant comorbidity associated with inflammatory diseases, including rheumatoid arthritis and psoriasis. Defining the contribution of psoriasis to the cause of lymphomas has been complicated by the overall rarity of this malignancy and the large clinical study patient base needed to establish statistically meaningful conclusions.

The risk of psoriatic patients developing lymphoid malignancies may be attributable to the pathophysiology or treatment of psoriasis. Abnormal immune activation has been demonstrated in psoriatic patients and might contribute to subsequent malignancy. A large, controlled cohort study found a modest increase in lymphomas, particularly Hodgkin's lymphoma and cutaneous T-cell lymphoma, among psoriatic patients compared with the general population, and a greater overall risk for these lymphomas was evident among patients with more severe psoriasis (i.e., those who received psoralen/phototherapy or systemic treatments, e.g., MTX, azathioprine, or cyclosporine). In addition to lymphoma, psoriatic patients have an increased risk for other malignancies, including those of the head and neck, solid organs (liver, pancreas, lung, breast, and kidney), and genitals, as well as non-melanoma skin cancer. The use of PUVA regimens has been implicated in the development of squamous cell carcinoma. Similarly, the use of cyclosporine in dermatologic regimens has been associated with an increase in non-melanoma skin cancers, particularly squamous cell carcinoma. Patients treated for more than 2 years with cyclosporine were shown to have a higher risk of developing malignancy than those who have not received cyclosporine. In addition, exposure to PUVA and to other immune suppressants was shown to contribute to the overall risk. Other antipsoriatic treatments, such as ionizing radiation and oral arsenic therapies, and the increased use of alcohol and tobacco, might be contributing factors for the increased incidence of solid tumors among psoriatic patients.

Psoriatic patients with diabetes are prone to develop digestive organ cancers. Chronic

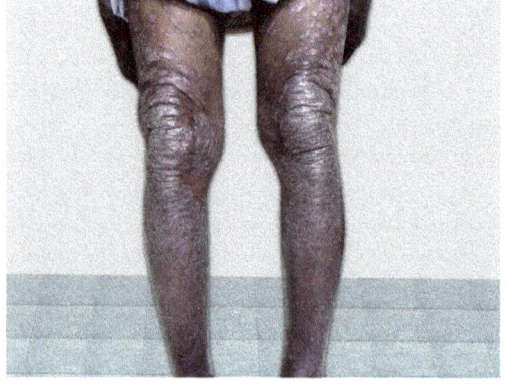

Fig. 8.14: Man developed lymphoma who was on immunosuppressive drugs for psoriasis for 5 years

inflammation acts as the driving force that enhances the risk of malignancy in psoriatics. Prevalent cancers in the population should be carefully monitored in the psoriatics over 40 years of age, especially for those with concomitant diabetes. Thus, there is increased risk of mortality for these psoriasis patients, when compared with the general population.[39]

COMORBIDITY IN CHILDHOOD PSORIASIS

Psoriatic children have a higher prevalence of obesity. It was also observed that overweight had different effects on childhood patients. Psoriasis in these children was more severe compared with psoriatic children of normal weight. There is a strong association between psoriasis and obesity in children, especially boys.[40] Increased incidence of hyperlipidemia, hypertension, and diabetes has also reported to be associated with psoriasis in children or adolescents. It may be considered that in an obese child, disease severity can be a marker of cardiovascular risk. Prevalence of comorbidities in persons in the age range 0–20 years with psoriasis was found to be more than those without psoriasis. Crohn's disease, hyperlipidemia, diabetes mellitus, arterial hypertension, rheumatoid arthritis, obesity, ischemic heart disease, ulcerative colitis were the comorbidities observed in childhood psoriasis.

Torres et al. observed that psoriatic children had a significantly higher prevalence and greater odds of excess adiposity compared to controls. A higher prevalence of MBS was observed in children with psoriasis compared to controls. Increased waist circumference, high blood pressure were observed in children with psoriasis. It was also observed that more atherogenic lipid profile was observed among psoriatic children without excess adiposity reinforcing the need for screening cardiovascular comorbidities in children with psoriasis. The authors suggest that these associations are in part genetically determined rather than uniquely acquired.[41]

CONCLUSION

Psoriasis is a debilitating chronic inflammatory disease that predisposes patients both young and old to serious comorbidities. Pediatricians and primary care physicians should be aware of potential cardiometabolic conditions and risk factors when treating patients with psoriasis. Young females with severe psoriasis suffer cardiovascular event five times more than their counterpart.[42]

- Antecedents of skin disorders and skin infection within the last year predisposes to development of comorbidities[43]
- Smoking was found to be an independent risk factor for psoriasis
- Obesity is a definite risk factor for psoriasis in the induction of comorbid conditions, no matter whether it is a cause or consequence, whether it is a child or an adult
- Positive association between psoriasis, diabetes, and insulin resistance has been observed in Indian patients as seen in developed countries.[10,44] This finding may well indicate that lifestyle and stress associated with such lifestyle plays a major role in the systemic associations, especially the metabolic comorbidities associated with psoriasis.

Certain predictive factors can help detect patients who will be at risk of developing comorbidities. In such patients, early therapeutic intervention will help prevent the onset of these comorbidities.

REFERENCES

1. Reich K. The concept of psoriasis as a systemic inflammation: implications for disease management. J Euro Acad Dermatol Venereol. 2012;26:3-11.
2. Hammadi A. Psoriatic Arthritis. Medscape [online] Available from http://emedicine.medscape.com/article/331037-overview. [Accessed October, 2015].
3. Cohen AD, Weitzman D, Dreiher J. Psoriasis and Hypertension: A Case-Control Study. Acta Derm Venereol. 2010;90:23-26.
4. Gelfand JM, Troxel AB, Lewis JD, Kurd SK, Shin DB, Wang X, et al. The risk of mortality in patients with psoriasis: results from a population-based study. Arch Dermatol. 2007:143:1493-9.
5. Park JV, Wheeler D, Grandinetti L. Psoriasis: Evolving treatment for a complex disease. Cleve Clin J Med. 2012;79(6):413-23.
6. Gelfand JM, Neimann AL, Shin DB, Wang X, Margolis DJ, Troxel AB. Risk of myocardial infarction in patients with psoriasis. JAMA. 2006;296:1735-41.
7. Ahlehoff O, Gislason GH, Jørgensen CH, Lindhardsen J, Charlot M, Olesen JB, et al. Psoriasis and risk of atrial fibrillation and ischaemic stroke: a Danish Nationwide Cohort Study. Eur Heart J. 2012;33(16):2054-64.
8. Ahlehoff O, Gislason GH, Lindhardsen J, Olesen JB, Charlot M, Skov L, et al. Prognosis following first-time myocardial infarction in patients with psoriasis: a Danish nationwide cohort study. J Intern Med. 2011;270:237-44.
9. Mehta NN, Yu Y, Pinnelas R, Krishnamoorthy P, Shin DB, Troxel AB, et al. Attributable Risk Estimate of Severe Psoriasis on Major Cardiovascular Events. Am J Med. 2011;124(8):775.e1-6.
10. Kumar P, Thomas J. Comorbid conditions in psoriasis – Higher frequency in females: A prospective study. Indian Dermatol Online J. 2012;3(2):105-8.
11. Altunay I, Demirci GT, Ates B, Kucukunal A, Aydın C, Karamustafalıoglu O et al. Do eating disorders accompany metabolic syndrome in psoriasis patients? Results of a preliminary study. Clin Cosmet Investig Dermatol. 2011;4:139-43.
12. Gyldenløve M, Storgaard H, Holst JJ, Vilsbøll T, Knop FK, Skov L. Patients with psoriasis are insulin resistant. 2015;72(4):599-60.
13. Boehncke WH, Boehncke S, Tobin AT, Kirby B. The 'psoriatic march': a concept of how severe psoriasis may drive cardiovascular comorbidity. Experimental Dermatology. 2011;20:303-7.
14. Boehncke S, Thaci D, Beschmann H, Ludwig RJ, Ackermann H, Badenhoop K, et.al. Psoriasis patients show signs of insulin resistance. Br J Dermatol. 2007;157:1249-51.
15. Damasiewicz-Bodzek A, Wielkoszyński T. Advanced protein glycation in psoriasis. J Eur Acad Dermatol Venereol. 2012;26(2):172-9.
16. Cowen M. Lung disease common in psoriasis patients. Br J Dermatol. 2008: Advance online publication. Available from http://www.medwirenews.com/52/76543/Consumer_Health/Lung_disease_common_in_psoriasis_patients.htm [Accessed October, 2015].
17. Yates VM, Watkinson G, Kelman A. Further evidence for an association between psoriasis, Crohn's disease and ulcerative colitis. Br J Dermatol. 1982;106:323-30.
18. Harty RF, Boharski MG, Harned RK, Agha FP. Psoriasis, dysphagia and esophageal webs or rings. Dysphagia. 1988;2:136-9.
19. Khardikova SA, Beloborodova Él. Clinical and functional disorders of the stomach-in patients with psoriasis in the presence of chronic opisthorchiasis. Med Parazitol (Mosk). 2011;2:22-5.
20. Valencak J, Trautinger F, Fiebiger WC, Raderer M. Complete remission of chronic plaque psoriasis and gastric marginal zone B-cell lymphoma of MALT type after treatment with 2-chlorodeoxyadenosine. Ann Hematic. 2002;81(11):662-5.
21. Michaëlsson G, Kraaz W, Hagforsen E, Pihl-Lundin I, Lööf L. Psoriasis patients have highly increased numbers of tryptase-positive mast cells in the duodenal stroma. Br J Dermatol. 1997;136(6):866-70.
22. O'Laughlin JC, Di Giovanni AM. Psoriatic enteropathy: Report of case and review of literature. J Am Osteopath Assoc. 1979;79(2):107-11.
23. Shuster S, Watson AJ, Marks J. Small intestine in psoriasis. Br Med J. 1967;3:458-60.
24. Korotky NG, Peslyak MY. Psoriasis as a consequence of incorporation of beta-streptococci into the micro-biocenosis of highly permeable intestines (a pathogenic concept). Vestn Dermatol Venereol. 2005;1:9-18.
25. Marks J, Shuster S. Dermatogenic enteropathy. Gut. 1970;11(4):292-8.
26. Park HS, Koh SJ, Park GY, Lee DH, Yoon HS, Youn JI, et al. Psoriasis concurrent with inflammatory bowel disease. J Euro Acad Dermatol Venereol. 2013;28(11):2-6.
27. Cho S, Cho SB, Choi MJ, Zheng Z, Bang D. Behçet's disease in concurrence with psoriasis. J EurAcad Dermatol Venereol. 2013;27(1):e113-8.
28. Willoughby CP, Banerji A, Bennett MK, Jewell DP. Gastrointestinal amyloidosis complicating psoriatic arthropathy. Postgrad Medical J. 1981;57:663-7.
29. Gisondi P, Giglio MD, Cozzi A, Girolomoni G. Psoriasis, the liver, and the gastrointestinal tract. Dermatologic Therapy. 2010;23:155-9.
30. Cassano N, Vestita M, Apruzzi D, Vena GA. Alcohol, psoriasis, liver disease, and anti-psoriasis drugs. Int J Dermatol. 2011;50(11):1323-31.

31. Langman G, Hall PM, Todd G. Role of non-alcoholic steatohepatitis in methotrexate-induced liver injury. J Gastroenterol Hepatol. 2001;16(12):1395-401.
32. Kelly JC. Psoriasis Linked to Autoimmune Diseases. Medscape. [Online] Available from http://www.medscape.com/viewarticle/773015 [Accessed October, 2015].
33. Wan J, Wang S, Haynes K, Denburg MR, Shin DB, Gelfand JM. Risk of moderate to advanced kidney disease in patients with psoriasis: population based cohort study. BMJ. 2013;347:f5961.
34. Singh NP, Prakash A, Kubba S, Ganguli A, Singh AK, Sikdar S, et al. Psoriatic nephropathy—does an entity exist? Ren Fail. 2005;27:123-7.
35. Wan J, Wang S, Haynes K, Denburg MR, Shin DB, Gelfand JM. Risk of moderate to advanced kidney disease in patients with psoriasis: population based cohort study. Br Med J. 2013;347:f5961.
36. Psoriasis and multi-organ failure. [online] Available from http://www.ehealthme.com/cs/psoriasis/multi-organ+failure#note_1 [Accessed June, 2015].
37. Vougas V, Dedemadi G, Noutsis K, Apostolou Th, Pantelidaki C, Drakopoulos S. Generalised Pustular Psoriasis (von Zumbusch type) following renal Transplantation. Report of a case and review of the literature. Hospital Chronicles. 2007;2(2):89-93.
38. Gottlieb AB, Dann F. Comorbidities in Patients with Psoriasis. Am J Med. 2009;122:1150.e1-9.
39. Paul CF, Ho VC, McGeown C, Christophers E, Schmidtmann B, Guillaume JC, et al. Risk of Malignancies in Psoriasis Patients Treated with Cyclosporine: a 5 y Cohort Study. J Inv Dermatol. 2003;120:211-6.
40. Boccardi D, Menni S, La Vecchia C, Nobile M, Decarli A, Volpi G, et al. Overweight and childhood psoriasis. Br J Dermatol. 2009;161:484-6.
41. Torres T, Machado S, Mendonça D, Selores M. Cardiovascular comorbidities in childhood psoriasis. Eur J Dermatol. 2014;24(2):229-35.
42. Gelfand JM, Troxel AB, Lewis JD, Kurd SK, Shin DB, Wang X, et al. The risk of mortality in patients with psoriasis: results from a population-based study. Arch. Dermatol. 2007;143(12):1493-9.
43. Huerta C, Rivero E, Rodríguez LA. Incidence and Risk Factors for Psoriasis in the General Population. Arch Dermatol. 2008;143:1559-65.
44. Pereira RR, Amladi ST, Varthakavi PK. A study of the prevalence of diabetes, insulin resistance, lipid abnormalities, and cardiovascular risk factors in patients with chronic plaque psoriasis. Indian J Dermatol. 2011;56(5):520-6.

CHAPTER 9

Investigations

INTRODUCTION

Diagnosis of psoriasis is essentially clinical except in variants like erythrodermic psoriasis, pustular psoriasis when they present for the first time where biopsy is mandatory to confirm the diagnosis. Linear psoriasis and persistent plaque psoriasis are common diagnostic challenges, if the classical features of psoriasis are lost. Under such situations, to establish the diagnosis and to rule out the differential diagnosis, biopsy is warranted. By and large, investigations per se in psoriasis are needed only under the following circumstances:

- To differentiate from close mimickers
- To rule out infection as a cause of psoriasis
- To assess the disease activity
- To assess patients with nail psoriasis
- To assess patients with psoriatic arthritis (PsA)
- To screen for comorbidity and systemic involvement
- To assess the patient's general condition during the acute presentation like erythrodermic psoriasis, pustular psoriasis
- To assess the patient for specific therapy
- Evaluation of drug therapy
- To assess the prognosis.

In view of the commonness with which psoriasis is associated with metabolic syndrome and other systemic comorbidities, apart from recording the body mass index (BMI), baseline investigations to be done in all patients with psoriasis above the age of 40 years will include:

- Complete blood count (CBC) including total count (TC), differential count (DC), erythrocyte sedimentation rate (ESR), hemoglobin, total red blood cells (RBCs), and platelets
- Blood sugar fasting and postprandial
- Fasting lipid profile
- Liver function tests (LFT)
- Uric acid levels
- Rheumatoid arthritis (RA) factor
- Antinuclear antibody (ANA)
- Renal function tests (RFTs) including urine analysis.

TO DIFFERENTIATE FROM CLOSE MIMICKERS

Biopsy and dermoscopy are two important investigations which help in the differentiation of psoriasis and diseases resembling psoriasis. Biopsy is the best investigation in case of doubt when the characteristic features of psoriasis are missing, especially in erythrodermic psoriasis. However, one must remember not all features of classical well-formed plaque of psoriasis can be seen in a patient with erythroderma.

Dermascopy is a useful tool with which diseases like pityriasis lichenoides chronica (PLC), lichen planus (LP), and seborrheic dermatitis of scalp can be easily differentiated. Psoriasis on dermoscopy shows diffuse dotted vessels whereas orange-yellowish structure less areas, focal dotted vessels and non-dotted vessels are the features seen in PLC.[1]

Lichen planus, shows a nonvascular feature or red lines along with gray-blue dots, comedo, milium-like cysts, while psoriasis shows a vascular feature (homogeneous red globules). Dermoscopic features of scalp psoriasis include red dots and globules, twisted-red loops, and glomerular vessels. In contrast, seborrheic dermatitis of the scalp shows arborizing vessels and atypical red vessels with the absence of red dots and globules. Investigation of vascular patterns can be valuable for the clinical diagnosis and differentiation of scalp psoriasis and seborrheic dermatitis.[2]

TO RULE OUT INFECTION AS A CAUSE OF PSORIASIS

Since chronic persistent plaque psoriasis in adults and guttate psoriasis in children are known to be associated with an occult streptococcal infection, throat swab culture, ESR, anti-streptolysin O (ASO) titer and C-reactive protein (CRP) levels will help in deciding on a course of antibiotic in children with guttate psoriasis and adults with persistent plaque psoriasis not responding to routine therapy.

TO ASSESS THE DISEASE ACTIVITY

It is important to assess the disease activity in order to monitor response to therapy. Since clinical assessment cannot be dependable at all times, markers serve as a useful tool in assessing the activity especially before and after treatment. Many markers are available to assess the disease activity in psoriasis. Most of these are done for research purpose. However, few markers like ESR, CRP, and ASO titer are still useful in day-to-day practice.

The following are various markers that can be tested in a patient with psoriasis.
- Markers of inflammation: antiprotease systems; and fibrinogen, ESR, CRP, haptoglobin, C3 and C4 complement
- Markers of neutrophil activation: Elastase, lactoferrin, and lipid peroxidation
- Markers of endogenous antioxidant: Total plasma antioxidant capacity (TAS), transferrin, ceruloplasmin, α 1-antitrypsin and α 2-macroglobulin.

These markers show a raised value in active psoriasis when compared to inactive psoriasis.

The role of CRP in inflammation and the significance of its values are debatable.

C-reactive protein was first defined by Tillett and Francis as a protein developed against carbohydrate component of streptococcus pneumonia capsule in the serum of patients with pneumonia and was named as carbohydrate reactive protein.[3]

C-reactive protein is a non-glycolized pentameric protein made by hepatocytes with a molecular weight of 118 kD. The molecule is known as a major acute phase reactant which increases rapidly after infections or tissue damage, widely used as a laboratory parameter for the follow-up of inflammatory and infectious disease activity and is accepted as a very sensitive inflammatory marker.[4]

Blood levels of CRP can increase up to 100 times in the first 24 hours and can decrease to normal levels soon after treatment or spontaneous healing. Therefore, CRP is a valuable laboratory parameter for infections, tissue damage, and inflammation. Standard measurements of CRP levels can detect plasma levels of 3–8 mg/L CRP levels and healthy individuals have blood levels of CRP under 2 mg/L. New laboratory methods for the measurement of CRP have been developed and these sensitive CRP measurements can detect lower levels of CRP in the plasma. The synthesis of CRP is mainly controlled by, interleukin-6 (IL-6) but IL-1 and tumor necrosis factor-α (TNF-α) may influence CRP levels as well and increase of CRP in blood and other body fluids is a constant result of these proinflammatory cytokines.[5,6]

In case of nail psoriasis, the following investigations are very useful, especially in isolated nail psoriasis.

The following investigations given in Box 9.1 will help in the diagnosis of nail psoriasis.

BOX 9.1: Investigations used in nail psoriasis

- Nail biopsy
- Dermoscopy
- Videodermoscopy
- Capillaroscopy
- Ultrasound
- Doppler technique
- Optical coherence tomography
- Confocal laser scanning microscopy
  ○ To exclude infections
- Nail clipping and potassium hydroxide examination, fungal culture
- Bacterial culture

Nail Biopsy

Longitudinal nail biopsy involving the full length of the nail will provide the maximum information. However, the extent of damage is much greater and hence, some prefer to select the site of nail to be biopsied depending on the clinical manifestation. The type of involvement and the preferable site of biopsy are given in Table 9.1.

Technique of Nail Biopsy

Since nail is made up of hard keratin and anatomically situated in the area of lesser vascular supply, care must be taken both with reference to the technique and anesthesia. The selected digit is anesthetized with a proximal ring block or a distal wing block and then exsanguinated. A tourniquet is then applied at the base of the digit to achieve complete hemostasis and a relatively avascular field, keeping in mind that the tourniquet should not be kept in place for more than 15 minutes at a stretch. A punch or an excision biopsy can be applied to any individual anatomical part of the nail unit, like the nail bed, nail plate, nail fold or matrix, whereas with a longitudinal nail biopsy, a part of all the parts of the nail unit are biopsied. The defect is then sutured using 3-0 to 6-0 silk. After completion

TABLE 9.1: Clinical findings and the site to be biopsied in nail psoriasis

Clinical feature	Site to be biopsied
Pitting	Proximal matrix
Dystrophy	Proximal matrix
Focal onycholysis	Distal matrix
Onycholysis	Nail bed
Subungual hyperkeratosis	Nail bed
Oil drop sign	Nail bed
Splinter hemorrhage	Nail bed

of biopsy, adequate hemostasis is secured and pressure dressing is done. The sutures are then removed after 10 days.[7]

Dermoscopy

Dermoscopy is a noninvasive, quickly applied and inexpensive test employing magnification up to 10 times that may aid in diagnosis of nail psoriasis

Dermoscopic description of common signs of nail psoriasis is as follows:[8]
- Pits: appear as irregular depressions surrounded by a whitish halo
- Salmon patches: appear as marks that are irregular both in size and shape with coloring that varies from red to orange
- Onycholysis: appears as an area that is either homogenously white or composed of multiple longitudinal striations, generally surrounded by a reddish orange stain
- Splinter hemorrhages: appear as longitudinal brown, purple or black marks
- Blood vessels-appear as dilated tortuous vessels seen in the distal nail bed.

Video-dermoscopy[9-11]

Video-dermoscopy represents an evolution of dermoscopy and is performed with a video-camera equipped with lenses providing magnification ranging from 10 to 1000 times. The images obtained are visualized on a monitor and can be stored on a personal computer. Using video-dermoscopy, the affected capillaries were dilated, tortuous, elongated, and irregularly distributed. The capillary density was different in each patient and positively correlated with disease severity.

Capillaroscopy[12]

Periungual capillaroscopy shows that capillary density in the periungual area is decreased in patients with psoriasis which is even lesser in patients with nail psoriasis. Avascular areas and coiled capillary loops in the periungual area are more common in patients with nail psoriasis.

New Diagnostic Techniques

Ultrasound[13]

In nails affected by psoriatic onychopathy, the nail plates may show hyperechoic parts or loss of definition, which can involve only the ventral plate or both plates. In later stages, a wavy thickened appearance of both plates may be visible. The nail bed appears thickened.

Doppler Study

Power Doppler technique can demonstrate increase in blood flow in the affected nail.

Optical Coherence Tomography[14]

Optical coherence tomography (OCT) works on the principle that infrared light reflected from nail is measured and the intensity is imaged as a function of position. The OCT probe is applied directly to the nail and scanned. OCT can also measure the thickness of the nail plate with a greater accuracy in comparison to ultrasound. This suggests that OCT has the potential to provide quantitative data regarding psoriatic nails and may become a more accurate and objective surrogate outcome measure for interventional trials in future.

Confocal Laser Scanning Microscopy[15]

It is a new noninvasive diagnostic tool which is becoming increasingly popular. It can visualize cell structures of the skin up to a depth of 300 μm *in vivo*. It works on the principle of increasing the optical resolution and contrast of a micrograph by using a spatial pinhole to eliminate out of focus light. Confocal laser scanning microscopy (CLSM) enables reconstruction of three-dimensional images of nails and is a promising tool in the diagnosis of nail psoriasis. Compared with the OCT images, which best allow the measurement of thickness of the entire nail plate and of the different layers of the nail unit, CLSM gives better information on the microscopic structures of the nail plate.

TO ASSESS EXTENT AND TYPE OF DAMAGE IN PSORIATIC ARTHRITIS

Psoriatic arthritis has been classically defined as an inflammatory arthritis associated with psoriasis. However, in comparison with other relevant inflammatory arthropathies in which a definite diagnosis is frequently possible only by means of laboratory investigations, in PsA, true laboratory diagnostic markers are lacking. Some markers are utilized more to differentiate other diseases than to characterize PsA.

Investigations including clinical assessment, human leukocyte antigen (HLA), hematologic, synovial fluid analysis, serologic, and imaging studies, although not specifically diagnostic in all, can be supportive both in the early detection of joint involvement and extent and type of damage. Investigations useful in PsA are given in Box 9.2.

Clinical Assessment

Measuring the ratio of the circumference of the affected digit to the circumference of the unaffected digit on the opposite hand or foot using a minimum difference of 10% could define a dactylitic digit. In a study conducted at UK, leeds dactylitis instrument (LDI) and LDI basic was used to measure the digital circumference. A tenderness score was also measured and the product was taken for analysis. This may be used as a simple tool to detect early features of dactylitis at the bedside. The LDI measures the ratio of the circumference of the affected digit to the circumference of the digit on the opposite hand or foot: using a minimum difference of 10% to define a dactylitic digit. The ratio of circumference is multiplied by a tenderness score and analyzed. The study showed circumferential soft tissue edema in the majority of cases studied.[16]

> **BOX 9.2: Investigations in psoriatic arthritis**
> - Clinical: scoring
> - Human leukocyte antigen
> - Erythrocyte sedimentation rate
> - C-reactive protein
> - Rheumatoid factor
> - Anti-cyclic citrullinated peptide
> - Synovial fluid analysis
> - Ultrasonography
> - X-ray
> - Skeletal scintigraphy
> - Computed tomography scan
> - Magnetic resonance imaging
> - Nuclear imaging studies

Human Leukocyte Antigen Test

Human leukocyte antigen-B27, though not specific, is strongly supportive of axial disease.

Hematologic Investigations

The determination of ESR and/or CRP is frequently disappointing in PsA, since they are both elevated in only half of the patients with PsA. However, ESR and/or CRP are considered reliable in the assessment of PsA. Furthermore, elevated levels of ESR have been proposed as one of the best predictors of damage progression and, in addition, a low ESR seems protective, while an ESR more than 15 mm/hour is one of the factors associated with an increased mortality in PsA.

Serological Tests

Although, a negative serology can rule out RA, the rheumatoid factor or the antibodies to cyclic citrullinated peptides (anti-CCP), may be useful to better identify RA in order to differentiate PsA. However, rheumatoid factor was found in 5-13% of patients with PsA, and anti-CCP may be observed in almost similar percentage.

Synovial Fluid Analysis

The synovial fluid effusion is much higher in PsA, in comparison with other arthropathies. When available, synovial fluid analysis may offer additive information useful for the diagnosis, such as the increased number of leukocytes, which underlines the inflammatory nature of the effusion even in a patient with normal serum levels of acute phase response. It was found that elevated IL-1 levels in synovial fluid of patients with early disease (<6 months), may be predictive of an evolution in polyarticular form at follow-up.[17]

With the advent of science and technology, many imaging studies have been found to be useful in the diagnosis of PsA.

Ultrasonography, X-Ray of the affected joint, skeletal scintigraphy, computerized tomogram (CT) scan and magnetic resonance imaging (MRI), nuclear imaging studies are currently available investigation for the diagnosis and management of PsA.

Ultrasonography is useful for assessing the extent of disease, but it is not the method of choice for monitoring bone involvement in PsA.

Ultrasonography can detect entheseal abnormalities even in clinically asymptomatic patients with psoriasis. Routine use of ultrasonography will help detecting early signs of PsA in asymptomatic patients with psoriasis may have the potential to positively influence disease prognosis and ultimately, clinical outcome. Ongoing studies address the value of sonography as a diagnostic and prognostic marker in PsA.

Perisynovial inflammation as well as enthesitis appears to be the most characteristic ultrasound findings in PsA, enabling the differentiation of the disease from overlapping conditions. Musculoskeletal ultrasound is increasingly used as a bedside tool for diagnostic and monitoring purposes in patients with PsA. The sonographic differentiation between PsA and RA may be challenging because the morphological appearance of synovitis is similar in both conditions. In contrast, perisynovial inflammation is a specific finding of early PsA, and enthesitis is more frequently detected in PsA than in RA. After initiation of effective therapies, a reduction of ultrasound signs of synovitis and enthesitis can be seen along with clinical improvement. While sonographic findings can be discordant from clinical results, their relevance is unclear, although it is a concern that ongoing subclinical inflammation results in worse structural outcomes.[18] Most important ultrasound findings in PsA are given in Box 9.3.

Ultrasonographic examination detected tenosynovitis of flexor and extensor Achilles

---

BOX 9.3: Most important ultrasound findings in psoriatic arthritis

- Perisynovial inflammation
- Enthesitis

tendonitis in patients with PsA. Psoriasis area severity index (PASI) score and CRP were significantly higher in psoriatic patients with ultrasonographically detected entheseal abnormalities compared to those with no ultrasonographic findings.[19]

X-rays of the hands and feet show significant changes in PsA. Early changes may be limited to periarticular soft tissue swelling and joint erosions similar to RA. Sites of entheseal attachments may show periostitis and new bone formation. Advanced cases, especially of the mutilating variety, may show widespread joint destruction, with "penciling" or narrowing of the heads of the metacarpals and metatarsals. Destruction of the central portion of the articular surface gives the "pencil-in-cup" appearance. With the destruction of the interphalangeal joints, especially the distal ones, bony ankylosis can occur (Figs 9.1 to 9.4). The radiographic appearance of PsA can be similar to that of RA. The distinguishing features of PsA are listed in Table 9.2.

Skeletal Abnormalities by X-ray

Bone scintigraphy in psoriasis has been in vogue as early as early 1970s and according to the results of the studies

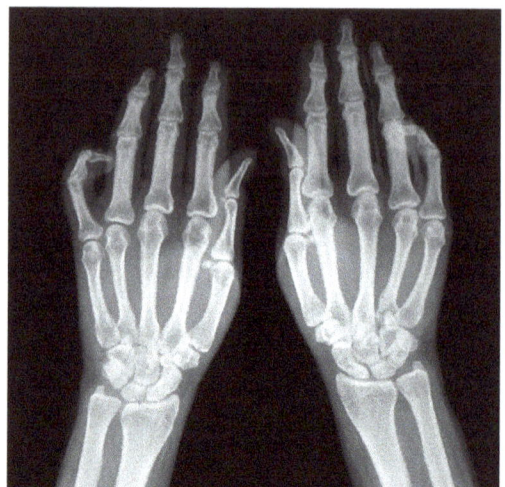

Fig. 9.2: Peripheral joint involvement in psoriatic arthritis

conducted, in addition to the clinically and roentgenologically defined PsA, in patients with psoriasis, osteopathy may exist, which can only be demonstrated by skeletal scintigraphy. It was also observed that these changes were found to be localized in bones adjacent to the joints. However, these changes can also be demonstrated in the region of extra-articular bones.[20]

Studies show that bone scintigraphy is more sensitive in the diagnosis of psoriatic bone involvement than clinical examination or conventional radiological imaging. Thus, bone scintigraphy may allow earlier diagnosis through the visualization and documentation of specific patterns and presence of disease in multiple sites. It also allows more discriminating selection of subsequent X-ray examinations to limit radiation exposure. Thus, bone scintigraphy can be regarded as the most important diagnostic tool in the assessment of PsA.[21] Whole-body scintigraphy shows the distribution of active joint disease. Abnormal radiotracer uptake precedes findings on plain radiographs.

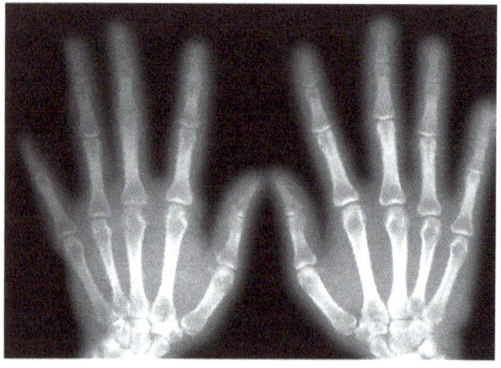

Fig. 9.1: Early psoriatic arthritis showing joint erosion

Investigations

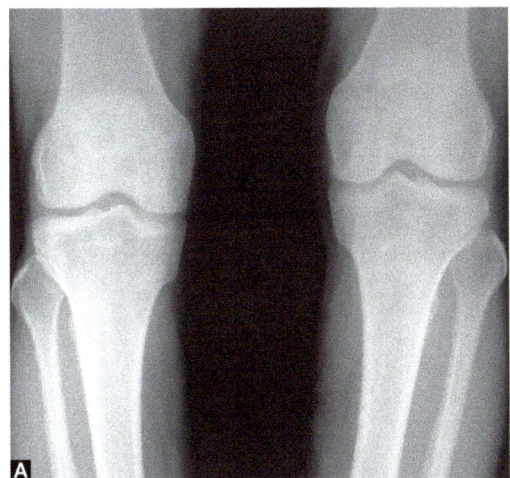

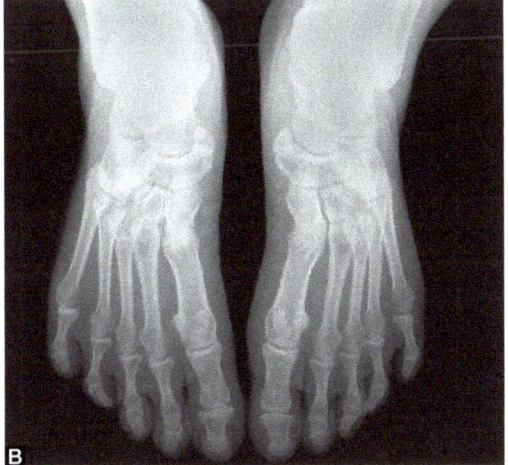

Fig. 9.3: X-ray of same patient as in Fig. 9.2 showing involvement of feet and knees

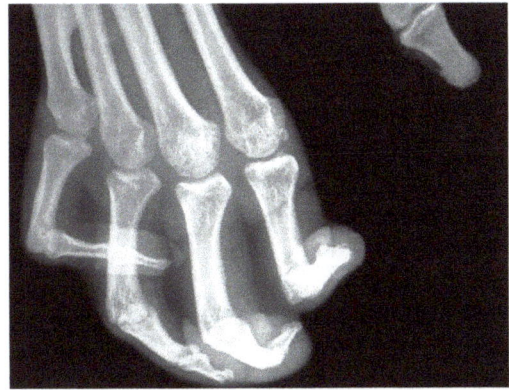

Fig. 9.4: Showing pencil in cup appearance

TABLE 9.2: Distinguishing features between psoriatic arthritis and rheumatoid arthritis

Findings	PsA	RA
Subcutaneous nodules	–	+
RA factor	–	+
Bony ankylosis	+	–
Periarticular bony proliferation	+	–
Osteopenia	–	+
Bone mineralization and has periosteal reaction and new-bone formation	Maintained	Lost
Sausage digit and spontaneous joint fusion	Common	Rare

RA, rheumatoid arthritis; PsA, psoriatic arthritis.

Computed Tomography Scan

In particular, CT scanning is useful in identifying inflammatory lesions, even when pre-existing degenerative disease is present; in demonstrating the articular surfaces of bone in an exact fashion; and, in some cases of sacroiliitis. CT scan can clearly demonstrate erosive changes that can appear equivocal or negative with radiography.

Magnetic Resonance Imaging

Findings on MRI are the most sensitive and specific for sacroiliitis and for other changes in the axial skeleton and the hands and feet. With MRI, it is possible to identify the early inflammatory phase of enthesitis before the development of erosion, as seen on radiographs. MRI can depict early cortical erosion, inflammatory granulation tissue and bone marrow edema. MRI scans have demonstrated that both tenosynovitis and synovitis contribute to the clinical picture of dactylitis. MRI images demonstrate widespread abnormalities in digits of people with PsA. Tender dactylitic digits have more abnormalities than other digits but the relationship between clinical and MRI scores is not strong.[16]

TO SCREEN FOR COMORBIDITY AND SYSTEMIC INVOLVEMENT

All patients should have their blood pressure and BMI read and recorded.

The following investigations must be carried out in all patients with psoriasis whereever possible which will detect the systemic involvement early aiding in early arrest of systemic consequences.
- CBC including hemoglobin, total leucocyte count, differential count, ESR, total RBC, and platelets
- Blood sugar: Fasting and postprandial, glycosylated hemoglobin
- Lipid profile
- Liver function test
- Uric acid
- RA factor
- Antinuclear antibody
- Renal function test including urine analysis.

Investigations that are to be done during acute stages like erythroderma include:
- Complete hemogram: Hemoglobin, total and differentials, ESR
- Peripheral smear
- Motion for occult blood
- X-ray chest, electrocardiogram
- Ultrasonography abdomen
- Serum electrolytes, creatinine
- Lactate dehydrogenase
- LFT including bilirubin and protein level
- Blood glucose
- γ globulin
- Immunoglobulin E (IgE)
- Lymph node biopsy should be considered in long standing or recurrent cases of erythroderma.

It is worthwhile remembering that laboratory findings observed in a case of gastrointestinal pathogen panel would be:

- Culture of the pus does not yield organisms
- There may be an absolute lymphopenia at the onset; quickly followed by polymorphonuclear leukocytosis
- The ESR is usually raised
- Plasma albumin, zinc, and calcium may be abnormally low
- Liver enzymes may be elevated.

TO ASSESS THE PATIENT FOR SPECIFIC THERAPY

It is mandatory to exclude tuberculosis, and other infection before initiating any immunosuppressive drugs including biologics.
- Complete blood count is to be done for all patients to be started on immunosuppressant drug
- RFT and LFT for those to be started on methotrexate (MTX)
- RFT should be assessed for those who are planned to be given cyclosporine, along with maintenance of blood pressure
- Lipid profile and LFT must be assessed in case of planning retinoid therapy.

Evaluation of Drug Therapy

While the patient is started on a drug-like MTX or biological agent, there is certain protocol to be followed while investigating the patients. These have to be meticulously adhered to and the results interpreted appropriately.

C-reactive protein has been found to be a useful investigation in assessing the efficacy of drugs used in treating psoriasis. Treatment with drugs like MTX and cyclosporine decrease CRP levels in PsA.[22,23] Interestingly, it was found that patients with higher CRP levels have a better response to cyclosporine therapy.[24]

Methotrexate

Premethotrexate evaluation:
- CBC with differential and platelet count
- Blood urea nitrogen and serum creatinine
- Urinalysis
- LFT including serum bilirubin
- Chest X-ray (if not taken in the last 6 months)
- Repeat every 2 weeks till 6 weeks there after every 2 months. X-ray repeated once a year
- Liver biopsy
- Pre-treatment liver biopsy in alcoholics is suggested before starting on MTX. However, this is not being routinely practiced as there are other options of therapy.

During treatment, liver biopsy is suggested if there is persistent elevation of aspartate transaminase (AST) and elevation of peptide of type III procollagen above 10 mcg/L in three samples in 1 year, or after a cumulative dose of 1.5 g of MTX.

In patients on MTX, noninvasive tests might help avoid liver biopsy. The use of noninvasive tests like transient elastography, fibro test, and serial procollagen III peptide level measurements can reduce the need for liver biopsy. Liver biopsy can be contemplated only, if two of the three tests show abnormality.[25]

Biological Agents

Screening tests recommended prior to starting etanercept usually include full blood count, liver enzymes, serum creatinine, urine analysis, pregnancy test if relevant (urine or serum), antibodies to hepatitis B virus (HBV) or hepatitis C virus (HCV), test for human immunodeficiency virus (HIV).

Tuberculosis screening includes chest X-ray, and Mantoux (intradermal test) or QuantiFERON-TB-Gold blood test.

The following protocol can be followed for monitoring patients on biological therapies:
- Annual screening for tuberculosis: Mantoux test, X ray chest alternatives include the QuantiFERON TB-gold blood test
- CD4+ T-lymphocyte count every 2 weeks for those who are on alefacept
- Complete metabolic panel with LFTs for each infliximab infusion and in those with any sign of hepatic injury
- CBC and metabolic panel every 3–6 months on all biological therapies
- Hepatitis screening and HIV testing when risk factors present in patients on all biological therapies
- Avoid all live and live-attenuated vaccines. Evaluation of CD4 lymphocyte count may be indicated in the event of development of opportunistic infection while on any immunosuppressant drug.

TO ASSESS THE PROGNOSIS

With the advancement in the field of genetics, there are many HLA and non-HLA genes found to be associated with certain disease outcome and treatment response. The following are some of the documented associations of psoriasis and HLA. Detection of these will help to manage the patient in a better way.
- Testing for HLA-B27 is useful in congenital erythrodermic psoriasis, where the etiology of erythroderma is not established. Positive HLA-B27 indicates spinal involvement
- HLA-B38, and HLA-B39 point to peripheral polyarthritis
- HLA-B39; HLA-B27 in the presence of HLA-DR7 and HLA-DQw3 may point to an increased risk for disease progression
- HLA-B22 if positive is supposed to be protective for disease progression
- HLA-Cw6 and HLA-DRB1*07 may imply a less severe course of arthritis

- MHC class I chain-related antigen A (MICA)-A9 variant positivity may denote 60% chance of developing PsA while
- MICA-A9 variant negativity indicates 70% chance of not developing PsA.

Biomarkers

Biomarkers have the potential to improve the evaluation and therefore, better assist management of psoriatic disease. There are still limited data available to validate candidate biomarkers in the different clinical forms of the disease. Promising candidate biomarkers for psoriasis include vascular endothelial growth factor (VEGF), β defensins and S100 proteins that can be found both in serum and in psoriatic plaques, and could be used in clinical practice to assess disease severity or as endpoints in studies of therapeutic interventions.[26]

The following table gives the list of various biomarkers available. These biomarkers can be used to diagnose cutaneous psoriasis, arthropathic psoriasis, to assess the association of comorbidities and to assess the response to therapy. Biomarkers in psoriasis are categorized in Table 9.3.

TABLE 9.3: Biomarkers in psoriasis

Tissue-associated biomarkers	Soluble biomarkers	Synovial fluid

• K1, K6, K10, K16,
 • VEGF
 • S100A8/A9
 • IL-6
 • IL-8
 • IL-18
 • TNF-α
 • IFN-γ
 • IL-17
 • IL-22
 • TLR
	• Serum/plasma
	 • CRP
	 • ESR
	 • VEGF
	 • hBD-2
	 • S100A8/A9
	 • IL-6
	 • IL-8
	 • IL-18
	 • TNF-α
	 • IFN-γ
	 • IL-17
	 • IL-22
	 • TGF-β1
	 • Leptin
	 • Resistin
	 • TIMP-1
	 • MMP-1
	 • CPII: C2C ratio
	 • MMP-3
	 • OPG
		• IL-1β
		 • IL-6
		 • IL-22
		 • Cell subsets:
		    ○ Th1
		    ○ Th17
		    ○ Th22
		    ○ NKT cells
		    ○ Osteoclast precursors
		 • Genetic markers:
		    ○ PSORS4 S100
		    ○ CNVDEFB4
		    ○ SNPs Il23r
		    ○ SNPs Il12b
		    ○ SNPs Il23a
		    ○ SNPs TNF-α encoding gene promoter
		    ○ NKG2D

VEGF, vascular endothelial growth factor ; CRP, C-reactive protein; ESR, erythrocyte sedimentation rate; TNF-α, tumor necrosis factor-α; IFN-γ, Interferon-γ; NKT cells, natural killer T cells; TIMP-1, tissue inhibitor of metalloproteinases-1; MMP-1, matrix metalloproteinase-1; OPG, osteoprotegerin; TGF-β1, transforming growth factor β 1; PSORS4, psoriasis susceptibility 4; SNPs, single nucleotide polymorphisms; NKG2D, natural-killer group 2, member D; IL, interleukin; TLR, toll-like receptors; Th, T helper cells; hBD-2, human β-defensin 2; CNVDEFB4, copy number variation of the defensin β 4; CPII:C2C, ratio between C-propeptide of type II collagen and collagen fragment neoepitopes.

Biomarkers of Cutaneous Psoriasis

A quantitative way of measuring the severity of psoriasis is by evaluation of histological changes in skin biopsies. Keratins can be used as biomarkers of psoriasis severity. Increased K16 expression in nonlesional psoriatic epidermis has been suggested as a marker of preclinical psoriasis. The candidate cytokine biomarker of disease severity supported by the greatest amount of evidence is IL-18.

Biomarkers for Psoriatic Arthritis

Vascular endothelial growth factor, the biomarker for active psoriasis and PsA, and could represent a factor predictive of disease progression. Serum IL-6 is proposed to represent a more specific marker than CRP and ESR in patients with PsA Patients with PsA have higher levels of IL-6 and IL-1 which was found to correlate with the number of joints affected by arthritis.

Other Markers

These include metalloproteinase-3, osteoprotegerin, and the ratio between C-propeptide of type II collagen and collagen fragment neoepitopes (CPII:C2C).

The serum level of the receptor activator of nuclear factor κB ligand reflects the extent of bone erosion and has been proposed as a predictive marker of progressive joint damage.

Circulating osteoclast precursors in patients with PsA have also been proposed as cellular biomarkers of disease severity because of their correlation with bone erosion. Increased expression of TNF-α, interferon-γ, IL-6, and IL-1β in the synovium from joints during disease, were found to be significantly reduced after therapy.

Human leukocyte antigen-Cw6 is an important marker for PsA. Other class I antigens are also associated with PsA, including HLA-B13, HLA-B57, HLA-B39, and HLA-Cw7. From linkage analysis studies, only one locus, i.e., psoriasis susceptibility (PSORS) 1 (PSORS8), seems to be specifically associated with PsA.

Biomarkers of Comorbidities

One of the most reliable predictive markers is CRP, which is a validated biomarker of cardiovascular disease. Leptin and resistin are considered as candidate biomarkers for prediction of development of insulin resistance and atherosclerosis in obese patients with psoriatic disease.

Biomarkers of Clinical Response to Biological Therapies

The most widely used soluble serum biomarker for the detection of the clinical response to biological therapies is CRP. Serum markers, such as CRP, VEGF, and resistin, were reduced by treatment in parallel with PASI score reduction that correlated significantly with downregulation of resistin.

Gene expression changes in lesional skin can also be used effectively as biomarkers of clinical response. In particular, downregulation of Th17 pathway genes.

CONCLUSION

Psoriasis is invariably diagnosed clinically needing biopsy only on certain clinical presentations where the close mimickers need to be excluded. Dermoscopy is a useful tool in the differentiation of psoriasis and diseases like PLC, lichen planus and seborrheic dermatitis of the scalp.

Investigations are to be done in all adults and in selected children with psoriasis to rule out metabolic comorbidities and to detect joint affection. By and large tests are done in order to exclude associations, complications and for planning treatment, follow-up and for research purposes.

REFERENCES

1. Errichetti E, Lacarrubba F, Micali G, Piccirillo A, Stinco G. Differentiation of pityriasis lichenoides chronica from guttate psoriasis by dermoscopy. Clin Exp Dermatol. 2015;40(7):804-6.
2. Kim GW, Jung HJ, Ko HC, Kim MB, Lee WJ, Lee SJ, et al. Dermoscopy can be useful in differentiating scalp psoriasis from seborrhoeic dermatitis. Br J Dermatol. 2011;164(3):652-6.
3. Steel DM, Whitehead AS. The major acute phase reactants: C reactive protein, serum amyloid P component and serum amyloid A protein. Immunology Today. 1994;2:81-8.
4. Blake GJ, Ridker PM. Novel clinical markers of vascular wall inflammation. Circ Res. 2001;89(9):763-71.
5. Ridker PM. C-reactive protein and other markers of inflammation in the prediction of cardiovascular disease in women. New Eng J Med. 2000;342:836-83.
6. Rohde LE, Hennekens CH, Ridker PM. Survey of C-reactive protein and cardiovascular risk factors in apparently healthy men. American J Cardiol. 1999;84:1028-32.
7. Grover C, Reddy BS, Uma Chaturvedi K. Diagnosis of nail psoriasis: Importance of biopsy and histopathology. Br J Dermatol. 2005;153:1153-8.
8. Farias DC, Tosti A, Chiacchio ND, Hirata SH. Dermoscopy in nail psoriasis. An Bras Dermatol. 2010; 85:101-3.
9. Micali G, Lacarrubba F, Massimino D, Schwartz RA. Dermatoscopy: Alternative uses in daily clinical practice. J Am Acad Dermatol. 2011;64:1135-46.
10. Micali G, Lacarrubba F. Possible applications of videodermatoscopy beyond pigmented lesions. Int J Dermatol. 2003;42:430-3.
11. Iorizzo M, Dahdah M, Vincenzi C, Tosti A. Video-dermoscopy of the hyponychium in nail bed psoriasis. J Am Acad Dermatol. 2008;58:714-5.
12. Ribeiro CF, Siqueira EB, Holler AP, Fabrício L, Skare TL. Periungual capillaroscopy in psoriasis. An Bras Dermatol. 2012;87:550-3.
13. Gutierrez M, Wortsman X, Filippucci E, De Angelis R, Filosa G, Grassi W. High-frequency sonography in the evaluation of psoriasis: Nail and skin involvement. J Ultrasound Med. 2009;28:1569-74.
14. Pierce MC, Strasswimmer J, Park BH, Cense B, de Boer JF. Advances in optical coherence tomography imaging for dermatology. J Invest Dermatol. 2004;123:458-63.
15. Hongcharu W, Dwyer P, Gonzalez S, Anderson RR. Confirmation of onychomycosis by in vivo confocal microscopy. J Am Acad Dermatol. 2000;42:214-6.
16. Healy PJ, Groves C, Chandramohan M, Helliwell PS. MRI changes in psoriatic dactylitis—extent of pathology, relationship to tenderness and correlation with clinical indices. Rheumatology. 2008;47(1):92-5.
17. Punzi L, Podswiadek M, Oliviero F, Lonigro A, Modesti V, Ramonda R, et al. Laboratory findings in psoriatic arthritis. Reumatismo. 2007;59 Suppl 1:52-5.
18. Husic R, Ficjan A. Christina Duftner, Christian Dejaco. Use of ultrasound for diagnosis and follow-up of psoriatic arthritis. EMJ Rheumatol. 2014;1:65-72.
19. De Filippis LG, Caliri A, Lo Gullo R, Bartolone S, Miceli G, Cannavò SP, et al. Ultrasonography in the early diagnosis of psoriasis-associated enthesopathy. Int J Tissue React. 2005;27(4):159-62.
20. Hahn K, Thiers G, Eissner D, Holzmann H. Bone scintigraphy in psoriasis (author's transl). [Article in German] Nuklearmedizin. 1980;19(4):178-86.
21. Holzmann H, Krause BJ, Kaltwasser JP, Werner RJ. Psoriatic osteoarthropathy and bone scintigraphy. [Article in German] Hautarzt. 1996;47(6):427-31.
22. Prodanovich S, Ma F, Taylor JR, Pezon C, Fasihi T, Kirsner RS. Methotrexate reduces incidence of vascular diseases in veterans with psoriasis or rheumatoid arthritis. J Amer Acad Dermatol. 2005;52(2):262-7.
23. Spadaro A, Riccieri V. Comparison of cyclosporin A and methotrexate in the treatment of psoriatic arthritis: A one-year prospective study. Clin Exp Rheumatol. 1995;13:589-93.
24. Ohtsuka T. The correlation between response to oral cyclosporin therapy and systemic inflammation, metabolic abnormality in patients with psoriasis. Arch Dermatol. 2008;300:545-50.
25. Lynch M, Higgins E, McCormick PA, Kirby B, Nolan N, Rogers S, et al. The use of transient elastography and FibroTest for monitoring hepatotoxicity in patients receiving methotrexate for psoriasis. JAMA Dermatol. 2014;150(8):856-62.
26. Molteni S, Reali E. Biomarkers in the pathogenesis, diagnosis, and treatment of psoriasis. Psoriasis: Targets and Therapy 2. 2012:55-66.

CHAPTER 10

Treatment

INTRODUCTION

Psoriasis, a common chronic inflammatory disease which is characterized by emissions and exacerbations, is associated with serious comorbidities including psoriatic arthritis (PsA), reduced quality of life (QoL), depression, malignancy, and cardiovascular comorbidities. The disease affects all ages including the newborn. Taking into consideration, the recurring nature of the disease, duration of therapy, especially early onset psoriasis, the side effects of drugs, and the cost involved in the tests to be performed, loss of number of working or earning days adding to the financial burden, psoriasis remains a cause for concern to the patient, parent, family, and the doctor alike. An effective therapy starts with counseling the patient and the parents. There are a number of different treatment options available for psoriasis. Typically, topical agents are used for mild disease, phototherapy for moderate disease, and systemic agents for severe disease.[1] Whether the patient is a child, adolescent or an adult, treatment options available, pros and cons of medication suggested, and the outcome should be explained. Above all, the recurring nature of the disease must be described. Adequate counseling is necessary before starting the patients on drug therapy. The treating doctor must take a long-term view. Severity of the disease and its importance in that particular individual must always be considered for an appropriate treatment. The details of the treatment must be commensurate with the patient's intelligence, physical capacity, job nature, affordability, and socioeconomic circumstances.

General measures like regular use of emollients, protein-rich diet, and avoidance of alcohol should be advised to patients before starting of treatment with specific drugs. It is worthwhile attending to patient's general, physical, and psychological health. Malnutrition, anemia, untreated arthritis, state of anxiety or depression, especially in the elderly patient, may to some extent lower the patient's tolerance of the disability. In most patients, severity of disease and psychosocial disability produced by the same do not always correlate. Rest, mild sedation, removal from a stressful environment, a holiday or a short stay as an inpatient in the hospital may all help to turn the therapeutic tide. The importance of talking to patients, trying to allay their concerns, coupled with advice on how to handle negative beliefs about their disease should be realized and sufficient time should be spent with the patients in counseling. Cognitive-behavioral therapy as an adjunct to pharmaceutical therapies is found to be effective in some patients.

This segment will review the treatment under the following headings:
- Symptomatic treatment
- Topical therapy
- Phototherapy
- Systemic therapy
- Biologics and other agents
- Treatment according to site or type
- Treatment of erythroderma
- Treatment of arthropathy
- Treatment of psoriasis in special populations
- Therapy of childhood psoriasis
- Novel drugs.

SYMPTOMATIC TREATMENT

Itching being the most common symptom, antihistamine is advised in symptomatic patients. The choice of antihistamine will depend on the patient's age, job nature, and other factors like associated systemic conditions. In some, sedative antihistamines are preferred in whom their job nature should be taken into consideration.

Pain is the most difficult symptom to treat, especially in case of PsA, which is dealt separately.

Patients with guttate, erythrodermic or pustular psoriasis may present to the emergency department. In each of these cases, restoration of the barrier function of the skin is of prime concern. Moisturizers, such as petrolatum jelly are helpful.

The simplest treatment of psoriasis is daily sun exposure, sea bathing, topical moisturizers, and relaxation. Daily application of moisturizing cream to the affected area is inexpensive and successful adjunct to psoriasis treatment. This will help to a great extent in reducing the steroid requirement. Application of emollients immediately after a bath or shower helps to minimize itching. Patients with photo koebnerization should be advised to avoid exposure to light.

TOPICAL THERAPY

For most patients, the initial decision point around therapy will be between topical and systemic therapy. However, even patients on systemic therapy will likely continue to need some topical agents. Topical therapy may provide symptomatic relief, minimize required doses of systemic medications, and may even be psychologically cathartic for some patients.[2]

Topical therapy is the mainstay for mild or localized disease with a psoriasis area and severity index (PASI) less than 10 or involvement of body surface area (BSA) of less than 20%.

Emollients, moisturizers, keratolytics, tar, anthralin, topical steroids, vitamin D analogs, calcineurin inhibitors, and retinoids are various topical preparations available for the treatment of psoriasis. The choice will depend upon the age of the patient, type of psoriasis, PASI score, site of involvement, other comorbidities and associations, tolerance, and affordability. Topical agents used in psoriasis are listed in Box 10.1.

Emollients

Emollients are the most commonly used topical agents in the management of psoriasis. White soft paraffin reduces transepidermal

BOX 10.1: Conventional topical agents used in psoriasis

- Emollients and moisturizers, fish oil
- Keratolytics
- Tars and anthralin
- Corticosteroids
- Vitamin D3 derivatives
- Calcineurin inhibitors
- Retinoids
- Newer drugs

water loss (TEWL), soothes and softens the skin and reduces scaling. They improve the barrier function of the skin and stratum corneum hydration, making the epidermis less amenable to trauma and stress, which is one of the trigger factors for the disease exacerbation. In adults, emollients are not effective as monotherapy in contrary to children, where it is wise to start treatment with emollients and allow the disease to evolve before embarking on any stronger medications having side effects. The major role for emollients and moisturizers is the supportive role in normalizing hyperproliferation, differentiation and apoptosis; furthermore, they exert anti-inflammatory effects, through physiologic lipids. Subsequently, an improved barrier function and stratum corneum hydration make the epidermis more resistant to external stress and reduce the induction of Koebner's phenomena.

Omega-3 polyunsaturated fatty acids compete with arachidonic acid as substrates for lipoperoxidases, which transform them into leukotrienes with low biological activity. As this process, in skin, may benefit psoriatic patients, it was shown that use of fish oil produced statistically significant improvement in erythema and scaling in psoriatic plaques.

Pazyar N et al. have studied the antipsoriatic effect of tea tree oil. Tea tree oil is considered an essential oil, obtained by steam distillation of the leaves and terminal branch-lets of *Melaleuca alternifolia*. Notably, terpinen-4-ol, the major tea tree constituent, has been found to have potent anti-inflammatory properties which may have a novel potential agent against psoriasis.[3]

Keratolytics

Keratolytics, such as salicylic acid and urea, reduce scaling and enhance absorption of other drugs. Salicylic acid can be used in lesions over the scalp, palms, and soles. Topical salicylic acid reduces the efficacy of ultraviolet B (UVB) phototherapy because of a filtering effect. It is to be avoided in children younger than 6 years of age because of the risk of percutaneous salicylate absorption leading to salicylism.

Tar

Coal tar is a complex mixture of substances produced by primary condensation during the carbonization of coal. Since standardization of tar preparation is impossible, there tends to be great variation in the biological activity of different preparations. This is one of the reasons why therapeutic results achieved in different centers using different preparations of tar may not be comparable. Tar has been used in topical therapy for more than a century. Its antimitotic effect is not consistently proved. Coal tar, which has antipruritic and anti-inflammatory effects, also suppresses deoxyribonucleic acid synthesis and acts as antiproliferative agent.[4,5] It can be used alone or in combination with other agents, such as corticosteroids, salicylic acid, and ultraviolet (UV) therapy. However, it is not to be used on face and flexures, and in children below 12 years of age. Tar causes irritation, when combined with ultraviolet light in the Goeckerman regimen. Tar is also known to induce chromosomal aberrations in peripheral lymphocytes and bring on release of heat shock proteins.[6]

Use of tar in psoriasis was popularized by Goeckerman. Goeckerman regimen incorporates daily application of 2–5% crude coal tar, combined with a tar bath and UV light. If used properly, tar gives good results in stable psoriatic plaques. Nearly, 80% of patients show clearance of lesion within 6 weeks. Many modifications of Goeckerman's regimen have been advocated, utilizing alcoholic extracts of tar in cream or ointment bases, tar gels which are easier to handle, but cruder the tar extract, the more effective it is. Concentrations of coal-tar solution up to 10% can be incorporated in various vehicles. Controversies about the role of tar and UV light have not yet been fully resolved as tar alone is found to be effective in treating psoriatic plaques as is UVB alone. It is worthwhile remembering that coal tar can sensitize the skin to ultraviolet A (UVA) but not to UVB and the phototoxicity induced is of photodynamic type.

Topical tar preparations including shampoos, creams, and other preparations, can be used once daily. Patients should be warned about the unpleasant odor and staining property of tar. Scalp preparations like shampoos are effective only, if the medication reaches the scalp and left in place for 5–10 minutes before rinsing.

New, advanced formula, such as sprays, foams, and nail lacquers provide opportunities to tailor treatment for individuals, which promotes patient adherence to medications. Combination of tar with other agents is preferred because of less of irritation caused when used as combination than used alone.

Tar can be considered as a safe topical agent, if used appropriately. Folliculitis is the most common side effect. Primary irritation is a common finding if used over sensitive skin like face, genitalia, and in the flexures. Tar may not be effective in unstable psoriasis due to its potential to cause irritation if used in unstable psoriasis. Allergic contact dermatitis is a rare complication of tar. Long-term use of tar can induce skin cancers. There is significantly greater risk of skin cancer in psoriatic patients treated with high-exposure coal tar and UV light therapy, than in matched patients treated with smaller dosage therapy. The risk increases in patients that are also on other immunosuppressive drugs. Prolonged use of tar should be avoided. Application of coal tar to the anogenital area including the scrotum and flexural skin is better avoided. Though the increased incidence of malignancy also depends on exposure to high-dose UVB, it is prudent to monitor patients who have received repeated intensive Goeckerman regimen and place them under regular surveillance. It may be considered that in some patients with difficult psoriasis, the benefits of repeated Goeckerman regimen may, however, outweigh the risk of skin malignancy, which should be easy to detect and treat. However, the responsibility lies with treating physician to make the correct choice of treatment and the duration. Pre-existing folliculitis, severe acne, known allergy to tar products, unstable psoriasis are contraindications to the use of tar. Erythrodermic or generalized pustular psoriasis (GPP) will infrequently tolerate even the weakest tars and, therefore, tar should not be prescribed during such acute stage of the disease.

Dithranol

Dithranol, also known as anthralin, (1, 8-dihydroxy-9-anthrone) was first introduced by Unna in 1916. Dithranol has anti-inflammatory and antiproliferative effects which are attributable to its ability to regulate keratinocyte differentiation and prevent T lymphocyte activation. When it was introduced, the preparation was unstable. Salicylic acid was used as an adjunct in stabilizing dithranol formulations which is used in the Ingram regimen. After a tar bath in which scales and the previous applications are removed, sub-erythema UVB is given, and the lesions are covered with dithranol paste. The initial concentration is 0.05% or 0.1%, increasing cautiously up to 4% according to response, and aiming to avoid irritation of the normal or psoriatic skin. The paste is kept in position with tubular gauze or stocking. After 18–22 hours, the cycle is repeated. This regimen can clear psoriasis in as short as 3 weeks. However, deep-brown staining that remains after therapy will be cosmetically disfiguring. Nevertheless, the stain will soon disappear after treatment is stopped. The staining of the bed linen and clothing is irreversible. Microcrystalline formulation of 1% dithranol that releases the active medication at skin surface temperature can reduce staining of fabrics significantly. However, staining of the skin can still occur. Aqueous gel-based liposome entrapped formulation of dithranol may be least irritant, and cause minimal staining. Allergic contact reaction is rare with dithranol, so are systemic side effects.

Dithranol is to be avoided over skin of the head and neck, flexures or genitalia. Eyes should be protected during treatment with dithranol from contact with the agent as it is highly irritant, if accidentally introduced into the eyes.

The drug accumulates in keratinocyte mitochondria, dissipates mitochondrial membrane potential, and induces apoptosis through a pathway dependent on respiratory competent mitochondria.[7] "Short-contact therapy" is the preferred method these days in which increasing concentrations of anthralin are applied for a short period (10–30 minutes) till a slight irritation develops, after which the dose and time are held constant till lesions clear.[8] 2-hour short-contact regimen using dithranol in Lassar's paste is as effective as a standard 24-hour Ingram regimen. Higher concentrations applied twice daily for 30 minutes provided no advantage over 2% dithranol in Lassar's paste applied for 2-hour once daily though the higher concentration could be tolerated well. A significant remission in 81% of children was observed with 1% concentration.[9] It can be combined with UVB phototherapy, as in Ingram regimen, to improve the response. Anthralin 1% or dithranol are rarely used for localized areas and can cause localized irritation.[10] The usage of dithranol has been reducing with advent of new more cosmetically acceptable topical preparations.

Combination of short-contact dithranol with broadband UVB (BBUVB) is more effective than short-contact dithranol or BBUVB used alone. However, dithranol in combination with narrowband UVB (NBUVB) (311 nm) is effective but, short-contact dithranol had a cumulative UVB sparing effect when used in combination with 311 nm NBUVB. Combination of dithranol with topical steroids ointment can produce more rapid clearing than when dithranol in Lassar's paste used alone. However, folliculitis is an important side effect one should look for, while combining with topical steroid along with dithranol.

Topical Steroids

Topical corticosteroids are of established value in psoriasis and still the mainstay of topical therapy in psoriasis. Topical steroids are useful in psoriasis of mild and moderate severity, where topical treatment is the first-line therapy, especially in the event of nonavailability of UVB therapy. In appropriate concentration and formula, topical corticosteroids are still used in treatment of plaques over the face, neck, flexures, and genitalia, even in children, however, topical calcineurin inhibitors are preferred in these sites for fear of side effects due to inadvertent use of topical corticosteroids. Diluted topical steroids are also used in unstable, erythrodermic and GPP, for a very short period in preference to tar or dithranol which can cause irritation. However, bland emollients are more suitable as the absorption of topical corticosteroids cannot be predicted in a breached skin. Topical corticosteroids have the merits of ease of application and removal, lack of irritancy, and the absence of staining of skin or linen. The hazards of therapy are now well known, and enhancement by polythene occlusion will magnify and hasten side effects. Topical steroids under occlusion do have a limited place in the management of recalcitrant psoriasis of the scalp, hands, feet, and other areas. Hydrocolloid dressing is found to be superior to plastic film used for occlusive therapy.

Topical steroids are the most suitable topical agents for the treatment of psoriasis among all age groups. They have anti-inflammatory, antiproliferative, immunosuppressive, and vasoconstrictive effects. High-potency corticosteroids should be avoided in children. Low-potency to mid-potency corticosteroids, class 5–7, are chosen for facial and intertriginous lesions, while mid-potency class 2–4, are chosen for extremities and the scalp.[11] Topical clobetasol has been approved for use in children ages 12 years and over in some formulations and can be quite effective for use in psoriatic lesions in adolescents[12] Their inadvertent and long-term use can lead to local infections, skin atrophy, telangiectasia, striae distensae, acneiform eruption, and purpura. Contact dermatitis to the molecule or the vehicle is not uncommon. Rebound and tachyphylaxis are to be remembered while using topical steroids for a prolonged period. It is always advisable to follow the fingertip unit and adhere to the schedule. Systemic side effects are more common in children than adults because of a higher skin surface or body mass ratio. Ointments are to be avoided in flexural, facial, and genital skin. Lotions are preferred for hairy scalp. They can also be combined with other topical agents, such as calcipotriol and tazarotene to enhance efficacy and reduce irritation.

Topical corticosteroids can be continued till the lesions become flat and inactive.

Skin atrophy can be avoided by adapting one or more of the following:
- Choosing the correct formula e.g., choosing foam and lotion for scalp and avoiding ointment over flexures and thin skin-like face
- Starting with a potent steroid and reducing the potency
- Intermittent use of topical steroid e.g., during weekends
- Combining with emollients.

Corticosteroid can be given intralesionally in resistant plaques of psoriasis. Triamcinolone hexacetonide (5 mg/mL) or triamcinolone acetonide (10 mg/mL) can be infiltrated intradermally into localized psoriatic lesions by needle injection. This is of particular value in troublesome, small, resistant lesions on the backs of hands, especially the knuckles, intensely pruritic small plaques or lichenoid lesions where systemic therapy is not required because of lesser involvement with reference to BSA. The remission is prolonged and repetition of the injection may not be required for several months. In psoriasis of fingernails, the nail fold can be injected, with triamcinolone acetonide, but the procedure may be painful and the results are as good as in psoriasis of skin.

More details on use of topical steroids in children are given in Chapter 5.

Topical Vitamin D Analogs

Topical vitamin D analogs have anti-inflammatory and antiproliferative actions. They also induce downregulation and correction of keratinocyte differentiation. Calcipotriol, calcitriol, maxacalcitol, and tacalcitol are the various vitamin D analogs useful in the treatment of psoriasis. When combined with betamethasone, the effect is better than either agent used alone. UVB phototherapy increases the efficacy of calcipotriol.[13] The most common adverse events are burning and stinging sensation, the drug is safe when the total dose does not exceed the recommended dose of not more than 75 g/week for children above 12 years and 50 g/week for children aging between 6 and 12 years. Over use of vitamin D analogs can lead to hypercalcemia. Calcitriol and its synthetic derivative calcipotriene are preferred for pediatric psoriasis, the latter being well-tolerated for sensitive skin.[14,15]

Calcineurin Inhibitors

Topical calcineurin inhibitors act as non-steroidal immune-modulatory drugs. They inhibit interleukin (IL)-2 production and subsequent T-cell activation and proliferation by blocking the enzyme calcineurin. Tacrolimus (0.03%, 0.1%) ointment and pimecrolimus (1%) cream are two drugs belonging to this class, which, although not Food and Drug Administration (FDA) approved, have proven efficacy. This has recently been documented for treatment of childhood psoriasis.[16,17] They can be used as steroid sparing agents and are also useful for sequential and rotational regimens, so as to avoid long-term adverse effects of topical steroids. They are useful for sites, such as face, flexures, and anogenital region where topical steroids cannot be used safely.[18] Use of topical calcineurin inhibitors in children under the age of 2 years is not recommended by the FDA.

Retinoids

Tazarotene is a third-generation retinoid that acts on keratinocyte differentiation, diminishing hyperproliferation and decreases expression of inflammatory markers. Skin irritation is the most common side effect and its use is thus usually restricted to thicker plaques in the non-intertriginous sites. Tazarotene 0.05% gel has been successfully used to treat nail psoriasis in a child in a single case report.[19] Short-contact therapy for 20 minutes will reduce the irritation caused by the drug without reducing the clinical response.

Combinations

The following are effective combination of molecules. The clinical response is better while using a combination than when they are used alone. Similarly, the side effects like irritation can be minimized by using combination. However, incidence of side effects like folliculitis can be more especially with combinations using potent steroids.
- Tar and corticosteroid
- Dithranol corticosteroid
- Calcipotriene and corticosteroids
- Keratolytics and corticosteroid.

Newer Topical Agents under Way

These molecules include neuropeptide-modulating agents, new nonsteroidal anti-inflammatory drugs (NSAIDs), mitogen-activated protein kinase 1/mitogen-activated protein kinase kinase 1 (MEK1/MEKK1) inhibitor, phosphodiesterase inhibitors, and pan-selectin antagonists. Box 10.2 gives the list of newer topical agents useful in psoriasis.

Neuropeptide-modulating Agents

Neuropeptide-modulating agents, such as capsaicin, somatostatin, and peptide T improve psoriasis K252a, a high-affinity nerve growth factor, receptor blocker, and CT327, a pegylated derivative of K252a, are being studied and found to show clinical and histological improvement of psoriasis.

New Nonsteroidal Anti-inflammatory Drugs

WBI-1001 [(2-isopropyl-5-[(E)-2-phenyl-ethenyl] benzene-1, 3-diol)] is a new anti-inflammatory, nonsteroidal, small molecule deriving from metabolites of bacterial symbionts of soil living nematodes. Its inflammatory action is due to significant inhibition of the expression of proinflammatory cytokines, such as tumor necrosis factor-α (TNF-α) and interferon-γ (IFN-γ). This topical synthetic compound has been developed for the treatment of chronic inflammatory skin diseases including psoriasis and atopic dermatitis.

LAS41002 and LAS41004 constitute novel interesting NSAIDs act on a corticosteroid receptor, thus determining both the suppression of inflammation and the inhibition of cellular proliferation.

PH-10, a preparation Rose Bengal disodium, is found to be effective in mild-to-moderate plaque psoriasis.

Janus-associated Kinase Inhibitors

Topical tofacitinib (CP-690, 550,) suppresses Janus-associated kinase 1 (JAK1) and JAK3 and, to a lesser extent, JAK2 and tyrosine kinase 2 (TYK2) signaling. It was developed as an immunosuppressive agent for the prevention of transplant rejection and for the treatment of immune-mediated diseases, such as rheumatoid arthritis, Crohn's disease, ulcerative colitis, and psoriasis. It was found that tofacitinib ointment to be well-tolerated and efficacious compared with vehicle for the treatment of plaque psoriasis.[20]

ASP-015K and INCB018424 were demonstrated to be effective, with a clinical improvement of the lesion score (lesion thickness, erythema, and scaling) greater than 50%.

Mitogen-activated Protein Kinase 1/ Mitogen-activated Protein Kinase Kinase 1 Inhibitor

Topical administration of E6201 (a novel kinase inhibitor of mitogen activated protein kinase) formulated as an ointment or cream was effective in reducing acute edema formation and neutrophil infiltration into mouse skin.

Phosphodiesterase Inhibitors

These include following:
- AN2728 [(5-(4-cyanophenoxy)-2, 3-di-hydro-1-hydroxy-2, 1-benzoxaborole)]

BOX 10.2: Newer topical agents useful in psoriasis

- Neuropeptide-modulating agents
- New NSAIDS
- Janus-associated kinase inhibitors
- MEK1/MEKK1 inhibitor
- Phosphodiesterase inhibitors
- Pan-selectin antagonists

NSAID, nonsteroidal anti-inflammatory drug; MEK1, mitogen-activated protein kinase 1; MEKK1, mitogen-activated protein kinase kinase 1.

- MK-0873
- M518101.

Pan-selectin Antagonists

- Bimosiamose or TBC1269 is found useful in plaque type psoriasis
- Efomycin M has been investigated in a mouse model, but clinical trials are still lacking.

PHOTOTHERAPY

It is well known that psoriasis improves during the summer months and UV irradiation has long been recognized as beneficial for the control of psoriatic skin lesions. UV radiation has antiproliferative effect, thereby slowing keratinization. Due to its anti-inflammatory effects, UV radiation induces apoptosis of pathogenic T-cells in psoriatic plaques. In choosing UV therapy, consideration must be given to the potential for UV radiation to accelerate photo damage and increase the risk of cutaneous malignancy. This must be particularly remembered while suggesting phototherapy for children. Phototherapy can be administered with UV radiation or light amplification by stimulated emission of radiation (LASER), both as an office procedure or home unit delivery. Whatever be the modality, the dermatologists should meticulously calculate the dose and monitor the patient for both clinical improvement and side effect.

The common modalities of light therapy used include:
- UVB
    - BBUVB
    - NBUVB
- Photochemotherapy with UVA—psoralen with UVA (PUVA)
- Combined therapy
- LASER.

Ultraviolet B

Phototherapy with UVB spectrum light (290–320 nm) has been used to treat psoriasis for at least the past 70 years. Phototherapy induces immunosuppression that involves induction of apoptosis in both T lymphocytes and keratinocytes, leading to decreased inflammation and epidermal hyperplasia. Exposure to UVB, alone or in combination with emollients or tar preparation is an effective therapy in the treatment of psoriasis. Successful clearance of psoriasis using UVB, with or without petrolatum, typically occurs within 6 weeks of treatment and weekly regimens range from 3 to 5 exposures per week, take an average of 25 doses to achieve clearance.

- BBUVB radiation (290–320 nm): This treatment is used in patients with extensive disease, alone or in combination with topical tar. The mechanism of action of UVB is likely through its immunomodulatory effects. Patients receive near-erythema-inducing doses of UVB at least three times weekly until remission is achieved, after which a maintenance regimen for 2 months is usually recommended to prolong the remission
- NBUVB phototherapy consists of a subset of the UVB spectrum, with a peak at 311 nm. This is an alternative to standard (BB: 290–320 nm) UVB in the treatment of psoriasis. Apoptosis of T cells is also more common with 311 nm than with BBUVB. The advantage of NBUVB being maximum clinical response with minimum erythema that is faster and more complete
- Home phototherapy: An alternative to office-based phototherapy is the use of a

home UVB phototherapy unit, prescribed by the treating clinician. This option may be preferred by patients who are not in close proximity to an office-based phototherapy center, whose schedules do not permit frequent office visits, or for whom the costs of in-office treatment exceed those of a home phototherapy unit. When use with adequate safety measures, they are as good as office unit, reducing time and travel.[21]

In a study conducted by Takahashi H et al., comparing the clinical efficacy of various psoriasis treatments among: (1) topical application of calcipotriol ointment twice daily; (2) topical application of calcipotriol ointment twice daily and NBUVB phototherapy once a week; (3) topical application of heparinoid ointment twice daily and NBUVB phototherapy more than twice a week; and (4) topical application of calcipotriol ointment twice daily and NBUVB phototherapy more than twice a week, it was found that combination of calcipotriol ointment plus NBUVB more than twice a week is superior to other treatment regimens, rapidly improving psoriasis lesions.[22] The pretreatment of psoriatic plaques with either petrolatum or crude coal tar may enhance the therapeutic outcome of NBUVB.[23] Similarly, it was observed that isotretinoin plus NBUVB can reduce number of phototherapy sessions and cumulative NBUVB dose.[24]

Psoriasis with thin scales responds best to NBUVB. Following are the indication of NBUVB:
- All types of moderate-to-severe psoriasis
- Where topical therapy is not sufficient to control disease or systemic drugs are contraindicated or poorly tolerated or ineffective
- Patients with comorbidities
- Children and pregnant women.

However, one must remember the contraindications to NBUVB.

Contraindications of Narrowband Ultraviolet B

Absolute contraindications include photodermatoses and cutaneous malignancy. Multiple atypical nevi are a relative contraindication. History of epilepsy, claustrophobia, cardiac insufficiency should be elicited and such patients should not be advised NBUVB.

Dosimetry: NBUVB can be given with a starting dose of 280–350 mJ in a frequency of 2–3 treatments a week with an increment of 20% at alternate sittings until clinical remission. However, the cumulative number of 450–500 sessions should not be exceeded and it is mandatory to screen them for malignancy once a year after 200 sessions.

Photochemotherapy

Photochemotherapy (PUVA) involves treatment with either oral or bath psoralen followed by UVA radiation (320–400 nm) under strict medical supervision. UVA penetrates deeper into the dermis than UVB and does not have the latter's potential for burning the skin. PUVA therapy can be oral PUVA, bath PUVA or topical PUVA.

In oral PUVA, 8-methoxypsoralen (MOP) is ingested at a dose 0.6 mg/kg 2 hours before irradiation, followed within 2 hours by exposure to UVA; this sequence is performed three times weekly, the dose is increased by increments of 0.5–1.5 J/cm^2 according to response until remission, then twice or once weekly as a maintenance dose. Higher clearance UVA doses (13–14 J/cm^2), higher cumulative doses (up to 200 J) and 10–12 weeks may be needed in selected cases.

With bath or topical PUVA, the psoralen capsules are dissolved in water [0.5 mL of 1.2% 8-MOP lotion in 2 L of water for final concentration of 3 mg/L or 5 mg of trimethylpsoralen (TMP) in 10 mL ethanol mixed with 15 L water], and affected skin (hands, feet or total body) is soaked for 15–30 minutes prior to UVA exposure. Pretreatment and posttreatment photoprotection (e.g., hat, sunscreen, sun protective goggles) are critical in preventing serious burn injury to the skin and eyes from being outside. PUVA is advisable for patients with disease involving more than 20% of the BSA, not controlled by conventional topical therapy. Treatment is given two to four times weekly. UVA dosage is increased by increments of 0.5–1.5 J/cm^2 according to response. PUVA therapy is contraindicated in children under 18 years. Similarly, pregnant women and those who are lactating should not be treated with PUVA therapy for fear of potential damage that can happen to the fetus and infant, respectively. Patients with photosensitive disorders like xeroderma pigmentosum and lupus erythematosus are not ideal candidates for PUVA therapy. Individuals with hepatic disorders are at increased risk of complications and hence, are better not given PUVA therapy. Pre-existing cutaneous malignancy is a contraindication to PUVA therapy as PUVA therapy by itself can induce malignancy. Patients with undue exposure to inorganic arsenic and those who are on radiotherapy should be exempted from PUVA therapy contraindications to PUVA therapy are given in Box 10.3.

PUVA should not be suggested for hairy scalp.

Of all the clinical types, psoriasis vulgaris responds best to PUVA therapy with a clearance rate as high as up to 90% have been. PUVA is also of value in GPP, erythrodermic psoriasis, palmoplantar pustulosis, and nail psoriasis, but success rates are much lower in these atypical patterns of disease. It would be advisable to give maintenance treatment

> **BOX 10.3: Contraindications to psoralen with ultraviolet light A therapy**
> - Exposure to inorganic arsenic
> - Radiotherapy
> - Cutaneous malignancy
> - Hepatic disorders
> - Photosensitive disorders
> - Xeroderma pigmentosum
> - Lupus erythematosus
> - Pregnancy
> - Lactation
> - Children under 18 years

for 2 months and stop PUVA, if remission is maintained.

Pretreatment emollients have long been thought to improve results with UVB. However, while thin oils do not impede UV penetration, emollient creams can actually inhibit the penetration of the UV and should not be applied before treatment. Gentle removal of plaques by bathing does help prior to UV exposure.

Since PUVA is associated with potential systemic side effects (erythema, pruritus, nausea, ocular damage, and increased risk of skin cancer) as well as death from accidental overexposure, it is generally not recommended as an option for home phototherapy.

Combination Therapy

The following combinations are used with success in the management of psoriasis that does not respond to conventional therapy:
- Etretinate or acitretin and PUVA
- Dithranol and PUVA
- Methotrexate (MTX) in combination with PUVA as in erythrodermic or pustular psoriasis

- Topical corticosteroids and PUVA
- Calcipotriol combined with PUVA
- Carcinogenicity is a risk while combining PUVA with cytotoxic drugs like MTX.

Hepatotoxicity should also be born in mind before combining PUVA with systemic drugs.
- Saltwater baths
  o Climatotherapy has also been used as a therapy for psoriasis, where bathing in sea water is combined with sun exposure
  o Balneophototherapy involves use of saltwater baths with artificial UV exposure.

Adverse effects associated with phototherapy include both acute adverse effects and cumulative, dose-related effects that occur with prolonged use. Early adverse effects associated with BBUVB and NBUVB phototherapy are typically limited to erythema and drying of the skin, with maximal erythema occurring between 8 and 24 hours following exposure. Blistering is more common with BBUVB phototherapy compared to NBUVB, due to the lower erythemogenicity of NBUVB. Late adverse effects due to cumulative UVB dose include premature aging (photo aging), wrinkling and leathery appearance, increased fragility of the skin, and increased risk of photocarcinogenesis.

Folate deficiency which is a theoretical possibility following UV exposure, more with UVA than UVB has not been proved beyond doubt in psoriasis patients treated with phototherapy. *In vitro* study, exposure of plasma to UVA led to a 30–50% decrease in the serum folate level within 60 minutes. However, folate deficiency secondary to UVA exposure has not been proven to occur *in vivo*.

Units with a built-in controlled prescription timer (CPT) are advisable to reduce, unauthorized use or inappropriate use.

Warning about Phototherapy

- Patient should avoid exposure to risky levels of UV rays for fear of developing cancer
- Proper protection should be given to the other parts of body that does not require radiation with sunscreen or clothing
- All photosensitizing products including drugs and perfumes should be avoided during phototherapy
- Periodic examination is mandatory to check for signs of skin cancer.

LASER

Excimer laser is another development in UV therapy for psoriasis and involves use of a high energy 308 nm excimer laser. The laser allows treatment of only involved skin; thus, considerably higher doses of UVB can be administered to psoriatic plaques at a given treatment compared with traditional phototherapy. LASER therapy results in faster responses than conventional phototherapy. UV-induced hyperpigmentation is a common sequel of excimer laser therapy which resolves after the discontinuation of treatment. A pilot study has reported 308 nm excimer lasers to be a safe and effective treatment for localized psoriasis in children as in adults.[25]

There is some evidence that a significant proportion of patients with psoriasis that is refractory to topical therapies may respond to laser treatment. Excimer lasers and EX-308 excimer laser system have been cleared by the FDA based on 510(k) applications for treatment of mild-to-moderate localized psoriasis. The potential benefits over standard UVB treatments are in terms of more rapid clinical response and more targeted therapy, avoiding the side effects of UV light exposure to unaffected skin. This procedure is usually repeated at least twice-weekly for 2–4 weeks.

Thus, the excimer laser may be considered as a treatment option for those patients in whom topical therapy has failed. According to published clinical studies, responses increase with up to 13 treatments, and the typical duration of response is 4–6 months. Additionally, clinical trials of the laser therapy selected patients with less than 10% of BSA affected because, in the clinical setting, it is not practical to treat more than 10% of BSA with the laser, because of the extended treatment time required due to the relatively small treatment spot size.

Pulsed dye laser (PDL) has been found to be effective in the treatment of plaque type psoriasis. It should be noted that the National Psoriasis Foundation (2007) states that PDL can be used to treat chronic localized plaque lesions. PDL combined with topical tazarotene 0.1% cream is an effective and safe therapy in the treatment of nail psoriasis.[26]

SYSTEMIC THERAPIES

Specific systemic therapy is frequently used in psoriasis to bring down the inflammation which is the main cause of systemic comorbidities. However, systemic therapy is rarely used in childhood psoriasis. In children, systemic therapy including retinoid, MTX, and cyclosporine, biologic is only used in severe forms of the disease, such as erythrodermic, pustular, and arthritic psoriasis. All these therapeutic options can be used as monotherapy or in various combinations.

The indication for systemic therapy is one or more of the following:
- Involvement of BSA more than 20%
- Psoriasis area and severity index more than 10
- Erythrodermic psoriasis, with or without metabolic complication
- GPP
- Psoriatic arthropathy

BOX 10.4: CSystemic drugs used in psoriasis
- Retinoids
- Methotrexate
- Cyclosporine
- Tacrolimus
- Hydroxyurea
- 6-thioguanine
- Azathioprine
- Fumaric acid esters
- Biologic agents

- Localized disease not responding to topical therapy alone or with significant psychological morbidity.

Systemic drugs used in psoriasis are listed in Box 10.4.

Retinoids

Systemic retinoids (derivatives of vitamin A) are utilized for patients with severe psoriasis, including pustular and erythrodermic forms, and in patients with human immunodeficiency virus (HIV)-associated psoriasis. The retinoid of choice in psoriasis is acitretin in a dose range of 25 mg every other day to 50 mg daily. When used in combination with UVB or PUVA therapy the response rates are higher with better tolerance and less UV exposure.

Monitoring for hypertriglyceridemia and hepatotoxicity are mandatory with retinoid therapy. Cheilitis and alopecia are common side effects. Being a teratogenic drug, it is to be avoided in patients in the reproductive age and pregnancy is contraindicated for 3 years after discontinuing the drug.

Etretinate and acitretin, belonging to second-generation retinoid, are the most commonly used systemic retinoid in children. The modes of action include modulation of the epidermal proliferation and differentiation, and anti-inflammatory activity. To begin with a low dose is started which can be increased up to 1 mg/kg/day and on improvement, tapered to 0.2 mg/kg body weight. The treatment continued for around 2–3 months postremission. Absorption is increased by milk or fatty foods and when dissolved in edible oils will enhance absorption.[27] The most common adverse effects are xerosis, cheilitis, epistaxis, and reversible alteration in liver enzymes and serum lipids. Premature closure of epiphysis limits its use in children. Retinoids are best avoided while treating girls.

Haushalter K et al. have revisited the pivotal acitretin trials to compare the efficacy of high-dose versus low-dose acitretin. Individualization of acitretin dosing is crucial to minimize side effects and should lead to improved adherence and efficacy. This analysis supports the utility of low-dose acitretin for psoriasis over extended treatment periods.[28]

Methotrexate

It is an antimetabolite agent and one of the most commonly used systemic agent for the treatment of psoriasis, because of its efficacy, affordability, and convenient dosing. It is usually given in a dosage of 0.2–0.4 mg/kg/week.[29] There are various studies documenting the successful use of MTX in various forms of juvenile psoriasis.

Methotrexate is well-tolerated by children. It is effective as a single weekly oral dose of 3.75–25 mg. Most of the children tolerate the drug well. Nausea, vomiting are the common side effects.[30] Serious adversities are a rare occurrence. When carefully monitored, MTX can be a safe and efficacious treatment option for severe forms of psoriasis in children. Obesity may be a relative contraindication, as associated nonalcoholic fatty liver disease is likely to increase hepatotoxicity.[31,32] As alcohol abuse greatly increases the risks of liver damage, therefore, patients receiving MTX, should be reminded regularly of the need to restrict or avoid alcohol intake.

Nausea is the most common side effect usually appearing within 12 hours of MTX ingestion lasting up to 3 days. It is usually mild, but in some patients, it is sufficiently severe enough to necessitate withdrawal of therapy. No measures are guaranteed to relieve symptoms. The subcutaneous administration has helped reduce problems with gastrointestinal intolerance.

Folic acid, supplementation has been found to be helpful in preventing folate deficiency, reducing myelotoxicity and improving tolerance of MTX. It is broadly recognized that folate supplementation should be initiated with MTX therapy although practice varies regarding the dose. Commonly, it is taken on the 6 days of the week when MTX is not taken. The minimum dosage recommended is 5 mg taken once weekly.

Although liver enzyme tests are an unreliable indicator of liver fibrosis, an acute rise in liver enzymes may indicate hepatic inflammation. If aspartate or alanine aminotransferase levels rise to greater than three times the upper limit of normal MTX would normally be discontinued.

A test dose of 5 mg should be given and if the full blood count is stable at 7 days, then MTX may be continued. Subsequent doses may be gradually increased, usually by 2.5–5 mg steps, according to clinical response and any accompanying toxicity. The aim of therapy should be to achieve sufficient control that it may be more readily managed with topical therapy and not to induce complete clearance of psoriasis. Most patients are adequately controlled on doses of 7.5–15 mg weekly and few patients require more than 20 mg. The maximum weekly dose should not exceed 30 mg. Lower doses are required in the elderly and those with renal impairment. Most forms of topical treatment can be continued while patient is on MTX. Systemic immunosuppressive drugs and UV radiation are not usually administered concurrently with MTX.

Nausea, vomiting, headache, and fatigue were significantly less common side effects in the patients who received MTX daily, but liver enzyme abnormalities were less common and clinical efficacy was greater in the patients who received MTX weekly.

Folic acid, 1 mg daily, protects against some of the common side effects seen with low-dose MTX, such as stomatitis. Folate does not appear to protect against pulmonary toxicity, and it is uncertain whether it protects against hepatic toxicity; monitoring for bone marrow suppression and hepatotoxicity are necessary during therapy. Concurrent use of other medications that interfere with folic acid metabolism, such as sulfa antibiotics, can increase the toxicity of MTX.

Risk factors for hepatotoxicity from MTX include:
- History of more than moderate alcohol consumption
- Persistent abnormal liver chemistry studies
- History of liver disease, such as chronic hepatitis B or C
- Family history of inherited liver disease (e.g., hemochromatosis)
- Diabetes mellitus
- Obesity
- History of significant exposure to hepatotoxic drugs (other than MTX) or chemicals
- Absence of folate supplementation during MTX therapy
- Hyperlipidemia.

Relative contraindications for MTX use will include:

- Renal dysfunction (dosage adjustments are needed)
- Significantly abnormal results on liver function tests
- Hepatitis
- Cirrhosis
- Significant pulmonary disease
- Blood dyscrasias (severe anemia, leukopenia, thrombocytopenia)
- Excessive alcohol consumption
- Active infectious disease [tuberculosis (TB) and pyelonephritis].

Indications for Considering Liver Biopsy

Patients without risk factors for hepatotoxicity should have liver chemistries drawn every 1–3 months. If five out of nine serum aspartate aminotransferase (AST) levels are elevated over the course of 12 months, or if the serum albumin level is decreased in the context of normal nutritional status and well-controlled psoriasis, a liver biopsy should be performed.
- Elevation of pretreatment aminoterminal peptide of procollagen type III (PIIINP) above 8.0 mcg/L
- Elevation of PIIINP above normal range (1.7–4.2 mcg/L) in at least three samples over a 12-month period
- Elevation of PIIINP above 8.0 mcg/L in two consecutive samples.

Indications for considering withdrawal of MTX:
- Elevation of PIIINP above 10 mcg/L in at least three samples in one 12-month period.

Methotrexate over dose: Suspected cases of MTX overdose or severe hematological toxicity should be treated with folinic acid. An initial dose of 20 mg, given intravenously should be followed by 15 mg given at 6 hourly intervals until the hematological abnormalities are improved (usually not more than 2–8 doses). If serum MTX is measured, a dose of 20 mg usually is sufficient for a MTX concentration of 0.5 µmol/L or less.

Systemic Calcineurin Inhibitors

The T-cell suppressor cyclosporine is effective in patients with severe psoriasis in the dose range of 3–5 mg/kg/day orally. Improvement is generally observed within 4 weeks.

Close monitoring is required since renal toxicity and hypertension are common and often limit the long-term use of cyclosporine in patients with psoriasis. cyclosporine is an effective drug in the management of childhood psoriasis and is generally well-tolerated.[33] It is used in a dose range of 3–5 mg/kg and is variably effective. In some patients, it is a true crisis buster. Nephrotoxicity, hypertension, and immunosuppression are the major side effects and hence, the drug is reserved only for severe cases.[34,35]

Long-term cyclosporine regimen can be justified in severe psoriasis not responsive to other treatments. When cyclosporine administration is required, obesity, pretreatment controlled hypertension, increased age (>70 years), and metabolic syndrome should be taken into consideration, as a significant correlation with occurrence of cyclosporine-induced side effects.[36]

Tacrolimus is found effective for treating moderate-to-severe psoriasis at a dose of at least 0.1 mg/kg/day.

Other immunosuppressive agents that are sometimes used in selected cases of severe psoriasis include hydroxyurea, 6-thioguanine, and azathioprine, which have a place in the treatment of psoriasis when other systemic modalities cannot be used, tacrolimus, which is similar to cyclosporine and requires larger studies before it can be considered an accepted alternative.

Hydroxyurea, a hydroxylated molecule of urea is commonly used to treat chronic myelogeneous leukemia and polycythemia vera. Studies suggest it can be used as an alternative to MTX in moderate-to-severe psoriasis. The efficacy and safety of hydroxyurea is equal to or better than MTX, and it can be used as a monotherapy or as an effective pair or in combination therapy or rotational therapy. Most studies have concentrated on the plaque form of the disease. However it was found useful in patients with pustular psoriasis in a dose of 1–2 g/day.[37]

A pregnancy category D drug, 6 Thiaguanine, a pregnancy category D drug is not FDA-approved drug for the use of psoriasis. The dosage is started at 80 mg two times/week; increased by 20 mg every 2–4 weeks; maximum dose is 160 mg three times/week. Contraindications include pre-existing liver disease, immunosuppression, anemia, leukopenia, and/or thrombocytopenia.

Azathioprine

Azathioprine has not been approved by the FDA for the use of psoriasis.

Allergy to azathioprine, pregnancy or attempting pregnancy, clinically significant active infection are absolute contraindications, while concurrent use of allopurinol and prior treatment with cyclophosphamide or chlorambucil are relative contraindications.

Thiopurine s-methyl transferase (TPMT) levels are generally used to guide dosing.

One suggested daily schedule guided by results of TPMT values 181.

- TPMT less than 5.0 U, do not use azathioprine
- TPMT 5–13.7 U, 0.5 mg/kg maximum dose
- TPMT 13.7–19.0 U, 1.5 mg/kg maximum dose

- TPMT more than 19.0 U, 2.5 mg/kg maximum dose.

Alternatively, start at 0.5 mg/kg, and monitor for cytopenia; if no cytopenia, can increase dose by 0.5 mg/kg/day after 6-8 weeks if necessary and increase by 0.5 mg/kg/day every 4 weeks and thereafter as needed; generally dosed at 75-150 mg/day.

Azathioprine has been used in the treatment of psoriasis with variable results, the dose being 2-5 mg/kg body weight (120-300 mg)/day for 2-24 weeks. Majority of the patients relapse in 1-6 months after stoppage of azathioprine. In a study conducted by Gupta, azathioprine pulse therapy (APT) has shown promising result with no recurrence of lesions for 40.14 + 22.56 months.

This azathioprine pulse therapy consisted of giving intermittent high dose (IHD) azathioprine 500 mg on 3 consecutive days, repeated every month in combination with continuous low dose azathioprine 100 mg orally given in between IHD. The regimen was divided into four phases.[38]
- Phase 1: APT was continued till the lesions cleared completely
- Phase 2: APT was continued for another 9 months
- Phase 3: Only daily azathioprine 100 mg was continued for another 9 months
- Phase 4: Azathioprine was stopped and patients were followed-up.

Apart from prolonged remission; the side effects following APT appear to be significantly mild and reversible. The most common side effect seen in all three phases was altered liver function tests. The other side effects included leucopenia, nausea, vomiting, weakness, giddiness, restlessness, uneasiness, loss of appetite, and hair loss which were mainly observed during phase 1.

Systemic Steroids

Systemic steroids are not used as a routine in the management of psoriasis for fear of dependence and flair following withdrawal. Psoriasis, being a disease characterized by remission and exacerbation, the requirement of steroid therapy will be for a prolonged period and hence, is not recommended for the treatment of psoriasis. However, patients with pustular psoriasis and erythrodermic psoriasis can be given a short course of systemic steroid to tide over the crisis and maintained with other systemic agents.

German analysis uncovered that corticosteroids were the most frequently prescribed systemic therapy among psoriasis patients, despite systemic corticosteroids not being outlined in European treatment guidelines.[39] It is advisable not to use systemic glucocorticoids due to the perceived potential for these drugs to induce a flare of psoriasis upon withdrawal.

Fumaric Acid Esters

Fumaric acid esters have been used to treat moderate-to-severe psoriasis. Reductions in disease severity after treatment with fumaric acid esters were similar to those observed with MTX therapy. Lymphopenia and progressive multifocal leukoencephalopathy (PML) have been reported in patients who continued to receive long-term fumaric acid ester therapy.

BIOLOGIC AND OTHER AGENTS

Biologic agents are important treatment options for moderate-to-severe plaque type psoriasis. The main T cell inhibitors include alefacept and efalizumab.

Cytokine inhibitors are capable of inhibiting either TNF-α or the ILs. TNF-α inhibitors include etanercept, infliximab, and adalimumab, while ustekinumab is an IL-12/23 inhibitor. All TNF-α inhibitors have the potential to activate latent infections and have also been associated with an increased risk of malignancies, including lymphoma and leukemia, and the development of new-onset psoriasis.

Etanercept, infliximab, adalimumab, ustekinumab, and alefacept, the agents so far found useful in psoriasis, should be considered only if the disease involves more than 10% of the BSA after excluding infections, and only when other drugs have failed or contraindicated.

Etanercept

The TNF-α inhibitor etanercept is of benefit in psoriasis. It is a dimeric fully human fusion protein consisting of two ligand binding domains of p75 tumor necrosis factor receptor fused to Fc portion of immunoglobulin (Ig) G1. This compound prevents the cytokine from binding to any cell surface receptor.

Etanercept was approved by the FDA for PsA and for adults with chronic moderate to severe plaque psoriasis. Given as subcutaneous injections in the dose of 25 mg weekly, 25 mg twice weekly or 50 mg twice weekly has a tissue half-life of 4.8 days and the bioavailability is 58%. Etanercept is well-tolerated.

Infliximab

Infliximab is chimeric mouse-human IgG1 antibody that binds soluble and trans-membrane TNF-α. Infliximab is of benefit in patients with moderate-to-severe plaque psoriasis and appears to act fast and is well-tolerated. The drug is given in the dose of 5 mg/kg at weeks 0, 2, 6, 14, and 22 given as slow intravenous administration for over 2 hours. Maintenance therapy with infliximab also appears to be effective. Maintenance dosing of infliximab is 5 mg/kg every 8 weeks. The impact of anti-infliximab antibodies on treatment efficacy in psoriasis remains unclear.

Adalimumab

Adalimumab, a humanized monoclonal antibody with activity against TNF-α, was originally used for patients with rheumatoid arthritis and is also effective for PsA. Adalimumab is approved by the FDA for treatment of adult patients with moderate-to-severe chronic plaque psoriasis who are candidates for systemic therapy or phototherapy. Adalimumab is given by subcutaneous injection 80 mg subcutaneous in first week followed by 40 mg subcutaneous in second week followed by 40 mg subcutaneous every other week.

Most patients do not require dose escalation and the safety results were similar between patients who dosage-escalated and those who did not. Adalimumab was effective and well-tolerated in patients with psoriasis previously treated with anti-TNF therapy.

Apart from injection site reactions, infections are the major side effect in patients treated with TNF-α inhibitors.

Cases of disseminated TB have been reported following TNF-α inhibitors therapy. If purified protein derivative greater than 5 mm should be considered positive and treatment should be started as for latent TB after evaluation with X-ray chest and other investigations. Tuberculosis is a rare but a severe complication of anti-TNF treatment and may develop in spite of chemoprophylaxis. The risk of TB in psoriasis patients in the present study is comparable to literature mostly based on rheumatology patients.[40] Upper respiratory infection, atypical fungal infections, hepatitis B, HIV is the other infections likely to develop with TNF-α inhibitors.

Congestive heart failure, demyelinating disorders mainly seen with etanercept which is reversible, lupus like disorder, nonmelanoma skin cancer, and lymphoma are other concerns while dealing with TNF-α inhibitors therapy.

Ustekinumab

Ustekinumab is a human monoclonal antibody that targets IL-12 and IL-23 also interferes with T cell differentiation and activation. In patients weighing less than 100 kg, the drug is given in the dose of 45 mg subcutaneously once initially and 4 weeks later with a maintenance dose: 45 mg subcutaneously once every 12 weeks. In patients weighing greater than 100 kg, the initial dose is 90 mg subcutaneously and 4 weeks later with the maintenance dose of 90 mg subcutaneously once every 12 weeks. Hypersensitivity, infections, and depression are the common side effects with ustekinumab. Uncommon drug-related adverse effects, such as reversible posterior leukoencephalopathy syndrome and a lymphomatoid drug eruption and cardiovascular complications have been reported. Ustekinumab offers patients rapid results and the convenience of four annual subcutaneous doses, with efficacy and safety profiles comparable with those of other biologics.

Ustekinumab is approved for the treatment of moderate-to-severe plaque psoriasis in adults who failed to respond to, or who have a contraindication to, or are intolerant to other systemic therapies including cyclosporine, MTX and PUVA.

The drug can be instituted alone or in combination with MTX, for the treatment of active PsA in adult patients, when the response to previous nonbiological disease-modifying antirheumatic drug (DMARD) therapy has been inadequate.

Ustekinumab treatment is associated with significant improvement in health-related quality of life and sexual difficulties due to psoriasis. There was greater reduction of sexual difficulties in those patients who had greater PASI improvement due to psoriasis. A similar pattern of improved sexual function was observed at weeks 24–28 in placebo cross over patients.

Alefacept

Alefacept was the first biologic used for psoriasis. It blocks clusters of differentiation 2 (CD2) found in memory T-cells and recombinant dimeric leukocyte-function-associated antigen (LFA)-3 fusion protein. The dosage used is 7.5 mg intravenous for 12 weeks and 5 mg intramuscular for 12 weeks. The recombinant protein alefacept is considered to be less effective for psoriasis than other biologic therapies. Hypersensitivity and HIV infection with CD4 count less than 250/μL were considered absolute contraindications while infections and malignancies are relative contraindications to the use of alefacept.

Injection site reactions, anaphylaxis, and angioedema were the common local side effects observed during treatment with alefacept. Dizziness, nausea, chills, infections, asymptomatic transaminitis, fall in CD4 and CD8 counts, malignancies were the systemic side effects observed. Long-term patient adherence to biologic therapy in patients with psoriasis is greatest with ustekinumab.

Efalizumab

Efalizumab is a recombinant humanized monoclonal antibody against LFA-1 that inhibits LFA-1 and intercellular adhesion molecule-1 interaction. Efalizumab interferes with immunological synapse and T cell activation. The recommended dose being 0.7 mg/kg subcutaneous followed by 1 mg/kg/week. Side effects reported include hypersensitivity, thrombocytopenia, and serious infections.

Worsening of psoriasis after discontinuation of therapy was one of the major drawbacks. The serious complication encountered with efalizumab was PML that subsequently resulted in banning of the drug.

Adalimumab and infliximab were associated with an increase in weight, while ustekinumab was associated with weight loss compared with etanercept.[41]

All patients on anti-TNF-α therapy who develop TB should discontinue therapy and receive anti-TB chemotherapy. In the case of infliximab, monitoring needs to be continued for 6 months after discontinuing treatment, due to the prolonged elimination phase of infliximab.

BI 655066

BI 655066, an anti-IL-23A mAb given intravenously or subcutaneously was found to be well tolerated and associated with rapid, substantial, and durable clinical improvement in patients with moderate-to-severe psoriasis, supporting a central role for IL-23 in psoriasis pathogenesis.[42]

Biologics in Children

The introduction of biologics in the armamentarium of anti-psoriatic drugs is indeed a giant leap in the management of refractory pediatric psoriasis where other drugs like retinoids, MTX, and cyclosporine cannot be used. Etanercept, an anti-TNF fusion protein, has been the one studied most extensively.[43-45] It has been found to be effective and well-tolerated in children and adolescents with moderate-to-severe plaque psoriasis.

Though etanercept was recommended for the treatment of pediatric psoriasis, possibility of increased risk of lymphoma and leukemia should be kept in mind while treating children. Etanercept should, therefore, not be used for children with a family history of lymphoma or leukemia, nor should it be prescribed for patients with Crohn's disease, unless there are no other viable options. However, with proper monitoring, it can be effective in children as young as 3 years old.

There are four case reports of the use of infliximab in childhood psoriasis with good results.[46-48] When providing a child with biologics, parents should be cautioned as to the side effects and potential life-threatening complications which can be associated. Being an immunosuppressive drug, the dosing of biologic agent is crucial ensuring that the child's immune system is not suppressed and allows for contacting infectious disease.

There are case reports in which adalimumab was prescribed to two adolescent patients with recalcitrant pustular psoriasis at a dose of 40 mg subcutaneously every 2 weeks, after the failure of etanercept and of other conventional systemic agents. In both cases, there was a favorable outcome.[49,50]

Infections and injection-site reactions were the most common adverse events. A multicenter double-blind randomized controlled trial (RCT) evaluating the efficacy and safety of adalimumab versus MTX in pediatric patients aged 4-17 years with chronic-plaque psoriasis is ongoing. It is possible that in the near future, adalimumab will be another attractive therapeutic alternative for adolescent psoriasis, although there are still several important issues to be determined.

There is a paucity of data regarding its efficacy and safety in children and adolescents, with only one published case reporting the successful administration of ustekinumab in a 14-year-old male patient with plaque psoriasis who failed to respond to conventional systemic agents as well as etanercept.[51] Ustekinumab's rapid onset of action as well as its convenient dosing schedule makes it a promising treatment option, although it is very early to recommend its universal adoption for the treatment of adolescent psoriasis. However, further multicenter studies will throw more light on the efficacy and safety of ustekinumab in children and adolescents. Administration of any of the above systemic drugs in a child should always be a team effort of dermatologist and pediatrician along with other specialist like gastroenterologist and hematologist, whenever necessary.

Body Weight and Biologics

Patients with psoriasis, in particular those requiring systemic treatment, tend to be above normal weight. Obesity is associated with psoriasis and contributes significantly to the increased cardiovascular risk in these patients. Most biologics used to treat psoriasis are fixed dosed treatments: etanercept, adalimumab, and ustekinumab. Apart from infliximab, dosing regimens do not account for weight, with the exception of ustekinumab, the dose of which should be doubled in patients weighing more than 100 kg. Infliximab response appears to be independent of body mass index.[52]

Reduced Treatment Response to Biologics

The response to various systemic therapies is not uniform in all patients at all times. Antidrug antibodies (ADAs) and genetic factors might have a role for lack of therapeutic response to drugs like anti-TNF-α agents, as previously suggested in patients with rheumatoid arthritis and inflammatory bowel disease.

Antidrug antibodies against biologic agents may be clinically significant and potentially alter a biologic drug's treatment efficacy. ADA development remains a challenge with biologic therapies and therefore, should be considered in psoriasis patients who experience diminished treatment response.[53]

The presence of −238G>A and −308G>A polymorphisms is associated with poor response to a 3-month therapy with etanercept. However, the data needs validation using larger cohorts.[54]

Future Therapies

An investigational oral calcineurin inhibitor, ISA247, has also shown efficacy in randomized trials in patients with moderate-to-severe plaque psoriasis, and may have less nephrotoxicity than cyclosporine.

Daclizumab, which is used for prevention of renal transplant rejection, and the cancer chemotherapeutic drug paclitaxel are also under investigation for use in severe psoriasis.

Interleukins in the helper T cells (Th17) pathway play a pivotal role in the pathogenesis of psoriasis and have become targets for drug development.

Briakinumab, another monoclonal antibody targeting IL-12/23, in moderate-to-severe plaque psoriasis, has exhibited efficacy superior to that of etanercept and MTX. However, concern has been raised regarding a potential relationship between briakinumab treatment and major cardiovascular adverse events.

Secukinumab, an anti-IL-17A monoclonal antibody, certolizumab pegol a humanized anti-TNF monoclonal antibody Fab fragment linked to polyethylene glycol are being tried in moderate-to-severe plaque psoriasis and PsA.

Other potential therapies include various small molecules that target the interruption of cellular signaling; such signaling is critical to propagation of the inflammatory response. Examples of small molecules that are being studied for the treatment of psoriasis include molecules that block JAK, lipids, and a protein kinase C inhibitor. Oral tofacitinib, a JAK inhibitor demonstrated efficacy for moderate-to-severe plaque psoriasis.

Apremilast, a phosphodiesterase 4 inhibitor, may be promising agents for the treatment of psoriasis.

The following are some useful tips while using systemic agents in the management of psoriasis:
- Methotrexate may be used for as long as it remains effective and well-tolerated.
- Cyclosporine is generally used intermittently for inducing a clinical response with one or several courses over a 3–6 months period
- Transition from conventional systemic therapy to a biological agent may be done directly or with an overlap if transitioning is needed because of lack of efficacy, or with a treatment-free interval, if transitioning is needed for safety reasons
- Combination therapy may be helpful
- Continuous therapy for patients receiving biologicals is recommended
- Switching biologicals because of lack of efficacy should be performed without a washout period while switching biologicals for safety reasons may require a treatment-free interval.

Dietary Supplement

Fish oil, rich in omega-3 fatty acids is the best-known dietary supplement. Oral and intravenous supplementation of omega-3 and, less effectively, omega-6 fatty acids have been found effective in psoriatic adults, possibly through alterations in production and alterations in arachidonic acid (20:4 omega 6) and docosapentanenoic acid.[55]

Indigo naturalis, a traditional Chinese medicine, can be formulated into topical ointment with anecdotal reports of good results in childhood psoriasis when used for 8 weeks.[56]

Supplementary treatment with omega-3 fatty acids complements topical treatment in psoriasis, and makes a significant contribution to reducing PASI and nail psoriasis severity index and improving dermatological life quality index; and to reducing scalp lesion and pruritus, erythema, scaling, and infiltration of the treated areas.[57]

TREATMENT ACCORDING TO TYPE AND SITE OF PSORIASIS

Treatments must be tailored to the age of the patient, QoL issues, type of psoriasis, and surface area affected. Patients may be grouped into mild, moderate, and severe disease categories. Limited, or mild-to-moderate skin disease can often be managed with topical agents, while patients with moderate-to-severe disease may need systemic therapy. The location of the disease and the presence of PsA and other comorbidities will also affect the choice of therapy. Psoriasis of the hand, foot, or face can be debilitating functionally or socially and may deserve a more aggressive treatment approach. Moderate-to-severe psoriasis is typically defined as involvement of more than 5–10% of the BSA (the entire palmar surface, including fingers, of one hand is approximately 1% of the BSA or involvement of the face, palm or sole, or disease that is otherwise disabling. Patients with more than 5–10% BSA affected are generally candidates for systemic therapy.

Application of topical agents other than emollients, to a large area is not usually practical or acceptable for most patients. The chances of treatment failure are high due to added cost, and inadequate clinical response which can lead to frustration in the patient-clinician relationship. The management of patients with extensive or recalcitrant disease is a challenge even for experienced dermatologists.

This portion will discuss the treatment of following types:
- Plaque type psoriasis
- Guttate psoriasis
- Pustular psoriasis
- Scalp psoriasis
- Inverse psoriasis or genital psoriasis
- Palmoplantar Psoriasis
- Nail psoriasis
- Mucosal psoriasis
- Genital psoriasis.

Plaque Type Psoriasis

Anthralin is an effective treatment of plaque psoriasis either with or without topical steroids. With the advent of newer drugs, the frequency of its use has come down. Topical steroids, calcipotriol, tazarotene are useful and safe if used properly. Salicylic acid can be used along with steroids in thick plaques. Psoriatic plaques that fail to respond to topical therapy may be improved by administration of intralesional corticosteroid injections. Triamcinolone (Kenalog) is often used for this purpose. The agent is injected directly into the dermis of a small, persistent plaque. The concentration is generally 3–10 mg/mL, depending on the size, thickness, and area of the lesion. The dose of triamcinolone is released gradually over 3–4 weeks; additional injections may be needed every 4–6 weeks to improve the response (Figs 10.1 to 10.3). Disadvantages of intralesional injections include pain during the injection and potential side effects of local atrophy and systemic absorption.[58]

Systemic agents like MTX and phototherapy may be needed in moderate-to-severe recalcitrant disease.

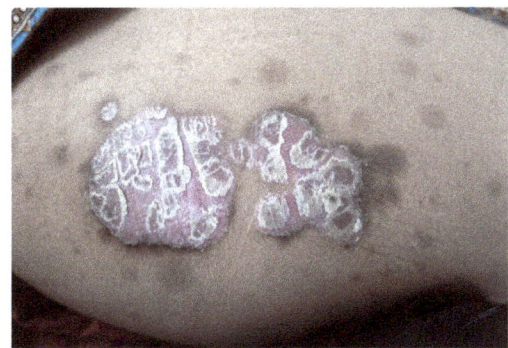

Fig. 10.1: Resistant plaque psoriasis before interleukin steroid therapy

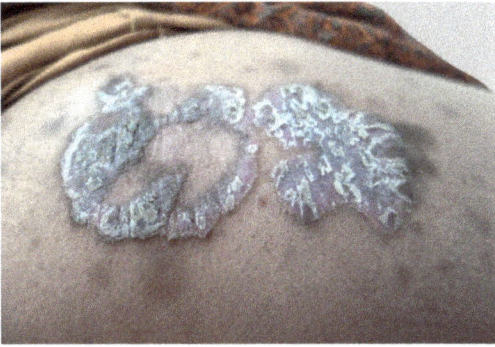

Fig. 10.2: Resistant plaque psoriasis after first dose of interleukin steroid therapy

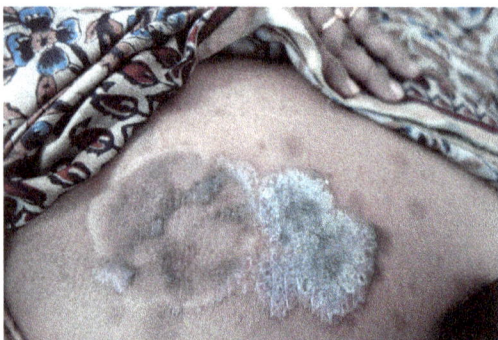

Fig. 10.3: Same as in Fig. 10.1 after second injection without any side effects

Guttate Psoriasis

Oral antibiotics are found to be useful in the treatment of guttate psoriasis. Systemic agents and phototherapy may be needed in moderate-to-severe disease. It should be remembered that guttate psoriasis can evolve into psoriasis vulgaris and hence, the child should be followed-up regularly.

Short-term antibiotic treatment is not effective in cases of acute guttate psoriasis. However, long-term antibiotic treatment seems to be more effective in controlling psoriatic relapse. This might be due to the elimination of antigenic stimulation caused by carried microorganisms.

In patients with acute guttate psoriasis, antibiotics can be added to conventional psoriasis treatment only if the presence of a streptococcal infection or a carrier state has been identified based on laboratory results. If there is no clinical or bacteriological evidence of an infectious episode precipitating the episode antibiotic treatment is unnecessary due to the lack of evidence supporting its benefits. Tonsillectomy can be advised, if there is definite evidence of tonsillitis which correlates with exacerbation of the disease, as tonsillectomy was shown to be effective only in uncontrolled studies.

Although both antibiotics and tonsillectomy have frequently been advocated both for patients with guttate psoriasis and for selected patients with chronic plaque psoriasis, there is to date no good evidence that either intervention is beneficial.

Topical emollients, drugs like coal tars, steroids or vitamin D creams are useful. Regular moisturizing should be encouraged. UVB therapy is to be considered, if the conventional treatment fails. Counseling is very important as most of the guttate psoriasis evolve into psoriasis vulgaris in future.

Pustular Psoriasis

If the disease is localized, topical agents like steroids will suffice. Treatment of palmoplantar pustulosis is dealt with under palmoplantar psoriasis.

All patients with GPP should be treated as inpatients. Maintenance of nutrition, fluid electrolyte balance, prevention of organ failure should be stressed. Multidisciplinary approach is mandatory depending on the extent of systemic involvement. Acitretin or isotretinoin (better avoided in adolescent girls) and dapsone can be tried depending on the biochemical parameters. Oral steroids are used only to tide over the acute crisis or in pregnant woman with impetigo herpetiformis. GPP responds well to MTX in children.[59]

Scalp Psoriasis

Topical steroid with or without salicylic acid as lotion applied at night followed by steroid or ketoconazole-based shampooing in the morning is helpful. For resistant plaques, tar-based shampoos will help. A combination with NBUVB or targeted phototherapy will give better results.

Inverse Psoriasis

Scientific evidence shows that involvement of the genital skin occurs in 29–40% of patients with psoriasis.

Short-term intermittent application of low-to-medium potent topical corticoids is useful as a first-line treatment option, which can be combined with vitamin D analogs or mild tar preparations. Mild topical coal-tar preparations are the second most advised topical therapy in adults and the first choice for children with napkin plaque psoriasis with or without topical steroids. Skin atrophy due to steroid and irritation or folliculitis due to tar preparation should be looked for and avoided. Zinc oxide, tacrolimus or 1% pimecrolimus cream, are regarded as third-line treatment options which can be used with safety in children. If used for a longer period, complications, such as local irritation, stinging, irritant or allergic contact dermatitis, candidiasis, and viral infections are the potential side effects. Topical cyclosporine is beneficial in genital psoriasis of the glans, penis and prepuce. If concurrent bacterial or fungal infections are present, they should be treated with topical antibiotics or antifungal drugs. Emollients should be advised to prevent friction and possible Koebner effect. Local treatment with topical dithranol and tazarotene should be avoided in the genital area. Systemic therapies are not used for isolated genital psoriasis. Dapsone has been shown to be an effective and convenient alternative for the treatment of inverse psoriasis in genital skinfolds, which can provide effective control of the disease.

Genital Psoriasis

Genital psoriasis can be difficult and frustrating to treat. However, it generally responds well to treatment. Due to the sensitivity of genital skin, treatment requires some special consideration. It is important to remember that response times to treatments vary among individuals.

Psoriasis in the genital region is very difficult to control. While it is easy to relieve the symptoms of itch and discomfort, treating the lesions effectively is more challenging. When treating genital psoriasis, it is important to keep the affected areas moisturized. When using moisturizers, any irritation that occurs may be due to sensitivity to some of the ingredients in them. Treatment of genital psoriasis should be individualized. There is limited published data for efficacy and safety of treatment options. The following suggestions for treatment of genital psoriasis are based on expert opinions and case reports:

- Emollients are an important part of the daily care of psoriasis in all parts of the body, including the genitalia. They help to make the skin more comfortable.

Topical Corticosteroid

A weak or moderate-potency topical corticosteroid cream may be used as required. Short-term intermittent use of moderate-to-potent corticosteroids may be necessary, but should be monitored to prevent side effects like atrophy, as there is increased absorption of topical steroids in genital skin. Depigmentation and infections both bacterial and viral are common side effects of prolonged usage of potent topical steroid. Prolonged use of high-potency steroids can also cause striae and development of resistance through tachyphylaxis can make topical corticosteroid less effective in the long-term. Topical steroid should never be stopped abruptly as this may trigger a rebound flare or precipitate pustular psoriasis.

Coal-tar Derivatives

Coal-tar preparations are better avoided over genital areas as they can cause irritation. Areas, such as the penis, the scrotum, the vulva are more prone to develop irritant dermatitis which may be further worsened, if the skin is cracked. However, mild topical coal-tar preparations can be used with caution when treatment with a weak topical steroid is insufficient. Mixing a tar with a steroid cream may reduce irritation caused by tar. Tar or ichthammol may be used with zinc oxide for napkin psoriasis.

Vitamin D Analogs

Topical vitamin D creams and ointments are effective in treating psoriasis and the newer types are less likely to cause irritation. However, some of them do have the potential to irritate sensitive areas, such as the genitalia. Vitamin D analogs, such as calcipotriol cream can be cautiously used alone or in combination with topical steroids. However, they may also irritate genital skin.

Immunomodulators

Calcineurin inhibitors (tacrolimus and pimecrolimus) are effective in treating genital psoriasis and do not have the side effect of thinning the skin that limits the use of topical steroids. Topical tacrolimus and pimecrolimus have the disadvantage of causing a burning sensation when applied and can reactivate sexually transmitted infections, such as herpes and viral warts. These may cause local irritation and stinging over the genital skin. They can also cause contact dermatitis, and increase the risk of candida infection.

Other Modalities

- Bland emollients can be used as required to reduce skin irritation and act as barrier cream
- Genital skin infections should be treated promptly
- Oral agents, such as MTX, cyclosporine, and acitretin are rarely necessary for genital psoriasis alone. They may be required in severe cases that fail to respond to topical treatments or for severe psoriasis on the rest of the body
- Dapsone has been shown to be an effective and convenient alternative for the treatment of inverse psoriasis in genital skinfolds, which can provide effective control of the disease.[60]

Ultraviolet light treatment is not usually recommended for genital psoriasis due to an increased risk of skin cancer in this area. Men with psoriasis undergoing UV light treatment are specifically advised to cover the genital area during treatment to reduce the risk of cancer.

Dithranol, tazarotene, UV rays (UVB phototherapy and photochemotherapy) and laser therapy should be avoided in the genital area.[61]

It is mandatory to re-evaluate therapy-resistant penile and vulval plaques clinically and histologically to rule out malignancy (penile intraepithelial neoplasia and vulval intraepithelial neoplasia).

Palmoplantar Psoriasis

Patients with palmoplantar psoriasis should be encouraged to wear good footwear made from natural fibers, should avoid minor trauma, resting the affected area where possible. Mild psoriasis of the palms and soles may be treated with topical treatments

like emollients, keratolytic agents, steroids, dithranol, and vitamin D analogs.
- Emollients
- Frequent application of thick, greasy barrier creams or ointments will moisturize the dry, scaly skin and help prevent painful cracking
- Keratolytic agents
- Keratolytics, such as urea or salicylic acid and tar will help remove thick scaling skin.

Topical Steroids

Ultra-potent steroids ointment should be applied initially daily for 2–4 weeks, if necessary under occlusion, to reduce inflammation, itch, and scaling. Maintenance use should be confined to 2 days each week (week end pulses) to avoid thinning of the skin and other local complications. This way tachyphylaxis can be best avoided.

Calcipotriol

Calcipotriol ointment is not very successful for palmoplantar psoriasis. It may cause an irritant dermatitis on the face if a treated area inadvertently touches it. Dithranol is too messy for routine use on hands and feet.

Phototherapy and LASER

- NBUVB and 308 nm excimer laser are found very useful in the treatment of palmoplantar psoriasis
- More severe palmoplantar psoriasis usually requires phototherapy or systemic agents
- Sytemic therapy.

Acitretin, MTX, and cyclosporine are useful for severe palmoplantar psoriasis. A variety of other medications that can help some subjects include colchicine, dapsone, and tetracycline antibiotics.

Biologics are occasionally effective when used for severe palmoplantar psoriasis. However, TNF-α inhibitors, such as infliximab, etanercept, and adalimumab may sometimes induce palmoplantar pustulosis as a side effect of treatment.

Alternate Therapy

Acupuncture is found useful in the management of palmoplantar psoriasis. Refined form of trauma, induced by needle piercing at certain points in acupuncture therapy, and may possibly be working through reverse Koebner's phenomenon.[62]

Nail Psoriasis

Psoriasis nail will frequently have super added fungal infection after treatment of which, topical corticosteroids, tazarotene or calcipotriene can be applied to the paronychial skin. Intralesional triamcinolone can also be used in the same region to reduce the subungual inflammation. Calcipotriol or tazarotene under occlusion covering the nail folds, plate, and under the nail plate are useful.

Dexamethasone iontophoresis may be a useful treatment of recalcitrant, difficult to treat severe nail psoriasis with significant impact on QoL.[63]

Mucosal Psoriasis

No therapy is usually needed to treat mucosa when shows involvement. However, topical steroids in an orabase can be used when needed. Candidal overgrowth is a common side effect of topical steroid application over the mucosa, which should be kept in mind while prescribing steroids for oral mucosa.

ERYTHRODERMIC PSORIASIS

Erythrodermic psoriasis can be considered as an acute dermatological emergency with multisystem involvement. Patients with erythrodermic psoriasis require hospitalization. Some of these patients may have unstable psoriasis and require close monitoring before deciding on the specific therapy. All such patients are preferably managed in the intensive care unit to take care of the fluid electrolyte balance and nutrition. A multidisciplinary approach is essential depending on the extent of system involvement. Emollients, wet dressings, and oatmeal baths can be used in concordance with systemic treatment to manage symptoms. Long-term maintenance therapy for psoriasis is required.

There is no high quality evidence to support specific recommendations for the management of erythrodermic psoriasis. Patients with severe, unstable disease should be treated with cyclosporine or infliximab due to the rapid onset and high efficacy of these agents. Patients with less acute disease can be treated with acitretin or MTX as first-line agents. Systemic glucocorticoids should be avoided except in cases of erythroderma due to impetigo herpetiformis where other drugs are contraindicated due to the potential for these drugs to induce a flare of psoriasis upon withdrawal of therapy. Infliximab is reported to be effective in erythrodermic psoriasis. Etanercept, adalimumab, and ustekinumab are other biologic agents found useful in erythrodermic psoriasis.

Erythrodermic psoriasis can be viewed as a condition with acute skin failure and treated accordingly. Maintenance of fluid and electrolytes, taking care of nutritional support to combat loss of protein and iron through scales and supplementation of calcium are important aspects of intensive care. The associated metabolic comorbidities should be born in mind while treating such patients which is also important while choosing the systemic therapy for treating psoriasis. Therapy should be based on acuity of disease and the patient's underlying comorbidities. Treatment of erythrodermic psoriasis should be approached and dealt in the following steps:

- Initial treatment
- Systemic medications
- Biologics
- Combination treatments
- Multidisciplinary approach
- Astute and sustained clinical observation.

It is advisable that all patients with erythroderma are advised hospitalization. This will give them physical rest and also alleviate emotional stress. This is followed by maintenance of fluids and electrolytes, temperature regulation, adequate nutritional supplements protein, iron, and calcium should be supplemented. All potential exacerbating agents should be avoided. While correcting dehydration, oral fluid should be encouraged and care must be taken to prevent fluid overload by intravenous fluid administration. Fluid overload if left unchecked can lead to pulmonary edema. Hypothermia in an erythrodermic patient may indicate sepsis. It is always advisable to go by the rectal temperature. Under such situations, tachycardia can be taken as an indirect clue to sepsis and increased body temperature. Protein loss and malnutrition can lead to pedal edema which can be a manifestation of anemia, renal and cardiac failure. Adequate nutritional supplements with protein, iron, and calcium are mandatory. Wherever possible, oral intake must be encouraged. While treating infection with antibiotics, it is better to avoid tetracycline and penicillin.

One must remember that erythrodermic psoriasis "throws off" the body chemistry and many a times the actual internal milieu is not reflected by the lab parameters.

The following are some clues to the effective management of erythrodermic psoriasis:

Bed Side Observation in the Management of Unstable Psoriasis or Erythroderma

Pulse, Temperature, and Respiration

- Pulse rate more than 120 in presence of septicemia or fever, a normal blood pressure may indicate negative fluid balance
- Erythrodermic patient may be febrile even in absence of infection
- Sudden onset hypothermia in a stable patient is a premonitory sign of septic shock
- Tachypnea may be the first sign of hypoxia from pneumonia or pulmonary edema.

Intake Output Chart

- A reduced urine output is an early indicator of hypovolemia or septicemia.

Intravenous fluid

Overzealous fluid correction will precipitate high output failure and lead to pulmonary edema.
General condition and diet:
- Altered sensorium, (anxiety or confusion) in an otherwise normal patient may be the first sign of sepsis
- Withhold periodic feeding, if residual gastric aspirate volume is more than 50 mL.

Investigations

- A low blood sugar may indicate testing very late after withdrawal of the sample
- A high blood sugar may be recorded if sample is taken while intravenous dextrose is on
- In the event of getting elevated urea and creatinine levels in a healthy individual, it is better to repeat investigation after adequate hydration
- Occult hypokalemia may exist despite normal serum potassium concentration. Hence, the clinical assessment should be meticulous and treatment given accordingly
- All complications pertaining to other systems should be promptly referred to concerned specialists and appropriately treated. Management of erythrodermic psoriasis is a multidisciplinary team work.

Bland emollients and cooling wet dressings are advisable at this stage. Topical steroid application has risk and disadvantage of increased percutaneous absorption. Sedative antihistamines are ideal for treating the itching. All patients with erythroderma should be evaluated for underlying infection and a safe and appropriate antibiotic administered. The role of steroids in the management of erythrodermic psoriasis is controversial. It is indicated to tide over the crisis in erythroderma due to GPP and impetigo herpetiformis. However, administration of systemic steroids can lead to a state of steroid dependence in some patients (Figs 10.4 and 10.5). In a patient who is already on systemic steroids, it is advisable not to withdraw systemic steroid abruptly.

Specific treatment of erythrodermic psoriasis includes systemic agents like cyclosporine, acitretin, and biologics. First-line agents include:

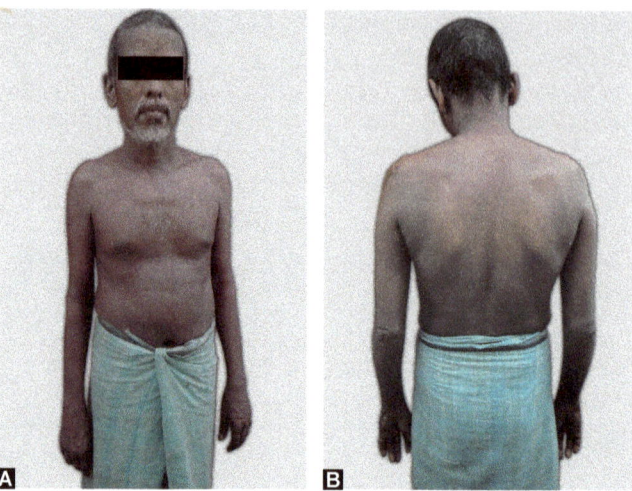

Fig. 10.4: Man with recurrent episodes of erythrodermic psoriasis while on methotrexate

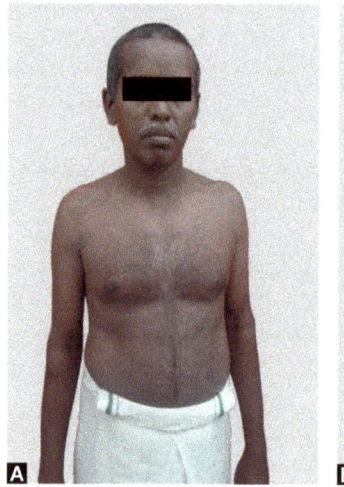 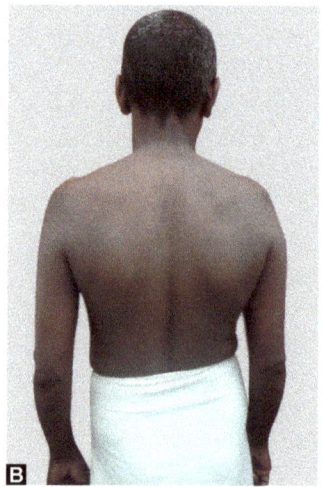

Fig. 10.5: Same as in Fig. 10.4 after treatment with systemic steroid, remission was maintained with methotrexate

- Cyclosporine and infliximab. These are most rapidly acting agents
- Acitretin and MTX. These usually work more slowly.

Second-line agents include:
- Etanercept is FDA approved and is well-tolerated
- Combination therapy is found to be more effective than a single-agent approach.

Intravenous immunoglobulin (IV Ig): Use of IV Ig in the management of erythrodermic psoriasis is not recommended as a routine as the cost is expensive to justify its use.

Certain don'ts to follow during the management of erythrodermic psoriasis are:
- Avoid fluid overload
- Avoid topical tar preparations and phototherapy in the early stage

- Avoid steroids as a routine unless in very ill patient or to tide over crisis
- Avoid tetracycline and penicillin.

Well managed case of erythrodermic psoriasis improves well. However, it is worthwhile remembering that hypocalcemia, oligemia, acute tubular necrosis of kidney are the frequent cause of death in acute skin failure due to GPP.

Multidisciplinary approach should be ideal whenever there is a need like treating the dermatogenic enteropathy, renal and cardiac complications.

After recovery from the acute state of erythroderma, all patients should be followed-up regularly an astute and sustained clinical observation is mandatory in order to treat the disease effectively and reduce the complications due to the drugs used and the disease apart from the metabolic complications.

ARTHROPATHIC PSORIASIS

Early diagnosis and treatment can help slow the disease and preserve joint function and range of motion.

The important steps in the effective treatment of PsA include good control of the skin disease, weight reduction, drugs, lifestyle modification and rarely, surgery. The holistic approach to management of PsA is depicted in Figure 10.6.

Good control of the skin disease is an important factor in the management of PsA. Advice on weight reduction is an important step in the management of PsA.

The following are early indicators of severe disease:
- Onset at a young age
- Having many joints involved
- Spinal involvement.

Goal of therapy in PsA is to:
- Improve QoL and signs and symptoms of disease:
  o Synovitis
  o Enthesitis
  o Dactylitis
  o Spondylitis
  o Skin and nail involvement
- Prevent joint damage and disability
- Avoid toxicity.

Nearly 40% of PsA patients are obese. Several studies have demonstrated that weight loss can improve response to medical treatments for both psoriasis and PsA.

Exercise and physical therapy are useful in better control of disease and may reduce requirement of drug intake. Treatments such as heat, exercise, and physical therapy may also help to relieve the pain and stiffness associated with PsA.

Drugs for the treatment of PsA are divided into three main categories:
- NSAIDs
- DMARDs
- Biologics.

Treatment varies depending on the level of pain. Those with very mild arthritis may require treatment only when their joints are

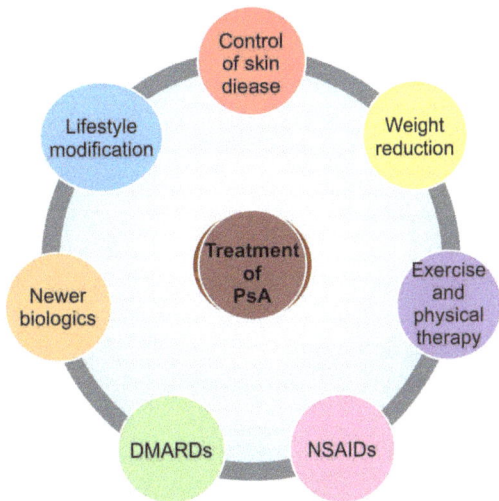

PsA, psoriatic arthritis; DMARDs, disease-modifying anti-rheumatic drugs; NSAIDs, nonsteroidal anti-inflammatory drugs.

Fig. 10.6: Holistic approach to management of psoriatic arthritis

painful and may stop therapy when they feel better.

Nonsteroidal Anti-inflammatory Drugs

Nonsteroidal anti-inflammatory drugs can help to control inflammation and to relieve the pain of PsA. NSAIDs must be taken continuously and at a sufficient dose to have an anti-inflammatory effect.

Nonsteroidal anti-inflammatory, must usually be taken for several weeks before their full degree of effectiveness as an anti-inflammatory effect is known. If the initial dose of a NSAID does not improve symptoms, a clinician may recommend increasing the dose gradually or switching to another NSAID.
- Nonselective NSAIDs include over-the-counter drugs, such as aspirin, ibuprofen, and naproxen, and a number of prescription-strength NSAIDs.
- Selective NSAIDs are the cyclo-oxygenase-2 inhibitors and are as effective as nonselective NSAIDs but the gastrointestinal injury and side effects are less when compared to the nonselective NSAIDS. It is also worth remembering that NSAIDs like ibuprofen and indomethacin themselves can worsen skin lesions of psoriasis.

Glucocorticoid Injections

Glucocorticoids can suppress inflammation and can relieve pain when injected into affected joints. Intra-articular injections have few side effects when compared to oral steroids, but there is a risk of joint infection. Some people experience a brief flare of pain after an injection.

If the arthritis does not respond, DMARD is to be prescribed. These include:
- Sulfasalazine
- MTX
- Cyclosporine
- Leflunomide
- Hydroxychloroquine
- Azathioprine may help those with severe forms of PsA.

Sulfasalazine

Sulfasalazine may be effective for the joint pain and skin lesions associated with PsA. However, not all patients benefit from sulfasalazine, and many patients cannot tolerate it due to gastrointestinal side effects. Patients who are allergic to sulfa drugs should not use sulfasalazine.

Methotrexate

Methotrexate is often recommended for people with multiple joint involvements due to PsA. Convincing evidence of its effectiveness has not been demonstrated and its disease-modifying effect of has not been proven well. MTX does not affect peripheral osteophyte formation in patients with PsA.

Cyclosporine

Cyclosporine is used to treat severe psoriasis and PsA. It may take 3–4 months before a response is seen. Adding cyclosporine to MTX may be more effective than either treatment alone. Side effects of cyclosporine like impaired kidney function and high blood pressure, and the advent of TNF inhibitors restrict the use of cyclosporine for PsA.

Leflunomide

Leflunomide can improve both skin and joint disease symptoms. It is recommended if the patient has not adequately responded to or has had side effects with MTX.

Possible side effects of leflunamide include diarrhea and elevated liver enzymes, and only about 40% of people with PsA benefit from this treatment.

Sometimes, combinations of these drugs may be used together.

Hydroxychloroquine

Hydroxychloroquine can reduce symptoms of arthritis due to its anti-inflammatory effect. However, it is better avoided as it can cause a flare of psoriatic skin lesions and sometimes precipitate erythroderma.

Azathioprine though is not superior to other medications in the treatment of PsA, it may be safely used and it provides an alternative therapy for patients with PsA.[64]

Biologics

Like MTX, the anti-TNF agents, such as adalimumab, etanercept, golimumab, and infliximab have the advantage of reducing both the skin lesion and joint involvement. Ustekinumab, has been recently approved by the FDA to be used alone or in combination with MTX for the treatment of adult patients (18 years or older) with active PsA. The approval was supported by findings from two pivotal phase 3 trials.[65]

Biologics target very specific components within the inflammatory pathway of psoriatic disease process. Most widely used and studied are those which block TNF-α, a potent proinflammatory cytokine. These include etarnercept, infliximab, and adalimumab all of which have received FDA approval for treatment of PsA.

In patients with active PsA, etanercept and infliximab significantly reduced the signs and symptoms of arthritis and disease progression. It improved skin and nail symptoms of psoriasis, enthesitis, and dactylitis thereby improving QoL.

In patients with active PsA, ustekinumab significantly reduced the signs and symptoms of arthritis improved physical function and reduced enthesitis and dactylitis. Safety profiles were similar between ustekinumab-treated and placebo-treated patients.

Indications for Biologic Agents in Psoriatic Arthritis

Indications for biologic agents in PsA include the following:
- Skin psoriasis:
  o Extensive psoriasis not responding to phototherapy, MTX, cyclosporine, and retinoids
- Nail psoriasis:
  o Not responding to phototherapy, MTX, cyclosporine, and retinoids
- Psoriatic Arthritis:
  o Peripheral arthritis
  o Not responding to NSAIDs, intra-articular injections, and traditional DMARD.
- Spondylitis:
  o Not responding to NSAIDs
- Enthesitis:
  o Not responding to NSAIDs and local cortisone injections
- Dactylitis:
  o Not responding to NSAIDs and local cortisone injections.

Intralesional Alefacept

The results from the pilot study conducted by Bhutani et al. demonstrated that alefacept appears to work intralesionally and this may be usable to predict systemic response. More importantly, these results strongly suggest that a biologic agent can work locally; a novel concept that contradicts the common notion that biologic agents must work "systemically".[66]

Certolizumab pegol has also been approved recently for the treatment of patients with active and progressive adult onset PsA. Patients treated with certolizumab pegol 200 mg every other week demonstrated greater reduction in radiographic progression compared with placebo-treated patients at week 24. It also resulted in improvement in skin manifestations in patients with PsA.[67]

Surgery can be resorted to repair or replace badly damaged joints.

There is limited evidence as to whether biologic therapy should be stopped or continued in patients with psoriasis and/or PsA who are undergoing surgical procedures. Current guidelines of care recommend a planned break from biologic therapy in those undergoing major surgical procedures. Continuing biologic therapy in psoriasis and PsA patients perioperatively did not increase the risk of postoperative complications. Interrupting biologic therapy perioperatively significantly increased the risk of disease flare. This study is limited by cohort size and requires replication, ideally in a prospective randomized controlled manner.[68] Treatment grid for PsA based on disease activity and impact [modified from group for research and assessment of psoriasis and psoriatic arthritis] is given in Table 10.1.

Choice of drug in various types of PsA is classified in Table 10.2.

TABLE 10.1: Treatment grid for psoriatic arthritis based on disease activity and impact (modified from group for research and assessment of psoriasis and psoriatic arthritis)

Severity of disease	Peripheral arthritis	Skin disease	Spinal disease	Dactylitis	Enthesitis
Mild	• <5 joints • No X-ray changes • No QoL impact	• BSA <5 • PASI <5	Mild pain No LoF	Absent or mild pain	1–2 sites No LoF
Moderate	• >5 joints • Mild X-ray changes • Mild QoL impact	• DLQI and • PASI <10 • N/R to Rx	LoF	LoF Erosive disease	>2 sites and LoF
Severe	• >5 joints • Damage seen in X-ray • Severe QoL impact	• BSA >10 • DLQI >10 • PASI >10	N/R to Rx	N/R to Rx	>2 sites, LoF and N/R to Rx

QoL, quality of life; BSA, body surface area; PASI, psoriasis area and severity index; DLQI, dermatology life quality index; LoF, loss of function.

TABLE 10.2: Choice of drug in various types of psoriatic arthritis

	Peripheral arthritis	Skin, nail disease	Axial disease	Dactylitis	Enthesitis
NSAIDs	+		+		
Intra-articular steroids	+				
Topicals		+			
Physiotherapy			+		
PUVA/UVB		+			
DMARD	+	+			
Biologics (anti-TNF antagonists	+	+	+	+	+

NSAIDs, nonsteroidal anti-inflammatory drugs; PUVA/UVB, psoralen with ultraviolet light A/ultraviolet B; DMARD, disease-modifying antirheumatic drugs; TNF, tumor necrosis factor.

Psoriatic Arthritis in Children

The main aim of treating juvenile PsA is to reduce joint inflammation, maintain mobility, and prevent deformity. Physiotherapy is as important as drug treatment. Daily exercises, hydrotherapy (supervised exercise in a warm pool), and day and night splints are all important for long-term joint mobility. The aim of treatment is for the child to have as normal and active a childhood as possible. In children with psoriatic arthropathy, MTX is the drug of choice.

TREATMENT OF PSORIASIS IN SPECIAL POPULATIONS

The treatment of psoriasis in pregnant women and patients with hepatitis B, hepatitis C, HIV virus infection, latent TB, and malignancy can be challenging. For those patients who cannot tolerate systemic drugs, phototherapy remains the choice of treatment. UVB therapy is the most safe and effective mode of therapy in most patients of this special population (Figs 10.7 and 10.8).

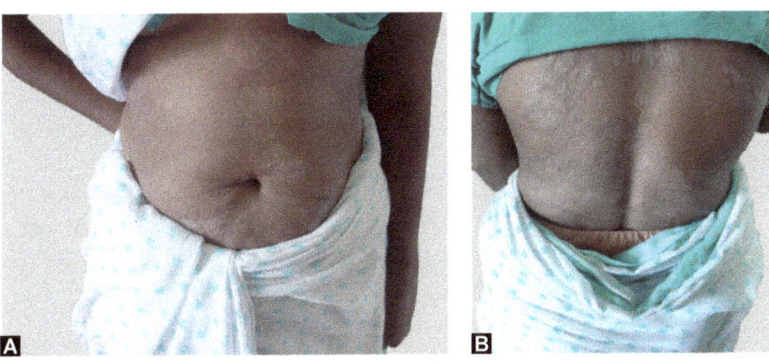

Fig. 10.7: Hypertensive with nonalcoholic fatty liver disease before treatment with ultraviolet B

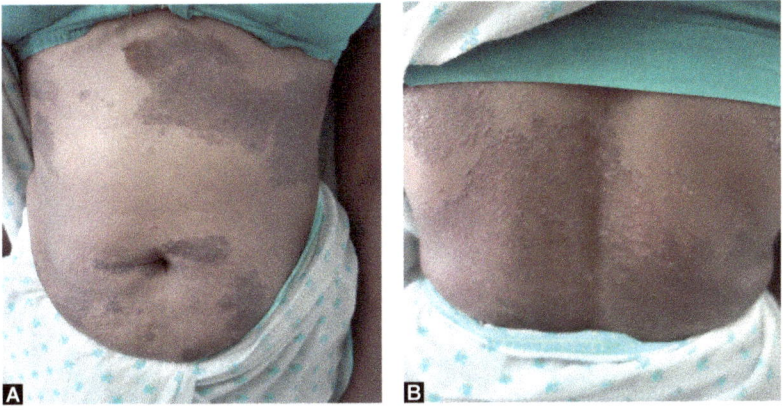

Fig. 10.8: Same patient as in Fig. 10.7 after ultraviolet B therapy

Psoriasis in Pregnancy and Lactation

(See Chapter 6)

Psoriasis and Hepatitis

There are enough studies to show that psoriasis is associated with hepatitis C virus (HCV) infection and not hepatitis B virus (HBV) infection. Treating psoriasis in patients with concomitant HCV infection presents a special challenge. Not only is psoriasis exacerbated by interferon therapy, the standard of care for HCV, but many psoriasis therapies are potentially hepatotoxic, immunosuppressive, or both, which has been generally thought to be a contraindication in chronic infections, such as HCV.

In limited psoriasis with HCV infection, topical therapies are first-line therapy and UVB phototherapy will be the second-line treatment. In moderate-to-severe disease, UVB phototherapies in combination with topical therapies are first-line and systemic therapies, such as acitretin and etanercept, are considered second-line therapy. Apart from screening for liver enzymes screening for hepatocellular carcinoma must be performed in all patients with HCV infection being treated with biologic therapies. Oral PUVA can be considered provide the liver functions can be maintained.

Patients with HBV infection should not be given MTX. As there are reports showing viral reactivation in patients treated with TNF inhibitors, it is advisable to screen all patients for HBV before initiating treatment with these biologics. For patients found to be seropositive, antiviral treatment is recommended with close follow-up.

Human immunodeficiency virus-positive patients who have psoriasis typically have severe symptoms, and particular care must be taken with any immunosuppressive therapy in this group. Studies, thus far, have not found serious adverse events in HIV-positive patients given TNF inhibitors, but the suitability of this treatment remains a matter of dispute.

Psoriasis in Tuberculosis Patient

All the TNF-α inhibitors are associated with an increased risk of developing active disease in patients with latent TB infection (LTBI), because of TNF-α playing a key role against *Mycobacterium tuberculosis*. Hence, exclusion of active TB and treatment of LTBI are clinical imperatives prior to starting this therapy. Apart from topical therapy, UVB and acitretin seem to be safer drugs in the treatment of psoriasis in a patient with TB infection. Isoniazid (INH) prophylaxis for newly identified LTBI in ustekinumab-treated patients with psoriasis was found to be safe.[69]

Psoriasis and Human Immunodeficiency Virus

Psoriasis occurs with at least undiminished frequency in HIV-infected individuals. The behavior of psoriasis in HIV disease is of interest, in terms of pathogenesis and therapy because of the background of profound immune dysregulation. It is paradoxical that, while drugs that target T lymphocytes are effective in psoriasis, the condition should be exacerbated by HIV infection.

Psoriasis in the setting of HIV disease may be mild, moderate, or severe. Standard therapies and zidovudine are effective in management. Survival does not seem to be adversely affected by the presence of psoriasis or its therapy.

Mild-to-moderate Disease

Topical therapy is the first-line recommended treatment. UVB can be considered as second-line therapy.

Moderate-to-severe Disease

- Phototherapy is the recommended first-line therapeutic agents
- Oral retinoids may be used as second-line treatment
- Refractory, severe disease: Cyclosporine, MTX, hydroxyurea, and TNF-α inhibitors may be considered and used with extreme caution
- Since skin lesions of patients with therapy-resistant acquired immunodeficiency syndrome (AIDS)- associated psoriasis have been reported to clear with oral zidovudine, this drug may be considered retinoid-resistant AIDS-associated psoriasis, where, MTX, cyclosporine, and PUVA may be contraindicated
- Oral gold was found to be safe and useful in a woman in the treatment of disabling PsA with HIV infection, in whom CD4 count during oral gold therapy showed a significant, sustained increase in CD4 cells.

Psoriasis and Malignancy

Psoralen with UVA, when given long-term, is associated with increased risks of cutaneous squamous cell carcinoma and malignant melanoma. MTX, cyclosporine, and mycophenolate mofetil are associated with an increased risk of lymphoproliferative disorders. TNF-α inhibitors may cause a slightly increased risk of cancer, including nonmelanoma skin cancer and hematologic malignancies. The increased risk of malignancy associated with psoriasis itself is a confounding factor. Topical therapy and UVB remain safe options for the treatment of psoriasis in patients with malignancy.

TREATMENT OF CHILDHOOD PSORIASIS

(For details, see Chapter 5)

Psoriasis in children is more or less similar to that in adults. However, there are some real differences between treating a child and an adult. Many of the systemic drugs used for adults may not be appropriate for children due to long-term or delayed side effects. Treatment should be carefully tailored according to the type and severity of the psoriasis, the areas of the skin affected and the patient's age and past medical history giving due importance to the family history as well.[70]

Infants

Treatment should be very conservative. Emollients or moisturizers can be a good first step. Oatmeal baths can help relieve the itching. The disease must be allowed to evolve before embarking on any specific therapy.

Children

For mild psoriasis, in addition to emollients, topical agents like steroids of appropriate strength, formula, and dose should be the ideal choice. Other drugs like vitamin D analog, calcineurin inhibitors are used where steroid are contraindicated. For moderate cases, regular BBUVB or NBUVB therapy can help clear the lesions. Antibiotics may help clear the bacteria that could have triggered the psoriasis only if there is clinical or laboratory evidence. Undue usage of antibiotics in children should be avoided.

Severe psoriasis can be treated with systemic drugs under careful monitoring.

Adolescent

Can be treated as above. One should always bear in mind that antimitotic like MTX should not be used as a routine in this age group. Being an emotionally turbulent stage of life, lot of time should be spent counseling these patients as well as their parents and care givers.

NEWER DRUGS

Most recent topical and systemic drugs under research will be discussed here.

Topical Drugs

Following are the novel topical medications currently in phase 2 and phase 3 clinical trials.[71]
- AN2728 (phosphodiesterase 4 inhibitor)
- AS101 (integrin inhibitor)
- Tofacitinib (JAK1 and JAK3 inhibitor)
- CT327 (tyrosine kinase inhibitor)
- DPS-101 (vitamin D analog)
- IDP-118 (steroid and retinoid combination)
- Ruxolitinib (JAK1 and JAK2 inhibitor)
- LAS41004 (steroid and retinoid combination)
- LEO 80190 (vitamin D3 analog and steroid combination)
- LEO 90100 (vitamin D analog and steroid combination)
- M518101 (vitamin D analog)
- MOL4239 and MOL4249 (phosphorylated signal transducer and activator of transcription 3 inhibitors)
- MQX-5902 (dihydrofolate reductase inhibitor)
- PH-10 (xanthine dye)
- STF115469 (vitamin D analog)
- WBI-1001 (proprietary product)
- AN2728.

AN2728 is a phosphodiesterase 4 inhibitor that blocks the inactivation of cyclic adenosine monophosphate, resulting in decreased production of inflammatory cytokines (e.g., IL-6, IL-12, IL-23, TNF-α).

AS101

AS101 is an integrin inhibitor, acting as stimulator of regulatory T cells and a redox modulator inhibiting the leukocyte integrins $\alpha_4\beta_1$ and $\alpha_4\beta_7$ that enable CD4$^+$ T cell and macrophage extravasation; it also limits expression of the inflammatory cytokines IL-6 and IL-17.

Tofacitinib

Tofacitinib, formerly known as CP-690,550 is a selective JAK1 and JAK3 inhibitor that limits expression of cytokines that promote inflammation (e.g., IFN-γ) and inhibits Th17 by down regulating expression of the IL-23 receptor. Epidermal keratinocyte proliferation in psoriasis is activated by Th17 cells that release IL-17 as well as Th1 cells that release IFN-γ and TNF.

CT327 (Tyrosine Kinase Inhibitor)

CT327 is a tyrosine kinase A inhibitor that affords a novel perspective in the treatment of pruritus by shifting the focus to sensory neurons.

DPS-101

DPS-101, a vitamin D analog, is a combination of calcipotriol and niacinamide. Calcipotriol increases IL-10 expression while decreasing IL-8 expression.[7] It curbs epidermal keratinocyte proliferation by limiting the expression of polo-like kinase 2 and early-growth response-1.[8] It also may induce keratinocyte apoptosis.[9] Niacinamide is the amide of vitamin B_3 and inhibits proinflammatory cytokines, such as TNF-α, IL-1β, IL-6, and IL-8.[10] In a dose-response phase 2b trial of 168 patients, DPS-101 demonstrated better results than either calcipotriol or niacin amide alone.[11]

IDP-118

IDP-118 is a combination of halobetasol propionate 0.01% (a topical corticosteroid) and tazarotene 0.045% (a selective topical retinoid) in a lotion formulation. In isolation, tazarotene is as effective as a mid to highly potent corticosteroid, but irritation may limit its tolerability. The use of combination treatments of mid to highly potent corticosteroids and tazarotene has shown enhanced tolerability and therapeutic efficacy.

Ruxolitinib (JAK1 and JAK2 Inhibitor)

Ruxolitinib formerly known as INCB18424 is a selective JAK1 and JAK2 inhibitor.

LAS41004

LAS41004 is an ointment containing the corticosteroid betamethasone dipropionate and the retinoid bexarotene that is being evaluated for treatment of mild-to-moderate psoriasis.

LEO 80190

LEO 80190 is a combination of the vitamin D_3 analog calcipotriol and the corticosteroid hydrocortisone. It was developed as a treatment for sensitive areas, such as the face and intertriginous regions.

LEO 90100

LEO 90100 contains the vitamin D_3 analog calcipotriol and betamethasone.

M518101

M518101 is a novel topical vitamin D_3 analog.

MOL4239 and MOL4249

MOL4239 and MOL4249 are phosphorylated signal transducers and activators of transcription 3 inhibitors. MOL4249 is more potent than MOL4239 with better lipid solubility.

MQX-5902

MQX-5902, a dihydrofolate reductase inhibitor, is a topical preparation of MTX tried for the treatment of fingernail psoriasis.

PH-10

PH-10, a xanthine dye in the form of topical aqueous hydrogel derived from Rose Bengal disodium. This new drug that may be beneficial in treating atopic dermatitis (AD) and mild-to-moderate psoriasis and can be a suitable topical therapy for patients with psoriasis AD overlap or coexistence.

STF115469

STF115469 is a calcipotriene tried as foam.

WBI-1001

WBI-1001 or 2-isopropyl-5-[(E)-2-phenylethenyl] benzene-1,3-diol, is a novel proprietary agent that inhibits proinflammatory cytokines like IFN-γ, TNF-α.

Newer Systemic Drugs

A number of novel targeted therapies including biologics as well as small molecule inhibitors targeting various cytokines and molecules involved in the pathogenesis of psoriasis are currently in different stages of development.[72]

These novel biological drugs include:
- Three IL-17 inhibitors: secukinumab, ixekizumab, and brodalumab
- Two IL-23 blockers: tildrakizumab and guselkumab
- Small molecule inhibitors: PDE4, apremilast
- JAK inhibitors: tofacitinib, baricitinib, and ruxolitinib.

Secukinumab

Secukinumab is a fully human monoclonal IgG1k antibody that selectively binds and neutralizes IL-17A. It is the first of the IL-17 antibodies to receive approval for the treatment of moderate-to-severe psoriasis. The speed of response, which was assessed as the median time to a 50% reduction in mean PASI score from baseline, was significantly shorter with secukinumab when compared with etanercept.

The incidences of adverse events were similar in the secukinumab and etanercept groups during both the induction period and the entire treatment period. The most common adverse effect noted in the secukinumab groups includes nasopharyngitis, headache, and diarrhea. However, candidal infections were more common with secukinumab than with etanercept.

Ixekizumab

- Ixekizumab is a humanized IgG4 anti-IL-17A monoclonal antibody
- Significant reductions in PASI scores were evident as early as week 1 and these reductions were sustained for 20 weeks (P<05). Phase 3 studies of ixekizumab currently are underway.

Brodalumab

Brodalumab, the third IL-17 blocker in the pipeline, is a human monoclonal antibody against IL-17RA, which blocks signaling of IL-17A and IL-17F as well as the IL-17A/F heterodimer, all of which are involved in the inflammatory process of psoriasis.

Results for this new IL-17 blocker are encouraging, but phase 3 data of brodalumab will need to be awaited.

IL-23 Blockers

Tildrakizumab

Tildrakizumab is a humanized IgG1 monoclonal antibody that blocks the p19 subunit of IL-23. Shows good results and the most common adverse effect noted was nasopharyngitis.

Guselkumab

Guselkumab is a human IgG1 monoclonal antibody in clinical development that specifically blocks the p19 subunit of IL-23 shows promising results in the treatment of psoriasis.

Small Molecule Inhibitors

In contrast to biologics, which mainly target soluble cytokine or cellular receptors, small molecule inhibitors target enzymes within signaling pathways. Small molecule inhibitors have some advantages over biologics in that they are relatively inexpensive to produce and can be administered orally; thus, they may be preferred by some patients over injectable drugs. PDE4 inhibitors and JAK inhibitors are some of the molecules that are undergoing clinical trials in psoriasis.

Apremilast

Apremilast is an oral small molecule PDE4 inhibitor that was approved by the FDA for the treatment of adult patients with active PsA; and for moderate-to-severe plaque psoriasis. PDE4 is a cyclic adenosine monophosphate-specific phosphodiesterase inhibitor, which is dominant in inflammatory cells. Inhibition of PDE4 increases intracellular cyclic adenosine monophosphate levels, thus downregulating proinflammatory cytokines, such as TNF-α, IFN-γ, IL-2, IL-12, and IL-23, and increasing the production of anti-inflammatory cytokines, such as IL-10.

The most common adverse effects noted were nausea and diarrhea, which were predominantly mild, occurring most commonly in the first week and resolving within a month. It was observed in studies done in patients with chronic obstructive pulmonary disease treated with roflumilast there was an increased incidence of depression and suicidal ideation.

Janus Kinase Inhibitors

Janus kinases are a family of intracellular tyrosine kinases that connect several cytokine receptors to the signal transducer and activator of transcription pathways. There are 4 JAK family members: JAK1, JAK2, JAK3, and TYK2. JAK1 and JAK2 have roles in IFN signaling, while JAK3 transduces signals from IL-2, IL-7, IL-15, and IL-21, which are T-cell growth and survival factors.

Tofacitinib

Tofacitinib is a novel oral signal transduction molecule that blocks the JAK3 pathway. This trial drug stays effective for psoriasis, even after a break in the treatment. Short-term treatment with oral tofacitinib results in significant clinical improvement in patients with moderate-to-severe plaque psoriasis and is generally well-tolerated.[73] Results show that tofacitinib can be a safe and effective treatment in patients with psoriasis, but further data from phase 3 studies will need to be awaited.

Ruxolitinib

Ruxolitinib, is an inhibitor of JAK1 and JAK2, which has been primarily studied as a topical agent for milder cases of the disease.

Many new drugs are currently on the horizon and will increase our armamentarium for treating psoriasis. Some of these agents promise greater levels of efficacy than currently used therapies. The topical agents currently in phase 2 and phase 3 clinical trials show promise in enhancing the treatment approach for better outcome. There is hope for more individualized treatment regimens with improved tolerability, better safety profiles with increased therapeutic efficacy. These new agents will certainly increase our options when choosing the most suitable treatment for a patient with psoriasis, but safety will remain a primary concern, and time and experience will tell whether efficacy outweighs any potential side effects.

CONCLUSION

Management of psoriasis is an art. Every patient should be explained about the disease and the drugs prescribed, with due stress on the side effects of the drugs. Though many modalities like topical and systemic therapies are available, phototherapy is found to be useful where most of the drugs are contraindicated. Biologics and other newer agents are a boon in the armamentarium of therapy for psoriasis. Drugs should be chosen according to the site or type of psoriasis keeping in mind the age and other associated comorbidities. Treatment of erythroderma involves interdisciplinary approach and has to be considered as a medical emergency in some patients. Every patient should be enquired for symptoms of arthropathy and treated accordingly. Treatment of psoriasis in special populations like pregnancy, those with chronic diseases, or HIV infection should be meticulously planned with the concurrence of the respective specialist. Therapy of childhood psoriasis is indeed very challenging as this group of patients are exposed to the medication not only topical and oral drugs but also phototherapy for a longer period in life than the adult population. Properly tailored treatment instituted at the right time with adequate monitoring and follow up should keep the disease under prolonged remission and prevent future complications as well as development of comorbidities.

REFERENCES

1. Menter A, Griffiths CE. Current and future management of psoriasis. Lancet. 2007:370:272-84.
2. Feldman SR. 2013. Treatment of psoriasis [online] Available from http:// www.uptodate.com/contents/treatment-of-psoriasis [Accessed November, 2015].
3. Pazyar N, Yaghoobi R. Tea tree oil as a novel antipsoriasis weapon. Skin Pharmacol Physiol. 2012;25(3):162-3.
4. Smith CH, Jackson K, Chinn S, Angus K, Barker JNWN. A double blind, randomized, controlled clinical trial to assess the efficacy of a new coal tar preparation (Exorex®) in the treatment of chronic, plaque type psoriasis. Clin Exp Dermatol. 2000;25:580-3.
5. Thami GP, Sarkar R. Coal tar: Past, present and future. Clin Exp Dermatol. 2002;27:99-103.
6. Borska L, Andrys C, Krejsek J, Hamakova K, Kremlacek J, Ettler K, et al. Genotoxic hazard and cellular stress in pediatric patients treated for psoriasis with the Goeckerman regimen. Pediatr Dermatol. 2009;26:23-7.
7. McGill A, Frank A, Emmett N, Turnbull DM, Birch Machin MA, Reynolds NJ. The anti-psoriatic drug anthralin accumulates in keratinocyte mitochondria, dissipates mitochondrial membrane potential, and induces apoptosis through a pathway dependent on respiratory competent mitochondria. FASEB J. 2005;19:1012-4.
8. Lebwohl M, Ali S. Treatment of psoriasis. Part 1. Topical therapy and phototherapy. J Am Acad Dermatol. 2001;45:487-98.
9. Zvulunov A, Anisfeld A, Metzker A. Efficacy of short contact therapy with dithranol in childhood psoriasis. Int J Dermatol. 1994;33:808-10.
10. Farber EM, Nall L. Childhood psoriasis. Cutis. 1999;64:309-14.
11. Kiken DA, Silverberg NB. Atopic dermatitis in children, part 2: treatment options. Cutis. 2006;78:401-6.
12. Kimball AB, Gold MH, Zib B, Davis MW. Clobetasol Propionate Emulsion Formulation Foam Phase III Clinical Study Group. Clobetasol propionate emulsion formulation foam 0.05%: review of phase II open-label and phase III randomized controlled trials in steroid-responsive dermatoses in adults and adolescents. J Am Acad Dermatol. 2008;59:448-54.
13. Rim JH, Choe YB, Youn JI. Positive effect of using calcipotriol ointment with narrow band Ultraviolet B phototherapy in psoriatic patients. Photodermatol Photoimmunol Photomed. 2002;18:131-4.
14. Oranje AP, Marcoux D, Svensson A, Prendiville J, Krafchik B, Toole J, et al. Topical calcipotriol in childhood psoriasis. J Am Acad Dermatol. 1997;36:203-8.
15. Liao YH, Chiu HC, Tseng YS, Tsai TF. Comparison of cutaneous tolerance and efficacy of calcitriol 3 microg g (-1) ointment and tacrolimus 0.3 mg g (-1) ointment in chronic plaque psoriasis involving facial or genitofemoral areas: a double-blind, randomized controlled trial. Br J Dermatol. 2007;157:1005-12.
16. Brune A, Miller DW, Lin P, Cotrim-Russi D, Paller AS. Tacrolimus ointment is effective for psoriasis on the face and intertriginous areas in pediatric patients. Pediatr Dermatol. 2007;24:76-80.
17. Mansouri P, Farshi S. Pimecrolimus 1 percent cream in the treatment of psoriasis in a child. Dermatol Online J. 2006;12:7.
18. Jain VK, Aggarwal K, Jain K, Bansal A. Narrow-band UV-B phototherapy in childhood psoriasis. Int J Dermatol. 2007;46:320-2.
19. Diluvio L, Campione E, Paternò EJ, Mordenti C, El Hachem M, Chimenti S. Childhood nail psoriasis: A useful treatment with tazarotene 0.05%. Pediatr Dermatol. 2007;24:332-3.
20. Ports WC, Khan S, Lan S, Lamba M, Bolduc C, Bissonnette R, et al. A randomised Phase 2a efficacy and safety trial of the topical Janus kinase inhibitor tofacitinib in the treatment of chronic plaque psoriasis. Br J Dermatol. 2013;169(1):137-45.
21. Nolan BV, Yentzer BA, Steven R, Feldman SR. A review of home phototherapy for psoriasis. Dermatol Online Journal. 2010;16(2):1.

22. Takahashi H, Tsuji H, Ishida-Yamamoto A, Iizuka H. Comparison of clinical effects of psoriasis treatment regimens among calcipotriol alone, narrowband ultraviolet B phototherapy alone, combination of calcipotriol and narrowband ultraviolet B phototherapy once a week, and combination of calcipotriol and narrowband ultraviolet B phototherapy more than twice a week. J Dermatol. 2013;40(6):424-7.
23. Abdallah MA, El-Khateeb EA, Abdel-Rahman SH. The influence of psoriatic plaques pretreatment with crude coal tar vs petrolatum on the efficacy of narrow-band ultraviolet B: a half-vs.-half intra-individual double-blinded comparative study. Photodermatol Photoimmunol Photomed. 2011;27(5):226-30.
24. Mortazavi H, Khezri S, Hosseini H, Khezri F, Vasigh M. A single blind randomized clinical study: the efficacy of isotretinoin plus narrow band ultraviolet B in the treatment of psoriasis vulgaris Photodermatol Photoimmunol Photomed. 2011;27(3):159-61.
25. Pahlajani N, Katz BJ, Lozano AM, Murphy F, Gottlieb A. Comparison of the efficacy and safety of the 308 nm excimer laser for the treatment of localized psoriasis in adults and in children: A pilot study. Pediatr Dermatol. 2005;22:161-5.
26. Huang YC, Chou CL, Chiang YY. Efficacy of pulsed dye laser plus topical tazarotene versus topical tazarotene alone in psoriatic nail disease: a single-blind, intrapatient left-to-right controlled study. Lasers Surg Med. 2013;45(2):102-7.
27. Pang ML, Murase JE, Koo J. An updated review of acitretin a systemic retinoid for the treatment of psoriasis. Expert Opin Drug Metab Toxicol. 2008;4:953-64.
28. Haushalter K, Murad EJ, Dabade TS, Rowell R, Pearce DJ, Feldman SR. Efficacy of low-dose acitretin in the treatment of psoriasis. J Dermatol Treat. 2012;23(6):400-3.
29. Cordoro KM. Topical therapy for the management of childhood psoriasis: Part I. Skin Therapy Lett. 2008;13(3):1-3.
30. Kumar B, Dhar S, Handa S, Kaur I. Methotrexate in childhood psoriasis. Pediatr Dermatol. 1994;11(3):271-3.
31. Collin B, Vani A, Ogboli M, Moss C. Methotrexate treatment in 13 children with severe plaque psoriasis. Clin Exp Dermatol. 2009;34(3):295-8.
32. Kalb RE, Strober B, Weinstein G, Lebwohl M. Methotrexate and psoriasis: National Psoriasis Foundation Consensus Conference. J Am Acad Dermatol. 2009;60:824-37.
33. Perrett CM, Ilchyshyn A, Berth-Jones J. Cyclosporin in childhood psoriasis. J Dermatol Treat. 2003:4(2):113-8.
34. Alli N, Góngφr E, Karakayali G, Lenk N, Artóz F. The use of cyclosporin in a child with generalized pustular psoriasis. Br J Dermatol. 1998;139:754-7.
35. Pereira TM, Vieira AP, Fernandes JC, Sousa Basto AJ. Cyclosporin A treatment in severe childhood psoriasis. Eur Acad Dermatol Venereol. 2006;20:651-6.
36. Borghi A, Corazza M, Mantovani L, Bertoldi AM, Giari S, Virgili A. Prolonged cyclosporine treatment of severe or recalcitrant psoriasis: descriptive study in a series of 20 patients . Int J Dermatol. 2012;51(12):1512-6.
37. Khondker L, Choudhury AM, Shah OR, Shahidullah, Khan SI, Ahmed ARS. Role of hydroxyurea in psoriasis-a review. J of Pakistan Association of Dermatologists. 2012;22(3):257-61.
38. Gupta R. Azathioprine pulse therapy in the treatment of Psoriasis. Journal of Pakistan Association of Dermatologists. 2013;23(2):120-5.
39. Gagnon L. 2014. Short-term systemic steroids for psoriasis efficacious despite 'dogma'. Dermatology times. [online] Available from http://dermatologytimes.modernmedicine.com/dermatology-times/RC/short-term-systemic-steroids-psoriasis-efficacious-despite-dogma?page=full. [Accessed June, 2015].
40. Ergun T, Seckin D, Bulbul BE, Onsun N, Zuleyha O, Unalan P, et al. The risk of tuberculosis in patients with psoriasis treated with anti-tumor necrosis factor agents. Int J Dermatol. 2015;54(5):594-9.
41. Ross C, Marshman G, Grillo M, Stanford T. Biological therapies for psoriasis: Adherence and outcome analysis from a clinical perspective. Australas J Dermatol. 2015.
42. Krueger JG, Ferris LK, Menter A, Wagner F, White A, Visvanathan S, et al. Anti-IL-23A mAb BI 655066 for treatment of moderate-to-severe psoriasis: Safety, efficacy, pharmacokinetics, and biomarker results of a single-rising-dose, randomized, double-blind, placebo-controlled trial. J Allergy Clin Immunol. 2015.
43. Paller AS, Siegfried EC, Langley RG, Gottlieb AB, Pariser D, Landellsl, et al. Etanercept treatment for children and adolescents with plaque psoriasis. N Engl J Med. 2008;358:241-51.
44. Trueb RM. Therapies for childhood psoriasis. Curr Probl Dermatol. 2009;38:137-59.
45. Kress DW. Etanercept therapy improves symptoms and allows tapering of other medications in children and adolescents with moderate to severe psoriasis. J Am Acad Dermatol. 2006;54:S126-8.
46. Pereira TM, Vieira AP, Fernandes JC, Antunes H, Basto AS. Anti TNF alpha therapy in childhood pustular psoriasis. Dermatol. 2006;213:350-2.
47. Farnsworth NN, George SJ, Hsu S. Successful use of infliximab following a failed course of etanercept in a pediatric patient. Dermatol Online J. 2005;11:11.
48. Menter MA, Cush JM. Successful treatment of pediatric psoriasis with infliximab. Pediatr Dermatol. 2004;21: 87-8.

49. Alvarez AC, Rodríguez-Nevado I, De Argila D, Rubio FP, Rovira I, Torrelo A, et al. Recalcitrant pustular psoriasis successfully treated with adalimumab. Pediatr Dermatol. 2011;28:195-7.
50. Callen JP, Jackson JH. Adalimumab effectively controlled recalcitrant generalized pustular psoriasis in an adolescent. J Dermatol Treat. 2005;16:350-2.
51. Fotiadou C, Lazaridou E, Giannopoulou C, Ioannides D. Ustekinumab for the treatment of an adolescent patient with recalcitrant plaque psoriasis. Eur J Dermatol. 2011; 21:117-8.
52. Puig L. Role of obesity in the outcome of obesity and psoriasis: body weight and body mass index influence the response to biological treatment. J Eur Acad Dermatol Venereol. 2011;25(9):1007-11.
53. Hsu L, Snodgrass BT, Armstrong AW. Anti-drug antibodies in psoriasis: a systematic review. Br J Dermatol. 2014;170(2):261-73.
54. De Simone C, Farina M, Maiorino A, Fanali C, Perino F, Flamini A, et al. TNF-alpha gene polymorphisms can help to predict response to etanercept in psoriatic patients. J Eur Acad Dermatol Venereol. 2015.
55. Grattan C, Burton JL, Manku M, Stewart C, Horrobin DF. Essential fatty- acid metabolites in plasma phospholipids in patients with ichthyosis vulgaris, acne vulgaris and psoriasis. Clin Exp Dermatol. 1990;15:174-6.
56. Lin YK, Yen HR, Wong WR, Yang SH, Pang JH. Successful treatment of pediatric psoriasis with Indigo naturalis composite ointment. Pediatr Dermatol. 2006; 23:507-10.
57. Balbás GM, Regaña MS, Millet PU. Study on the use of omega-3 fatty acids as a therapeutic supplement in treatment of psoriasis Clin Cosmet Investig Dermatol. 2011;4:73-7.
58. Pardasani AG, Feldman SR, Clark AR. Treatment of Psoriasis: An Algorithm-Based Approach for Primary Care Physicians. Am Fam Physician. 2000;61(3):725-33.
59. Parimalam K, Nithya P, Saratha KP, Mythili PC, Manoharan K. Effect of methotrexate in juvenile generalized pustular psoriasis. JAMS. 2012;1(3):28-31.
60. Guglielmetti A, Conlledo R, Bedoya J, Ianiszewski F, Correa J. Inverse Psoriasis Involving Genital Skin Folds: Successful Therapy with Dapsone. Dermatol Ther. 2012; 2(1):15.
61. Meeuwis KA, De Hullu JA, Massuger LF, Van de Kerkhof PC, Van Rossum MM. Genital psoriasis: a systematic literature review on this hidden skin disease. Acta Derm Venereol. 2011;91(1):5-11.
62. D'Souza V. Beating palmoplantar psoriasis away. Ind J Dermatol. 2012;57(3):241-2.
63. Le QV, Howard A. Dexamethasone iontophoresis for the treatment of nail psoriasis. Australas J Dermatol. 2013;54(2):115-9.
64. Lee JC, Gladman DD, Schentag CT, Cook RJ. The long-term use of azathioprine in patients with psoriatic arthritis. J Clin Rheumatol. 2001;7(3):160-5.
65. Dermwire Practical Dermatology. (2013). Stelara receives FDA approval to treat active psoriatic arthritis. [online] Available from bmctoday.net/practicaldermatology/dermwire/view.asp?20130923-stelara_receives_fda_approval_to_treat_active_psoriatic_arthritis. [Accessed November, 2015].
66. Bhutani T, Kamangar F, Zitelli K, Chiang C, Gattu S, Nguyen T, et al. Intralesional injections of alefacept may predict systemic response to intramuscular alefacept: results from a pilot study. J Dermatolog Treat. 2013;24(5):348-50.
67. van der Heijde D, Fleischmann R, Wollenhaupt J, Deodhar A, Kielar D, Woltering F. Effect of different imputation approaches on the evaluation of radiographic progression in patients with psoriatic arthritis: results of the RAPID-PsA 24-week phase III double-blind randomised placebo-controlled study of certolizumab pegol. Ann Rheum Dis. 2014;73(1):233-7.
68. Bakkour W, Purssell H, Chinoy H, Griffiths CEM, Warren RB. The risk of post-operative complications in psoriasis and psoriatic arthritis patients on biologic therapy undergoing surgical procedures. J Euro Acad Dermatol Venereol. 2015.
69. Tsai TF, Ho V, Song M, Szapary P, Kato T, Wasfi Y, et.al. The safety of ustekinumab treatment in patients with moderate-to-severe psoriasis and latent tuberculosis infection. Br J Dermatol. 2012;167:1145-52.
70. Shah KN, Cortina S, Ernst MM, Kichler JC. Psoriasis in childhood: effective strategies to improve treatment adherence. Dovepress. 2015;5:43-54.
71. Feely MA, Smith BL, Weinberg JM. Novel psoriasis therapies and patient outcomes, Part 1: topical medications. Cutis. 2015;95(3):164-8, 170.
72. Mansouri Y, Goldenberg G. New systemic therapies for psoriasis. Cutis. 2015;95(3):155-60.
73. Papp KA, Menter A, Strober B, Langley RG, Buonanno M, Wolk R, et al. Efficacy and safety of tofacitinib, an oral Janus kinase inhibitor, in the treatment of psoriasis: a Phase 2b randomized placebo-controlled dose-ranging study. British J Dermatol. 2012;167(3):668-77.

CHAPTER 11

Complications and "The Psoriatic March"

INTRODUCTION

Complications due to psoriasis are not uncommon. These are either due to the disease or drugs used for the treatment and can be limited to the skin or may at times involve other systems as well. Secondary infection of psoriatic plaques, eczematization are common local complications. Arthritis can be considered as a part of psoriasis or result as a complication of chronic severe psoriasis. Systemic amyloidosis is a rare complication of psoriasis. Recently, there is an increase in the prevalence of comorbidities due to the persistent inflammation due to psoriasis.

COMPLICATIONS

Complications in psoriasis by themselves are though rare, they may result from the persistence of inflammation. Association of certain diseases themselves can be considered as complication as they at times worsen as psoriasis worsens. Complications in psoriasis can be viewed as:

- Cutaneous complications
- Metabolic and systemic complications
- Arthropathic complications
- Ocular complications
- Psychosocial complications
- Complications due to treatment.

Cutaneous Complications

Itching, eczematization, and infections are common complications encountered in day-to-day practice. Intensity of itching can range from complete absence to severe pruritus. It is more common in unstable forms. Itching can be very intense in erythrodermic psoriasis which is sometimes difficult to control. Since degree of itching reflects the emotional state of the patient and, if severe, may be a symptom of anxiety or depression.

Eczematization of the plaque is very common in anatomical sites like the palms and soles. That apart, irritant topical application can lead to eczematization which is then difficult to make a diagnosis.

Secondary bacterial infection of psoriatic lesions is rarely a problem except during surgical wounds. However, *Staphylococci* are carried by 50% of psoriatics, especially on the lesions. Carriage of *Staphylococci* may prove to be a problem, if a surgical procedure is to be carried out through a psoriatic plaque. Because of exfoliation, these patients may disseminate infections in hospital wards. Fissuring in flexural psoriasis may get secondarily infected. Itching can be considered as a symptom which by it in some individual can be very severe, especially in unstable forms. Whereas, pustular and erythrodermic patterns are accompanied by sensations of burning or tightness. Secondary infection of psoriatic lesions is a problem during topical steroid therapy used under occlusive dressings, which can lead to folliculitis and furunculosis.

It is not uncommon to see flexural psoriasis to be secondarily infected by candida overgrowth. Superadded dermatophytes infections are not uncommon with psoriatic nails.

Metabolic and Systemic Complications

Obesity, diabetes, hypertension, and dyslipidemia are common comorbidities resulting from psoriasis. A significant incidence of hyperthyroidism and hypothyroidism and the presence of thyroid antibodies have been found in association with palmoplantar pustulosis. A greater tendency to develop diabetes has also been documented. Various arthropathies are also associated, including chronic recurrent multifocal osteomyelitis, sternoclavicular involvement, pustular arthroosteitis, axial and peripheral arthritis. Some patients have antigliadin antibodies.

Patients with severe psoriasis can develop folate deficiency.

Nephritis and Renal Failure

The role of streptococcal infection, especially in the throat, in provoking acute guttate psoriasis is well-known, a case of concomitant onset of diffuse psoriasis and mesangiocapillary glomerulonephritis has been reported. Renal failure due to acute tubular necrosis may rarely result from the oligemia after loss of albumin into and from the skin in acute pustular psoriasis.

Hepatic Failure

Severe abnormalities of liver function may occur in erythrodermic or pustular psoriasis, and are likely to be related to drugs, alcohol intake, and oligemia.

Apical pulmonary fibrosis has been established as a nonarticular complication of psoriatic spondylitis as well as chronic plaque psoriasis.

Secondary amyloidosis is a rare sequel of arthropathic, generalized pustular and severe nonpustular forms which may be an additional cause of renal failure in association with psoriasis.

The prevalence of polycystic ovary syndrome (PCOS) in women with psoriasis is remarkably greater than in age-matched and body mass index-matched control women. Psoriasis is linked with metabolic syndrome, insulin resistance (IR), and nonalcoholic fatty liver diseases, which are also common features, found to be associated with PCOS. Whether there is a missing link between psoriasis and subfertility is to be probed and explored. Systemic and metabolic complications of psoriasis are listed in Box 11.1.

Generalized pustular psoriasis is known to develop complications and morbidity more frequently than other forms of psoriasis.

Occasionally, acute respiratory distress syndrome may complicate generalized pustular psoriasis.

Other complications in pustular psoriasis may include the following:
- Secondary bacterial skin infections, hair loss (telogen effluvium), and nail loss
- Malabsorption and malnutrition

> **BOX 11.1: Systemic and metabolic complications of psoriasis**
> - Obesity
> - Diabetes
> - Hypertension
> - Dyslipidemia
> - Liver disease
> - Hyperthyroidism and hypothyroidism
> - Folate deficiency
> - Arthropathies
> - Chronic recurrent multifocal osteomyelitis
> - Antigliadin antibodies
> - Nephritis and renal failure
> - Organ failure in erythroderma
> - Apical pulmonary fibrosis
> - Secondary amyloidosis
> - Subfertility

- Hypoalbuminemia secondary to loss of plasma protein into tissues
- Hypocalcemia
- Renal tubular necrosis as a result of oligemia
- Liver damage as a result of oligemia and general toxicity
- Telogen effluvium
- Amyloidosis
- Inflammatory polyarthritis.

Death in untreated pustular psoriasis may occur as a result of cardiorespiratory failure.

Arthropathic Complications

Approximately, one-half of patients with early-onset psoriatic arthritis PsA develop erosive joint damage within 2 years of onset. In addition, PsA patients have an increased mortality rate, with cardiovascular complications reported to be the most common cause of death. PsA patients can experience sleep apnea and a reduced quality of life and increased functional disabilities compared with the general population, and the reduction in quality of life is greater in those with higher scores of psoriasis area and severity index.

Ocular Complications

Ophthalmic complications of psoriasis affect almost any part of the eye. Psoriatic eye findings may include conjunctivitis, dry eye, episcleritis, and uveitis, all of which may precede articular changes. Uveitis, seen in up to 25% of PsA patients, may be recognized by the presence of conjunctival injection, photophobia, pain, lid swelling or otherwise unexplained visual changes.

A clinically distinct form of bilateral uveitis that is prolonged can develop in patients with PsA and in patients with psoriasis.

Ocular involvement of psoriasis may be easily missed. Early recognition is of paramount importance as the natural course may lead to loss of vision. Physicians should maintain a high index of suspicion that ophthalmic symptoms in patients with psoriasis may be related to their underlying disease, even though signs and symptoms are often vague.

Psychosocial Complications

Alcoholism is known to exacerbate psoriasis, however, heavy drinking was found significantly more commonly in male patients with severe psoriasis than in other groups with the disease, and could be a symptom of stress caused by severe skin disease.

Complications Due to Treatment

Topical therapy is considered relatively safe. However, they are not without causing side effect, if not properly used. Topical steroid therapy under occlusive dressings, can lead to cutaneous atrophy, and secondary infection with bacteria, fungi, and virus apart from hypopigmentation and comedone formation in some individuals.

Salicylic Acid

Apart from causing irritation, percutaneous salicylate absorption can lead to salicylism.

Tar when applied in higher concentration can cause irritation, or when combined with ultraviolet light in the Goeckermann regimen.

Anthralin apart from causing skin irritation can stain the skin and clothes.

Vitamin D analog sometimes can cause burning and stinging sensation and hypocalcemia.

Tazarotene, although topical, is a category X medication. Side effects include desquamation, erythema, burning, stinging, dry skin, skin irritation, skin pain, irritant or contact dermatitis and photosensitivity.

Systemic agents used in psoriasis as well as drugs used for other illness, are known for their adverse effects, requiring judicious follow up. When there is an adverse cutaneous drug reaction in a patient with psoriasis, the drug reaction component resolves on withdrawal of the offending drug, exposing the original psoriatic morphology (Figs 11.1 to 11.3).

Common side effects of retinoid include xerosis, cheilitis, epistaxis, and reversible

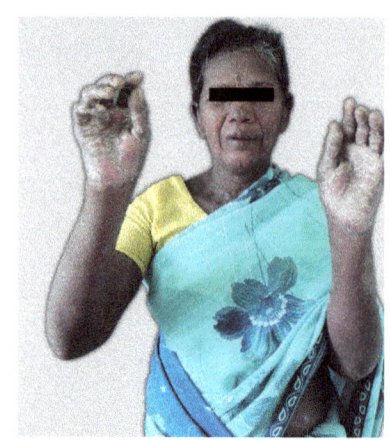

Fig. 11.2: Same woman as in Fig 11.1, showing improvement on treatment

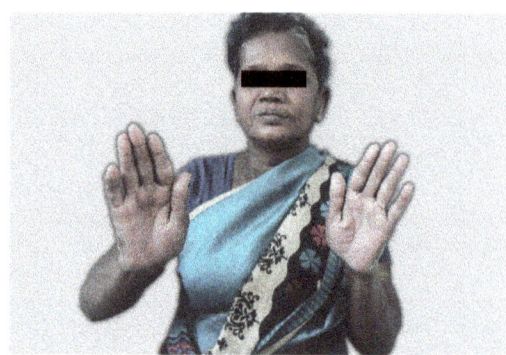

Fig. 11.3: Same woman as in Fig 11.1, complete resolution of drug reaction showing residual lesions of palmar psoriasis

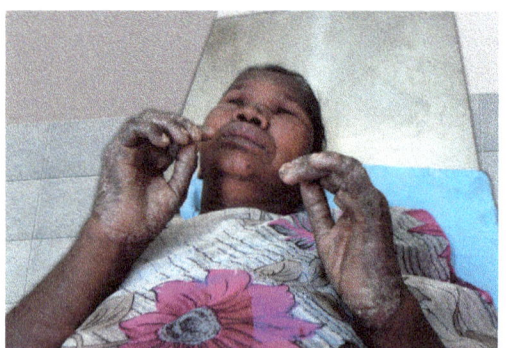

Fig. 11.1: Adverse cutaneous drug reaction in a psoriatic, note the facial involvement

alteration in liver enzymes and serum lipids. Premature closure of epiphysis limits its use in children.

The following drugs cause immunosuppression and hence, lead to increased proneness for infection:
- Methotrexate can cause myelotoxicity; hepatotoxicity, and pulmonary fibrosis
- Cyclosporine is known for its nephrotoxicity. It can also induce systemic hypertension
- Biologics are found to be associated with increased risk of malignancies, including

lymphoma, leukemia, and development of new-onset psoriasis. Reversible posterior leukoencephalopathy syndrome and a lymphomatoid drug eruption, and cardiovascular complications were reported with the use of ustekinumab.

THE PSORIATIC MARCH

The "March of psoriasis" has been used to describe the process in a step-wise manner, beginning with genetic, and possibly environmental, factors that initiate disease-specific pathways involving the immune system. This leads to expression of psoriasis and subsequent comorbidities as a consequence of chronic inflammation (Fig. 11.4). Cardiovascular risk being the one most elaborately studied in this aspect. The common factor, the vasculature and the IR lead to a cascade of events marching to affect the corresponding effector organ, depending on the degree of resultant impairment.

The systemic inflammation associated with psoriasis enhances IR, causing endothelial dysfunction, atherosclerosis, and eventual coronary events. The innate and adaptive immune responses are both responsible for disease pathology, resulting in changes to the epidermis and vasculature. Although the 'march of psoriasis' is described in a step-wise manner, the inflammatory processes involved may drive the development of cardiovascular risk factors concomitantly with the presentation of psoriasis.

Biomarkers indicating a state of systemic inflammation have been observed to be elevated in the blood of psoriasis patients, including C-reactive protein, vascular endothelial growth factor (VEGF), and indicators of platelet activation, such as P-selectin. Of these, it was noted that VEGF

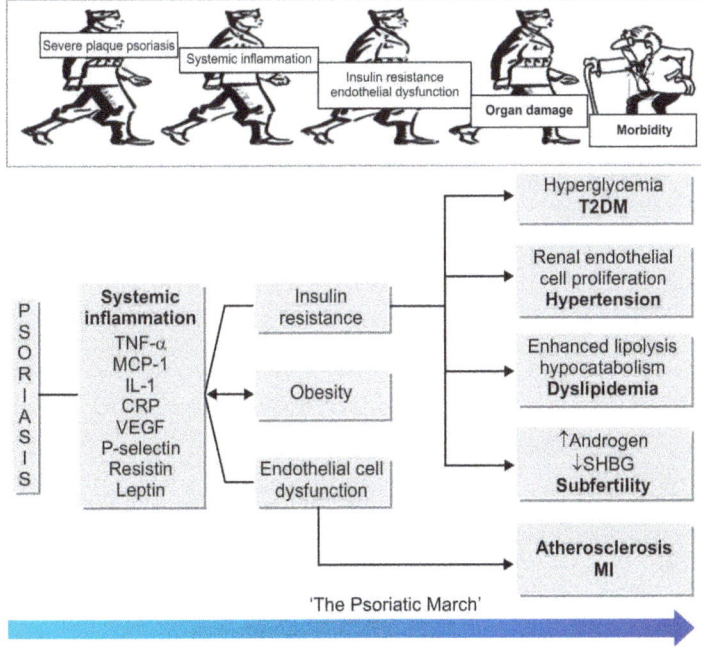

TNF, tumor necrosis factor; MCP-1, monocyte chemoattractant protein-1; IL, interleukin; CRP, C-reactive protein; VEGF, vascular endothelial growth factor; T2DM, type 2 diabetes mellitus; SHBG, sex hormone binding globulin; MI, myocardial infarction.

Fig. 11.4: "The Psoriatic March"

never drops to levels as low as in non-psoriatic controls, but remains somewhat elevated even in the absence of clinical signs of psoriasis. This persistently elevated levels of VEGF support the concept of psoriatic march even in the absence of clinical activity of the disease indicating that all psoriasis need to be treated vigorously in order to prevent organ damage. The elevated levels of resistin and leptin functioning as insulin antagonists lead to insulin resistance.

The resulting insult is simplified for better and easy understanding:

- IR leads to hyperglycemia. With the β cells in the pancreas producing more of insulin, further contributes to hyperinsulinemia. This often remains undetected and can contribute to development of type 2 diabetes mellitus
- Renal endothelial cell proliferation with extramedullary matrix deposit induced by IR through a cascade of events results in glomerular sclerosis and hypertension. Hypertension by itself can have its effect on all organs including the central nervous system leading to stroke
- In insulin-resistance states, enhanced lipolysis and increased fatty acid flux from adipose tissue, hypersecretion and hypocatabolism of chylomicron and very low density lipoprotein (VLDL) remnants, and de novo lipogenesis are three major sources of tryglyceride (TG), the main substrate regulating apolipoprotein B secretion as VLDL. Altered metabolism of TG-rich lipoproteins is crucial in the pathophysiology leading to dyslipidemia associated with IR.
- IR and the resultant hyperinsulinemia via increased levels of androgenic enzymes and reduced sex hormone binding globulin leads to androgen excess. Anovulation and polycystic ovary caused by androgen excess may lead to subfertility
- Endothelin are identified to be produced by keratinocytes. The levels of endothelin 1 are significantly elevated in psoriasis. This along with the reduced production of nitric oxide creates an imbalance predisposing the endothelium toward an atherogenic milieu.

Timely and appropriate systemic therapy will certainly reduce the pace of March though cannot fully stop the progress and organ damage.

CONCLUSION

Both cutaneous and systemic complications should be looked for in every patient with psoriasis. Topical steroid-induced complications are very common and can be easily averted by judicial use of the steroid molecule. Metabolic and systemic complications including arthropathic complications are on the rise and all attempts should be made to screen patients and detect these as early as possible which will help better management and reduce morbidity. Ocular complications are not uncommon and should be suspected as early recognition will certainly prevent loss of vision. Every patient, be it child or adult, should be given effective counseling to prevent psychosocial complications and appropriate referral is of paramount importance to actively manage the same. In the current era of biologics and immunosuppressant therapy for psoriasis, enough precautions have to be taken to avoid complications due to treatment.

REFERENCES

1. Boehncke WH, Boehncke S, Anne-Marie Tobin, Kirby B. The 'psoriatic march': a concept of how severe psoriasis may drive cardiovascular comorbidity. Experimental Dermatology. 2011;20:303-7.
2. McDonald I, Connolly M, Tobin MN. A review of psoriasis, a known risk factor for cardiovascular disease and its impact on folate and homocysteine metabolism. J Nutr Metab. 2012;2012:965385.

CHAPTER 12

Psychological Aspects, Course and Prognosis, Follow-up and Rehabilitation

INTRODUCTION

Persons with psoriasis have a definite impairment of quality of life (QoL). Being a chronic disease, psoriasis has tremendous financial ramification which adds further to the impairment of QoL. These factors significantly affect the way the person sees himself/herself. Counseling patients with psoriasis will certainly improve the mental and psychological status, thereby improving the compliance to therapy. The foremost step in the treatment of psoriasis is to establish a strong patient-doctor relationship. All the care givers of patients with psoriasis should be empathetic while dealing with them. Counseling for the relatives is as important as it is for the patient.

PSYCHOLOGICAL ASPECTS

Psoriasis is a common dermatologic disorder with psychiatric comorbidity that often goes undetected and untreated. Psoriasis has higher associations with psychiatric illness than do other dermatologic conditions. We found that psoriasis patients suffer psychiatric and psychosocial morbidity that is not commensurate with the extent of cutaneous lesions. Biologic therapies and nonpharmacologic psychosocial interventions show promise in treating comorbid psychiatric illness.[1] Psoriasis has a tremendous impact on QoL. Studies have shown that psoriasis detracts more from QoL than any other condition except depression and that's including life-threatening illnesses, such as heart disease and diabetes. Psoriasis has a significant negative impact on patients' QoL. Psoriasis has been linked to the depression and suicidal tendencies in the patients. The costs associated with decrements in QoL, lost productivity, and work absenteeism may be enormous, increasing overall costs associated with the disease management. Studies show that up to 75% of patients believed that psoriasis had moderate-to-large negative impact on their QoL, with alterations in their daily activities and at least 20% of psoriasis patients had contemplated suicide. Psoriasis adversely affects the working ability in the work spot in addition to causing extra expenditure toward the medication while the working days have reduced in number due to abstinence from work. Studies show that physical and emotional effects of psoriasis were found to have a significant negative impact at patients' workplace as measured by the validated scales including work productivity assessment index, Short Form-8 Health Survey, hospital anxiety and depression (HADS), and past medical or psoriasis history.[2]

Psoriasis patients often experience difficulties like maladaptive coping responses, problems in body image, self-esteem, self-concept and also have feelings of stigma, shame, and embarrassment regarding their appearance. Various factors may be attributed to the lower QoL in psoriasis patients.

The following are some of the problems leading to lowered QoL in patients with psoriasis:
- Hopelessness in terms of cure for the condition
- Unexpected outbreak of symptoms interfering with future plans
- Lack of control over the disease
- Social and psychological difficulties created by their environment
- Feel of humiliation during the need to expose their bodies like while swimming, intimate relationships, using public showers, or living in conditions that do not provide appropriate privacy
- Need to hide the disease, thus severely affecting the self-confidence
- Failure of appreciation by their own doctors and relatives of negative impact of psoriasis on their life
- Social difficulties and friction with family members due to the disease
- Other people reacting to their disease or anticipation of the same
- Limitations in daily activities, occupational and sexual functioning.

There are different indices in practice to assess the QoL.[2]

Psoriasis-specific measures:
- Psoriasis index of QoL (PSORIQoL)
- Psoriasis life stress inventory (PLSI)
- Psoriasis disability index (PDI)
- Psoriasis area and severity index (PASI) and simplified PASI (SAPASI).

Skin-specific measures:
- Questionnaire on experience with skin complaints (QES)
- Dermatology life quality index (DLQI).

Generic QoL measures:
- Short form-36 (SF-36)
- Subjective well-being scale (SWLS)
- EuroQoL 5D (EQ-5D).

Mixed QoL measures:
- Salford psoriasis index (SPI)
- Koo-Menter psoriasis instrument (KMPI).

Psoriasis-specific Measures

Psoriasis Index of Quality of Life

This is a 25-item version of the PSORIQoL. This version was found to be reliable having a good reproducibility and is expected to work in a uniform manner across patient samples, irrespective of age and gender.

Psoriasis Life Stress Inventory

The PLSI is a 15-item questionnaire that provides a measure of the daily hassles of psychosocial stress associated with having to cope with everyday events in living with psoriasis. Scores on this scale range from 0 to 45. The PLSI also permits patients to be classified as a function of their distribution of scores into two groups: those patients who react significantly to the stress associated with having psoriasis (score of >10); and those patients who are not significantly affected with having psoriasis-related stress (score of <10).

Psoriasis Disability Index

The PDI is a 15-item scale that specifically addresses self-reported disability in areas of daily activities, employment, personal relationships, and leisure and treatment effects. The items are concerned with the practical effects of psoriasis in everyday life.

Psoriasis Area and Severity Index and Simplified PASI

Psoriasis area and severity index is the most widely used measure of severity in the research as well as the clinical setting. This makes it an important tool in gauging the impact of the disease on QoL, though other instruments to measure QoL are encouraged. Since PASI or SAPASI do not measure the impact of psoriasis on patients' QoL directly, use of other QoL scales is recommended.

Skin-Specific Measures

Questionnaire on Experience with Skin Complaints

The short form of the QES with 23 items is a valid instrument for examination of social and psychic burdens of psoriasis. The recording of stigmatization feeling and of QoL determines different supplementary aspects of the illness-related stress of patients with chronic skin diseases.

Dermatology Life Quality Index

The DLQI is a compact self-reported questionnaire to measure health-related quality of life (HRQoL) over the previous week in patients with skin diseases. It consists of 10 items covering symptoms and feelings. Each item is scored on a four point scale, with higher scores indicating greater impairment in HRQoL.

Generic Quality of Life Measures

Short Form-36

The SF-36 health survey is a widely used generic, 36-item, self-reported health status questionnaire assessing 8 domains of health status, (1) physical activities; (2) social activities; (3) usual physical role activities; (4) bodily pain; (5) general mental health; (6) usual emotional role activities; (7) vitality; (8) general health perceptions. A score from 0 to 100 is calculated for each subscale, with higher scores indicating better HRQL. The SF-36 may be the best characterized measure for comparing QoL differences across different diseases. The SF-36 was used to show that the impact of psoriasis is as great as that of other major medical disorders.

Subjective Well-being Scale

The SWLS is a short 5-item instrument designed to measure global life satisfaction. The scale has been validated and correlates with other measures of subjective well-being (SWB). The SWLS was developed to assess satisfaction with the respondent's life as a whole, without assessing satisfaction with specific life event.

EuroQoL 5D

The EQ-5D is a standardized generic instrument developed for describing and valuing health states. It specifically refers to health status at the time of questioning.

Mixed Quality of Life Measures

Salford Psoriasis Index

The SPI is derived from combining a score of current severity of psoriasis based on the PASI, a score indicating psychosocial disability, and a score based on historical information. The resultant three-figure signs, psychosocial disability, interventions (SPI) is a similar paradigm to the tumor, nodes, metastasis classification used for cancer staging. The SPI provide an holistic assessment of overall disease severity.
- S—Signs: a 0-10 measure of physical severity derived from the PASI
- P—Psychosocial disability: measured as 0-10 on a visual analog scale
- I—Interventions: a cumulative historical record of systemic therapies, episodes of erythroderma, etc.

The SPI is represented as three figures and is a guide to the difficulty of treating any one patient at a certain time. There are many instruments to measure QoL for psoriasis and psoriatic arthritis (PsA). It does not appear that one will cover all the issues that QoL encompasses.

Koo-Menter Psoriasis Instrument

The KMPI is a diagnostic algorithm and a formal measure, to aid in identifying patients with significant impact on QoL warranting systemic therapy. In addition, the KMPI can be used to document and justify treatment decisions for health care payers.

Quality of Life and Psychological Aspects of Psoriasis

Although psoriasis generally does not affect survival, it certainly has a number of major negative effects on patients, demonstrable by a significant detriment to QoL. Stress in the form of pathological worry has a deleterious effect in response to therapy. The exact mechanism by which psychological distress exacerbates or triggers psoriasis is poorly understood. May be that psychological stress has the potential to regulate the immune response, and there is emerging evidence that abnormal neuroendocrine responses to stress may contribute to the pathogenesis of chronic autoimmune diseases, as has been described for rheumatoid arthritis (RA). It is likely that, in some patients with psoriasis, there is an abnormal hypothalamic–adrenal axis response to acute stress. The QoL measures take into account the effect of the treatment on the patient. QoL data fulfills the role of measuring the intangible changes in a patient's life that determine treatment success. Living with psoriasis often has emotional and social consequences.
- Patients may feel embarrassed by having visible plaques and that can lead to depression to such an extent as to stay withdrawn from society (Figs 12.1 to 12.3)

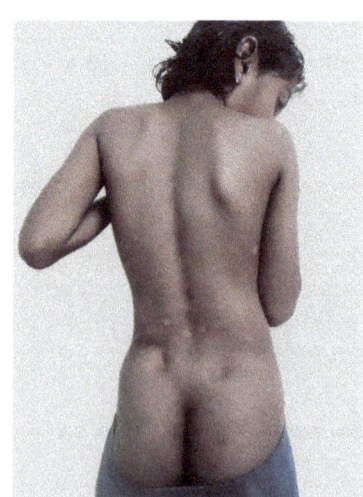

Fig. 12.1: Depression leading to social isolation in an adolescent with psoriasis

Psychological Aspects, Course and Prognosis, Follow-up and Rehabilitation

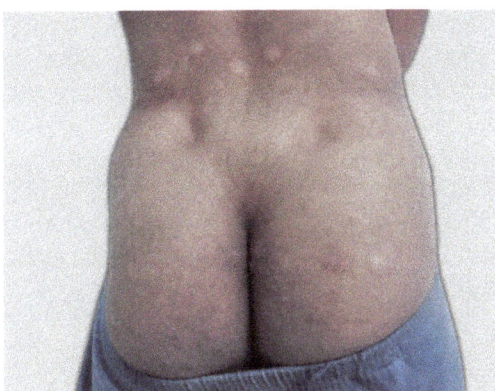

Fig. 12.2: Note the psoriatic plaques in the same patient as seen in Fig. 12.1

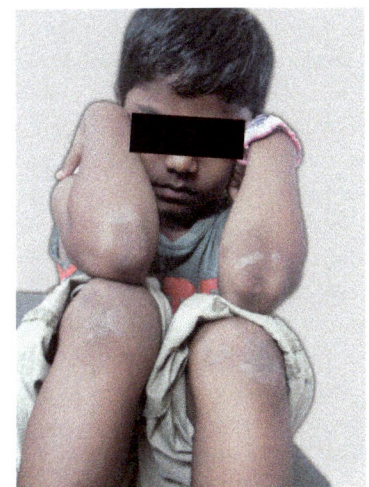

Fig. 12.3: Young depressed boy with psoriasis

- Symptoms may become so severe that patients have to leave their jobs, further increasing the risk of psychological and emotional problems in addition to the economical strain
- Several surveys have shown that a significant number of patients with psoriasis report a negative mental and physical impact that is similar to several chronic conditions including cancer, hypertension, heart disease, depression, and diabetes.

Oxidative Stress Index and Psoriasis

Studies show that psoriasis patients had higher HADS scores, higher oxidative stress index (OSI) and total oxidant capacity (TOC) levels, and lower total antioxidant capacity (TAC) levels compared with the control group. Comparison among four groups with/without psoriasis and higher or lower HADS scores revealed statistically significant differences with regard to TAC. TAC, TOC, and OSI levels did not differ significantly in psoriasis patients with regard to higher or lower HADS scores. Based on the findings of this study, the presence of either psoriasis or higher HADS scores in the control subjects was associated with increased oxidative stress, whereas presence of higher HADS scores did not lead to further increase in oxidative stress in psoriatic patients.[3] Human leukocyte antigen-Cw6 is found to be linked to depression in psoriatic patients.[4]

In 2009, Ortonne et al. devised the nail psoriasis QoL scale-10 (NPQ10) to evaluate the impact of nail psoriasis on QoL. The scale correlated well with the DLQI. A valid and reliable questionnaire consisting of 10 questions was prepared with all the questions specifically targeting the impact of nail psoriasis on QoL. The questionnaire was answered by 1,309 patients and showed that 86% patients considered nail psoriasis as bothersome, 87% as unsightly, and 59% as painful. Such an impact of nail psoriasis definitely warrants an insight into its clinical manifestations and treatment options by a present day dermatologist.[5]

Not only dermatologists, but also general practitioners and other health care providers should assess the severity and impact the condition has on a person at first presentation, and before referral for specialist's advice.

This assessment should cover the impact the disease has on the physical, psychological, and social well-being of those with the condition.

The severity of disease should also be assessed, as should the presence of comorbid conditions.

Risk factors for cardiovascular comorbidities should be discussed with people who have any type of psoriasis. The patient's care taker or the parent, as the case may be, should be adequately informed about the consequences.

Tailored advice and healthy lifestyle information and support for behavioral change should be provided. All possible measures must be taken to advice on lifestyle modification and to prevent comorbidities, especially obesity and type 2 diabetes mellitus.

Psoriasis affects in a cumulative way the QoL of both patients and their close relatives. Regarding family dermatology life quality index (FDLQI), 90% of the participating family members, responded that their relative's psoriasis affected their own QoL indicating the impact of the disease in the family members as well.[6]

According to Armstrong AW et al. who studied the relationship between psoriasis and sexual behavior in US women found that psoriasis was associated with a significantly reduced number of sexual partners in nonheterosexual women. They conclude stating psoriasis may differentially impact sexual behavior based on sexual orientation in women.[7]

Quality of Life in Psoriatic Arthritis

Quality of life and functional capacity were found to be significantly reduced in patients with PsA compared with psoriasis patients without arthritis or healthy controls.[8] The use of the original HAQ appears to be sufficient, as it has been found that the addition of features did not alter the level of disability noted by patients with PsA.[9] The impact of the disease in patients with PsA appears to be similar to that of patients with RA according to Sokoll et al.[10] Husted et al. demonstrated that patients with PsA have less vitality than those with RA. Thus, the severity of the disease has an impact on the functional status and QoL of patients with PsA.[11] Studies have shown improvement in patients treated with drugs.

COURSE AND PROGNOSIS

Course and prognosis of psoriasis still remains unpredictable despite the enormous development that has taken place in the understanding of the disease and its consequences. It is not possible to predict either the duration of the disease or the period of remission. Though guttate psoriasis tends to carry a better prognosis, most of them eventually end up in psoriasis vulgaris sooner or later. At the other extreme, erythrodermic and pustular forms carry an appreciable mortality and arthropathic forms a considerable morbidity. Early onset and a family history of the disease appear to worsen the prognosis. Stress in any form seems to precipitate, exacerbate or worsen psoriasis.

Relapse is the rule, however completely the lesions are treated and by whatever method. Despite the advent of new biological agents, it has not been possible to assure any patient a complete cure. If only the clinician is able to prevent the March of psoriasis and reduce the incidence of resultant comorbidity will there be justification in treating any given patient, be it an infant, child, adolescent or an adult young or old.

FOLLOW-UP AND REHABILITATION

Psoriasis by itself is a disease that causes a lot of psychological stress and vice versa.

Psoriasis was recently shown to have a great impact on QoL even in affected children. Like atopic dermatitis, urticaria, and acne, psoriasis in the pediatric age group can lead to a severe emotional burden to the extent of impairing the HRQoL. A study on children and adolescents aged between 5 and 16 years found that in children with psoriasis, the values were as high as in children with atopic dermatitis and higher than in children with urticaria or acne.[12]

Medication adherence and compliance are essential for disease management and can significantly improve outcomes and quality of patient care. The literature suggests that up to 40% of patients do not use their medication as intended. Adherence in the treatment of psoriasis can improve QoL by improving the outcome and thereby patient's confidence. A better understanding of the determinants of adherence can improve the outcomes of psoriasis treatment and lead to higher patient satisfaction and quality of care.[13] In a study conducted by Balata N et al. to evaluate the use of text messages (TM) in improving treatment adherence and several patient outcomes, such as QoL, disease severity, patient–perceived disease severity, and the patient–physician relationship. TM interventions seemed to be a very promising tool for the long-term management of patients with psoriasis, leading to an increased compliance to therapy, positive changes in self-care behaviors and better patient–physician relationship allowing improved clinical outcomes and better control of the disease.[14] The afflicted children must learn to cope with life and to adapt to their individual health situation. They must be counseled to choose a profession suitable to them in future. Rehabilitation of psoriatic children and adolescents can also supplement therapy of and prevent the disease.[15]

Therapy goals of rehabilitation will include:
- Regular treatment of the skin under proper supervision clubbed with climate therapy, nutritional therapy, and psychological interventions
- Help in coping with the disease with respect to the psychosocial consequences of psoriasis
- Help in finding an occupation.

Accurate assessment of people with psoriasis will ensure they can access the right treatment as early as possible whether in primary or specialist care.

Psoriasis patients must be given enough time in the consultation chamber either by the physician or a counselor, who takes time to explain the patients to cope with the disease with ease and learn to live with the disease at the same time try to control it. This will not only improve the QoL of the patient but also reduce the financial burden in the form of treatment. Following are some of the aspects that can be given importance:
- Good nourishment
- Effective management of day-to-day stress
- Planning regular holidays
- Clothing
- Sun exposure
- Build self-esteem.

Good nourishment: A balanced protein rich diet and complete abstinence from alcohol will go a long way in maintaining the remission.

Effective management of day-to-day stress: Regular meditation and or exercise will alleviate the anxiety and reduce stress, thereby will prevent an exacerbation.

Planning regular holidays to places with adequate sunshine and ample relaxation will help calm the skin and mind.

Wearing ideal clothing and to be cautious during winter.

Loose fitting cotton cloth will be comfortable and help avoid friction due to tight fitting garments.

To get exposed to sun light as much as possible and using moisturizers liberally will help prevent an exacerbation.

To build self-esteem, patients must be made to believe that they are not their disease. They should be helped to find a support group of people (locally or online) who are coping positively with their condition. Periodic meeting in person with such group will be beneficial to all in a positive manner.

Physicians' Role[16,17]

Management of psoriasis must start with counseling. Counseling will improve the mental and psychological condition of the patients. Aim of the counseling should include increasing personal control, encouraging active coping strategies, restructuring negative thoughts about the disease and encouraging patients to express emotions, seek social support, and distract themselves. As in treatment of other medical conditions, establishing a strong physician-patient relationship is the foundation of effective psoriasis treatment. Due to the recurring nature of the disease, patients are more likely to be frustrated with the disease and with the care they receive or have received in the past. Establishing a bond and trust between patient and physician will encourage patients to be more complaint to their physician's recommendations concerning treatment and will potentially improves treatment compliance and outcomes. Physician must communicate a sense of empathy and understanding that will assure the patient of the physician's competence in managing psoriasis. Adequate time must be spent with the family members explaining the noncontagious nature of the disease. The relatives and friends must be motivated to treat patients with psoriasis as any other person. They must understand that psoriasis, has a significant negative impact on patient's QoL.

CONCLUSION

Psoriasis is a serious condition and is associated with significantly lower QoL. Studies have utilized different measures available to assess QoL of psoriasis patients. Most commonly used measures were psoriasis specific, such as PASI and DLQI followed by generic measures, such as SF-36. Pharmacological interventions along with patient counseling and education may be an effective strategy to improve QoL among psoriasis patients. Lack of head-to-head comparisons of available treatment options limits conclusions regarding superiority of one agent over another in improving QoL in psoriasis patients.

"We, the health care providers have the duty to see that every patient with psoriasis is helped to live his/her normal span of life in perfect health."

REFERENCES

1. Rieder E, Tausk F. Psoriasis, a model of dermatologic psychosomatic disease: psychiatric implications and treatments. Int J Dermatol. 2012;51:12-26.
2. Bhosle MJ, Kulkarni A, Feldman SR, Balkrishnan R. Quality of life in patients with psoriasis. Health Qual Life Outcomes. 2006;4:35.
3. Karababa F, Yesilova Y, Turan E, Selek S, Altun H, Selek S. Impact of depressive symptoms on oxidative stress in patients with psoriasis. Redox Rep. 2013;18:51-5.
4. Gudjónsson JE, Kárason A, Antonsdóttir AA, Rúnarsdóttir EH, Gulcher JR, Stefánsson K, et al. HLA-Cw6-positive and HLA-Cw6-negative patients with Psoriasis vulgaris have distinct clinical features. J Invest Dermatol. 2002;118(2):362-5.
5. Ortonne JP, Baran R, Corvest M, Schmitt C, Voisard JJ, Taieb C. Development and validation of nail psoriasis quality of life scale (NPQ10). J Eur Acad Dermatol Venereol. 2010;24:22-7.

6. Tadros A, Vergou T, Stratigos AJ, Tzavara C, Hletsos M, Katsambas A, et al. Psoriasis: is it the tip of the iceberg for the quality of life of patients and their families. J Eur Acad Dermatol Venereol. 2011;25(11):1282-7.
7. Armstrong AW, Follansbee MR, Harskamp CT, Schupp CW. Psoriasis and Sexual Behavior in U.S. Women: An Epidemiologic Analysis Using the National Health and Nutrition Examination Survey (NHANES). J Sex Med. 2013;10(2):326-32.
8. Husted JA, Gladman DD, Farewell VT, Long JA, Cook RJ. Validating the SF-36 health survey questionnaire in patients with psoriatic arthritis. J Rheumatol. 1997;24:511-7.
9. Husted J, Gladman DD, Long J, Farewell VT. A modified version of the Health Assessment Questionnaire (HAQ) for psoriatic arthritis. Clin Exp Rheumatol. 1995;13:439-44.
10. Sokoll KB, Helliwell PS. Comparison of disability and quality of life in rheumatoid and psoriatic arthritis. J Rheumatol. 2001;28:1842-6.
11. Husted JA, Gladman DD, Cook RJ, Farewell VT. Responsiveness of health status instruments to changes in articular status and perceived health in patients with psoriatic arthritis. J Rheumatol. 1998;25:2146-55.
12. Beattie PE, Lewis-Jones MS. A comparative study of impairment of quality of life in children with skin disease and children with other chronic diseases. Br J Dermatol. 2006;155:145-51.
13. Augustin M, Holland B, Dartsch D, Langenbruch A, Radtke MA. Adherence in the treatment of psoriasis: a systematic review. Dermatology. 2011;222(4):363-74.
14. Balato N, Megna M, Di Costanzo L, Balato A, Ayala F. Educational and motivational support service: a pilot study for mobile-phone-based interventions in patients with psoriasis. Br J Dermatol. 2013;168(1):201-5.
15. Sticherling M, Augustin M, Boehncke WH, Christophers E, Domm S, Gollnick H, et al. Therapy of psoriasis in childhood and adolescence–a German expert consensus. J Dtsch Dermatol Ges. 2011;9:815-23.
16. Renzi C, Tabolli S, Picardi A, Abeni D, Puddu P, Braga M. Effects of patient satisfaction with care on health-related quality of life: a prospective study. J Eur Acad Dermatol Venereol. 2005;19:712-8.
17. Renzi C, Picardi A, Abeni D, Agostini E, Baliva G, Pasquini P, et al. Association of dissatisfaction with care and psychiatric morbidity with poor treatment compliance. Arch Dermatol. 2002;138:337-42.

Index

Page numbers followed by *f* refer to figure, *t* refer to table, and *b* refer to box.

A

Abdominal obesity 157
Acitretin 121, 138, 139
   hepatotoxicity 166
   safety in pregnancy 143*t*
Acrodermatitis continua of hallopeau 51
Acropustulosis 68
Acute generalized exanthematous pustulosis (AGEP) 52, 134
   differentiation from pustular psoriasis 134
Acute generalized pustular psoriasis 51
Acute generalized pustular psoriasis of Von zumbusch 50*f*
Adalimumab 204
   safety in pregnancy 143*t*
Adiponectin 32, 159, 160
Adult onset psoriasis (AOP) 97
AGEP *See* Acute generalized exanthematous pustulosis (AGEP)
Alcohol
   role in psoriasis 18
Alefacept 205
   dose in psoriasis 205
   safety in pregnancy 143*t*
Amyloidosis
   due to psoriasis 80
Angiotensin-II 155
Annular psoriasis 76*f*
Anthralin 137
   in plaque type psoriasis 209
Antimalarials 15
Apical pulmonary fibrosis
   due to psoriasis 80

Apremilast 227
Arthritis mutilans 86
Arthropathic psoriasis 113
   choice of drug in 220*t*
   holistic approach to management 217
   treatment 217
      biologics 219
      cyclosporine 218
      glucocorticoid injections 218
      hydroxychloroquine 219
      leflunomide 218
      methotrexate 218
      nonsteroidal anti-inflammatory drugs 218
      sulfasalazine 218
AS101 224
Atherosclerosis, in psoriasis 154
   inflammation role in 155
Auspitz sign 42*f*, 44
Autoimmune diseases 166
Azathioprine 202
   dose in psoriasis 202

B

BBUVB 195
Beau's lines 68
Behçet's disease 164
Beta (β) blockers 15
   role in psoriasis etiopathogenesis 15
BI 655066 206
Bimosiamose 195
Biologic agents 138, 139, 203
   breastfeeding during therapy with 141
   evaluation of drug therapy 183

   in children 206
   in psoriatic arthritis 219
   reduced treatment response to 207
Biologic therapy 139
Biomarkers, in psoriasis 184
   cutaneous psoriasis 185
   of comorbidities 185
   psoriatic arthritis 185
Blaschko's linear psoriasis. 48
Brodalumab 226
Bupropion 15

C

Calcipotriene
   safety in pregnancy 143*t*
Calcipotriol 138
   palmoplantar psoriasis 213
Calcitriol
   safety in pregnancy 143*t*
Calcium channel blockers 15
Candidal intertrigo 60
Capillaroscopy
   periungual 177
Capillaroscopy12 177
Captopril 15
Cardiovascular disease, in psoriasis 154, 156
Caspase recruitment domain-containing protein 15 (CARD15) 13
Catalase (CAT) 26
Ceruloplasmin 175
Childhood psoriasis 38, 171
Chronic obstructive pulmonary disease 161*f*
   in psoriasis 161
Classical flexural psoriasis 105*f*

Classical palmoplantar psoriasis 102f
Classical spongiform pustule 25f
Coal-tar derivatives 212
Coal tar, in psoriasis 137, 189
  preparations 190
  prolonged use 190
Confocal laser scanning microscopy 177
Congenital erythrodermic psoriasis (CEP) 57, 94, 111f
Congenital psoriasis 42, 98, 109
Congenital psoriatic erythroderma 98
C-reactive protein (CRP) 32, 155, 175
Crohn's disease 78, 161, 164, 167
CT327 (tyrosine kinase inhibitor) 224
CUSP syndrome 147
Cutaneous psoriasis biomarkers 185
Cyclosporine 121, 123, 138, 139
  complications 234
  evaluation of drug therapy 182
  hepatotoxicity 166
  safety in pregnancy 143t
Cytochrome C concentrations 26

D

Dermascopy 175, 177
  lichen planus 175
  psoriasis 175
  seborrheic dermatitis 175
Dermatology life quality index 239
Diabetes 158
Dithranol, in psoriasis 137, 190
DPS-101 224
Drug-provoked psoriasis 14
  clinical presentation 14
  drug-aggravated psoriasis 14
  drug-induced psoriasis 14
  drugs associated 15b
  features of 15t
  true 15

E

Eating disorders (EDs) 158
Eczema 26

Eczematization
  due to psoriasis 79
Eczematous dermatitis 54
EDs See eating disorders (EDs)
Efalizumab 206
  dose in psoriasis 206
  safety in pregnancy 143t
Elephantine psoriasis 46
Emollients 188
Endothelin-1 155
Enthesitis 84
Erythroderma 14
Erythrodermic psoriasis 54, 76, 214
  clinical features 54
  crimson red erythema 55f
  forms 54
  histology 24
  in children 56
  treatment 214
  zebra-like manifestations 76
Estradiol 18
Etanercept 204
  dose in psoriasis 204
  in pediatric psoriasis 206
  safety in pregnancy 143t
Etretinate 121
Euroqol 5D 239

F

Fetuin-A 32
Fibroblasts 28
Flexural psoriasis 59
  female 60f
  male 60f
  with candidal intertrigo 60f
  with psoriasis vulgaris 60f
Flexural psoriasis 106f
Fluoxetine 15
Follicular psoriasis 76f, 148
  with phrynoderma 114f
Fumaric acid esters 203

G

Gastric secretory function 162
Gastrointestinal and hepatobiliary system, in psoriasis 161
Generalized plaque psoriasis 14
Generalized pustular psoriasis 50f, 51, 74

Genital psoriasis 69
  anus and surrounding skin 73
  buttocks crease 73
  clinical features 70
  female genitals 72
  male genitals 72
  pubis 72
  treatment 211
  upper thighs 73
Gestational pustular psoriasis 133
Ghrelin 32
Gliadin 161
Glyburide 15
Granulocyte colony-stimulating factor 15
Graves' disease 167
Guselkumab 226
Guttate psoriasis 11, 13, 46, 47f, 101
  characteristics of 101
  cw0602 allele 11
  histology 24
  lesions in 46
  salmon-pink papules in 46
  streptococcal throat infection 13
  treatment 210

H

Hashimoto's disease 167
Helper t type 2 (TH2) cell 11
Hepatic failure
  due to psoriasis 79
Hepatitis C virus infection 161
High-density lipoprotein cholesterol 157
HIV-associated psoriasis 145
  keratoderma in 147f
  oral gold in 149
  treatment 149
  zidovudine in 149
HLA-b27 183
HLA-b39 183
HLA-bw6 11
HLA-cw6 5, 11, 183
HLA-dqw3 183
HLA-dr7 183
HLA-drb1 183
Human immunodeficiency virus (HIV) infection 145
  Rieter's syndrome in 147f

Human leukocyte antigen (HLA)
 class I 11
Human leukocyte antigen (HLA)
 class II 11
Hydroxyurea 138
Hyperkeratosis 20, 21f
Hypertension 157
 in psoriasis 153, 154f
Hypertriglyceridemia 157
Hyperuricemia
 role in psoriasis 17

I

IDP-118 225
IL-13 11
IL-23 blockers 226
IL-23r 11
Immune-mediated inflammatory
 disease (IMID) 151
Impetigo herpetiformis, in
 pregnancy 18, 133, 134f
 clinical features 133
 course and prognosis 134
 investigations 135
 safety of drugs in 136
 treatment 135
  cyclosporine 135
  narrow-band ultraviolet light
   B phototherapy 136
  oral corticosteroid 135
  ultraviolet B (UVB)
   phototherapy 136
Increased insulin
 resistance 157
Infantile psoriasis 42, 98, 110
Inflammatory arthritis 30
Inflammatory biomarkers 32
Inflammatory bowel diseases, in
 psoriasis 164
Inflammatory linear verrucous
 epidermal nevus (ILVEN) 47
Infliximab 204
 dose in psoriasis 204
 in pediatric psoriasis 206
 safety in pregnancy 144t
Infundibulo folliculitis 48
Insulin-like growth factor-1 28
Insulin resistance 156, 158
 pathogenesis of 159
Interferon 15
Interleukins 15

Intertrigo with sharply
 marginated erythema 41f
Intralesional alefacept 219
Inverse psoriasis 59
 treatment 211
Itching
 due to arthritis 79

J

Janus-associated kinase
 inhibitors 194
Janus kinase inhibitors 227

K

Kawasaki disease 46
Keratinocytes 21, 27
 psoriatic 28
Keratins 31
Keratolysis punctata like
 lesions 40f
Keratolytics, in psoriasis 189
Koebner's phenomenon 12, 13,
 38, 67, 189
Kogoj's micropustules 19, 96
Koo-menter psoriasis
 instrument 240

L

Las41004 225
Laser, in psoriasis 198
Late cornified envelope genes
 (LCE3C and LCE3B) 11
Latent psoriasis 73
Leo 80190 225
Leo 90100 225
Leptin 32, 159, 160
Leukonychia 68
Lichen planus psoriasis 78
Linear psoriasis 47, 105
 lesions in 47
Lipid-lowering drugs 15
Lithium-provoked psoriasis 15,
 16
 pathogenesis 16
Localized pustular psoriasis 48,
 49f, 50
Lymphoepithelial kazal-
 type inhibitor (LEKTI)
 antibody 97

Lymphomas, in psoriasis 170
 risk of 170

M

M518101 225
Malondialdehyde (MDA) 26
Markers of endogenous
 antioxidant, in psoriasis 175
Markers of inflammation, in
 psoriasis 175
Markers of neutrophil activation,
 in psoriasis 175
MBS *See* metabolic syndrome
Metabolic syndrome 157
Metalloproteinase-1 32
Methotrexate 121, 123, 138, 200
 complications 234
 evaluation of drug
  therapy 182
 indications for considering
  withdrawal 201
 liver biopsy indicatrions 201
 premethotrexate
  evaluation 183
 relative contraindications
  for 123
 risk factors for
  hepatotoxicity 201
 safety in pregnancy 144t
Methotrexate hepatotoxicity 166
Mild psoriasis 73
Mimicking lichen simplex
 chronicus 59f
Mitogen-activated protein
 kinase 1/mitogen-activated
 protein kinase kinase 1
 (MEK1/MEKK1) 193, 194
Mitogen-activated protein (MAP)
 kinase pathway 159
Moderate psoriasis 74, 74f
Moderate-severe
 psoriasis 74, 75
MQX-5902 225
Mucosal psoriasis 64
 treatment 213
Munro's microabscesses 19, 20f,
 96
Mycophenolate mofetil 138
Myocardial infarction, in
 psoriasis 154–156
 role of inflammation in 155

N

Nail biopsy 176
Nail pitting 41, 42f
Nail psoriasis 64, 84, 213
   clinical feature 176t
   dermoscopy in 177
   diagnosis of 69
   doppler study 177
   histology 25
   investigations in 176b
   investigations used in 70b
   manifestations 68
   onycholysis 177
   optical coherence tomography (OCT) 177
   pits 177
   salmon patches 177
   splinter hemorrhages 177
   technique 176
   treatment 213
   ultrasound 177
Nail psoriasis severity index 69
Napkin psoriasis
   characteristics of 102
NBUVB 195
   contraindications 196
   indication 196
Netherton syndrome (NS) 96
Neuropeptide-modulating agents 194
Neurotensin 18
   induced vascular endothelial growth factor (VEGF) 19
Nitric oxide (no) 26, 155
Nonalcoholic fatty liver disease (NAFLD) 165
Nonpustular psoriasis
   differential diagnosis 25
Nonsteroidal anti-inflammatory drugs 17, 194
Nonsteroidal anti-inflammatory drugs provoked psoriasis
   pathogenesis 17

O

Obesity and psoriasis 157
Ocular psoriasis 64
Onycholysis 68, 66f
Osteopontin (OPN) 27
Ostraceous psoriasis 46, 76

P

Palmoplantar psoriasis 61
   histology 25
   treatment 212
Palmoplantar pustulosis (PPP) 14, 37, 50
Pan-selectin antagonists 195
Parakeratosis 19, 20, 21f
Paronychia 69
Pediatric-onset psoriasis (POP) 97
   topical therapy 115
Pediatric psoriasis 94
   age of onset 97
   along blaschko's lines 107
   arthropathic psoriasis 113
     treatment 125
   biologics 123
   calcineurin inhibitors 119
   classification 94
   coal tar 116
   congenital erythrodermic psoriasis
     treatment 125
   congenital psoriasis 109
   cyclosporine 123
   dietary supplement 124
   dithranol 116
   due to avitaminosis 114f
   emollients 116
   epidemiology 95
   erythrodermic psoriasis 108
     scalp involvement 110f
   etiopathogenesis 95
   exacerbating factors 98
   gene for 95
   grading 99
   guttate psoriasis 101
     treatment 124
   infantile psoriasis 110
   inverse psoriasis
     treatment 125
   keratolytics 116
   laser 124
   linear psoriasis 105, 108f
   methotrexate 123
   mucosal psoriasis 108
     treatment 125
   nail psoriasis 107
     treatment 125
   napkin psoriasis 102

     treatment 125
   pathology 96
   phototherapy 121
   plantar psoriasis 101
   plaque psoriasis 99, 109, 112f
     treatment 124
   psoriasis vulgaris 108f
   psychosocial impact of 126
   pustular psoriasis 112
     clinical patterns of 112
     treatment 125
   retinoids 120
   scalp
     treatment 124
   scalp psoriasis 101
   systemic therapies 121
   topical corticosteroids 117
     side effects of 117
   topical vitamin d analogs 118
   treatment 115, 223
     children 223
     infants 223
Penicillin 15
Periumbilical erythema 41f
PH-10 225
Phosphodiesterase inhibitors 194
Photochemotherapy (PUVA) 196
   contraindications 197
   dithranol and 197
   oral 196
   psoriasis vulgaris 197
Photosensitive psoriasis 13
Phototherapy and laser
   palmoplantar psoriasis 213
Phototherapy, in psoriasis 195
   warning 198
Pimecrolimus 138
Pityriasis amiantacea 102, 105f
Pityriasis rosea 47
Pityriasis rubra pilaris 48, 148
   categories 148
Plantar psoriasis 61f, 101
   affecting the entire sole 62f
   characteristics of 101
   early stage of 61f
   of palm 62f
Plaque psoriasis 2, 13, 55f, 99
   facial involvement 99
   HLA genes associated 6
   sites involved 99
Plaque type psoriasis 42, 44, 99

affecting the extensor
        surface 45f
    persistence of 45f
    treatment 209
Plasminogen-activator-inhibitor 1
        (PAI-1) 160
Platelet-derived growth factor
        (PDGF) 28
Poriatic arthritis sine psoriasis 86
Prostacyclin 155
Protein tyrosine phosphatase N22
        (PTPN22) 6
PsA *See* psoriatic arthritis
P-selecti 155
Psoriasiform epidermal
        hyperplasia 96
Psoriasis 1
    according to site of
        involvement 58
    and duodenum 162
    and esophagus 162
    and hypothyroidism 167f
    and human immunodeficiency
        virus 145
    and malignancy 170
    autoimmune diseases in 166
    autoimmune diseases in 168b
    based on type of disease 44
    based upon disease
        manifestation 73b
    B-hemolytic streptococci 46
    biomarkers 31, 155, 184t
        cellular 31
        genetic 31
    cellular changes in the skin 10
    clinical spectrum of 44b
    clinical variants 43
    complications 79b, 231
        arthropathic
            complications 233
        cutaneous
            complications 231
        due to treatment 233
        hepatic failure 232
        metabolic and systemic
            complications 232
        ocular complications 233
        polycystic ovary syndrome
            (PCOS) 232
        psychosocial
            complications 233
        renal failure 232

systemic and metabolic
    complications of 233b
diaper rash 5
disease association 77
    lichen planus 78
    vitiligo 78f
dry scaly plaque of 72f
environmental risk factors 39b
etiological factors
    drugs 14
    estradiol 18
    genetic factors 10
    infection 13
    obesity 19
    role of infection 13b
    stress 18
    sunlight 17
    trauma 13
follow-up and
    rehabilitation 242
gastrointestinal tract
    manifestations 167b
genes involved 5, 11
grading 42
hepatobiliary
    manifestations 167b
histology 23
history 1
    components 21
history and evaluation 36
immunologic evolution 29
immunopathogenesis 27, 27f
joints involvement 30
in children 42
infection 13b
    HIV assocaiation 14
    malassezia association 14
    streptococcal association 13
infections associated 6
infertility in women 142
intraoral manifestations of 162
investigations 174
involving groin 70f
isomorphic response in 42f
jejunum and small
    intestine 163
lactation during 142
liver and gall bladder in 165
loci of the susceptibility
    region 12t
management in pregnancy and
    lactation 137

phototherapy 138
    systemic therapies for 138
    topical therapies 137
markers of comorbidity 32
medications assocaiated 6
molecules differentially
    regulated in 12t
multiorgan failure due to 169
nail dystrophy in 65f
nail involvement in 67b
nail onychomycosis 65f
new topical agents 194b
oxidative stress and
    enzymes 26
paronychia in 67f
pathogenesis 19
pathogenesis as multisystem
    disease 26
pathology 19
pregnancy outcomes 141
prevalence 4
    in adolescence 5
    in childhood 5
prognosis 242
    investigations 183
psoriasis-specific
    measures 238
psychological aspects 237
renal disease and 168
resembling eczema 63f
salmon pink plaques 46f
secondary gastrointestinal
    amyloidosis due to 164
signals of 39, 41b
skin-specific measures 239
symptoms of 37
systemic diseases in 152f
systemic drugs used in 199b
    indication 199
topical steroids 191
topical therapy 188
treatment 187
    human immunodeficiency
        virus 222
    in hepatitis 222
    in malignancy 223
    in pregnancy and
        lactation 222
    in tuberculosis patient 222
    newer drugs 224
triggered by β-blocker 39f
type I 37

type II 37
with guarded prognosis 74
Psoriasis area and severity index
and simplified PASI 239
Psoriasis disability index 239
Psoriasis follicularis 76
Psoriasis gyrate 75
Psoriasis index of quality of
life 238
Psoriasis inflammation 156
Psoriasis life stress inventory 238
Psoriasis pustulosa 99
Psoriasis vulgaris 19, 23, 99
histology 23
Psoriatic arthritis 30, 79, 80, 178
asymmetrical 82f
biomarkers 185
bone erosion 30
classification 81
classification criteria for
psoriatic arthritis
(CASPAR) criteria 87
clinical assessment 178
clinical findings of 84, 85b
asymmetric oligoarthritis 85
dactylitis 85
distal interphalangeal joint
arthritis 85
enthesitis 84
nail psoriasis 84
skin 84
spondylitis 86
symmetric polyarticular
arthritis 86
clinical manifestations 81
arthritis mutilans 86
computed tomography
scan 181
course of disease in 88
definite 89
diagnostic criteria 86, 89
differentiation from
osteoarthritis 85t
differentiation from
rheumatoid arthritis 84,
181t
forms 89
hematologic investigations 178
human leukocyte antigen
test 178
immune pathogenesis 30
in children 89, 221

investigations 178, 178b
magnetic resonance
imaging 181
minor criteria 89
oligoarthritis 82f
onset 80
predictors of disease
progression in 88
probable 89
quality of life in 242
risk factors 80
sacroiliitis 82
serological tests 179
symmetrical 82
symptoms of 81
synovial fluid analysis 179
synovial tissue in 30
types 81
ultrasound findings 179b
X-rays 180
involvement of feet and
knees 181
peripheral joint
involvement 180f
Psoriatic arthritis screening and
evaluation (PASE) 87
Psoriatic arthropathy 153
Psoriatic cutaneous lymphocyte-
associated antigen 13
Psoriatic erythroderma 74
Psoriatic
gastrointestinopathy 163
Psoriatic march 3, 231, 235
Psoriatic nephropathy 168
Psoriatic onycho-
pachydermoperiostitis 69
Psoriatic skin 10
changes observed 28b
Psoriqol *See* psoriasis index of
quality of life
Pustular psoriasis 48, 78, 112
childhood 52
circinate type of 53
complications 232
differentiating features of 52t
drugs precipitating 52b
histology 24
in pregnancy 18
localized form of 54
nail dystrophy in 66f
of infancy 53
treatment 210

types of 50f
with arthropathy 83f
Pustular psoriasis of
pregnancy 133
PUVA
safety in pregnancy 144t

Q

Questionnaire on experience with
skin complaints 239

R

Reactive oxygen species (ROS) 27
Recurrent infundibulo
folliculitis 48
Reiter's syndrome 25, 147
diagnosis in HIV infected
patient 147
scalp scales 148f
Reiter's syndrome 77f
Resistin 32, 159, 160
Retinoids 121, 199
in psoriasis 193
Reverse Koebner reactions 38
Rheumatoid arthritis. 166
Rupioid psoriasis 46, 76
Ruxolitinib 225, 227

S

Salicylic acid 189, 234
complications 234
in plaque type psoriasis 209
Salmon patch 68
Scalp psoriasis 42, 58
Auspitz sign 58f
characteristics of 101
mimicking seborrhoeic
dermatitis 59
psoriatic corona 58f
treatment 210
Sclerosing cholangitis 165
Secondary gastrointestinal
amyloidosis, in psoriasis 164
Secondary renal amyloidosis 168
Secukinumab 226
Selenium (SE) 27
Severe psoriasis 74, 75f
Severe seborrheic dermatitis 40,
114f

Sezary syndrome 54
Short-contact dithranol
  with broadband UVB
  (BBUVB) 191
Short form-36 239
Single transducer and activator
  of transcription 2 gene
  (STAT2) 11
Sjogren syndrome 167
Skin-derived antileukoproteinase
  (SKALP) 29
Spinulosic psoriasis 48
Splinter hemorrhages 68
Spondyloarthropathies 30
Spongiform pustule 20f
Spotted lunula 68
STF115469 225
Subjective well-being scale 239
Subungual hyperkeratosis 68
  with onycholysis 41f
Superoxide dismutase (SOD) 26
Surgical hypoparathyroidism 17
Symptomatic treatment, in
  psoriasis 188
Synovitis, acne, pustulosis
  palmaris, hyperostosis and
  osteomyelitis (SAPHO)
  syndrome 78
  dermatologic
    manifestations 78
Systemic calcineurin
  inhibitors 202
Systemic involvement, in
  psoriasis
  investigations in 182
Systemic steroids 203

T

Tacrolimus 138
Tazarotene 120
  complications 234
  safety in pregnancy 144t
  side effect 120
Terbinafine 15
Tetracyclines 17
  provoked psoriasis
    pathogenesis 17
Thiopurine s-methyl transferase
  (TPMT) 202
Tildrakizumab 226
Tinea amiantacea 105f
Tofacitinib 194
  mode of action 194
Tofacitinib 224, 227
Tonsillectomy
  in guttate psoriasis 210
Topical corticosteroids 117, 191,
  211
  choice of potency of 117t
  palmoplantar psoriasis 213
  potency of 118
  safety in pregnancy 144t
  side effects of 119t
  United Kingdom system of
    classification 119b
  United States system of 118b
Topical therapy, in psoriasis 188
  conventional therapy 189b
Topical vitamin D analogs, in
  psoriasis 193
Total antioxidant status (TAS) 26,
  175
Transepidermal water loss
  (TEWL) 188
Transferrin 175
Transforming growth factor-α
  (TGF-α) 28
Treated psoriasis 26
  histology 26
Tumor necrosis factor α-induced
  protein 3 gene (TNFα-IP3) 11

U

Ulcerative colitis 164
Ultraviolet B (UVB)
  phototherapy 189
Unstable psoriasis 57
  fiery red erythema 58f
  intense pruritus 58f
  severe itching 57f
Ustekinumab 205
  dose in psoriasis 205
  in pediatric psoriasis 207
  plaque psoriasis 205
UVA 195
UVB 195
  BBUVB 195
  NBUVB 195
  safety in pregnancy 144t

V

Vascular endothelial growth
  factor (VEGF) 155
Video-dermoscopy 177
Vitamin D analog 212
  complications 234

W

WBI-1001 194, 225
  inflammatory action of 194
Wickham's striae 47
Woronoff's ring 46

Z

Zidovudine 149

www.ingramcontent.com/pod-product-compliance
Lightning Source LLC
Chambersburg PA
CBHW040539220526
45473CB00016B/2973